Remembering to Live

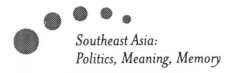

Southeast Asia:
Politics, Meaning, Memory

Seeking to raise the visibility of Southeast Asia
in scholarly circles and among general readers, the
broad scope of this series covers history (memory) and
culture (meanings), especially when these topics also
elucidate issues of power (politics).

COEDITORS: DAVID CHANDLER AND RITA SMITH KIPP

KIM N. B. NINH
A World Transformed: The Politics of Culture in
Revolutionary Vietnam, 1945–1965

PETER ZINOMAN, EDITOR
Dumb Luck: A Novel by Vu Trong Phung

M. CAMERON HAY
Remembering to Live: Illness at the Intersection of
Anxiety and Knowledge in Rural Indonesia

HEATHER L. CLAUSSEN
Unconventional Sisterhood: Feminist Catholic
Nuns in the Philippines

Remembering to Live

Illness at the Intersection of
Anxiety and Knowledge
in Rural Indonesia

M. Cameron Hay

ANN ARBOR

THE UNIVERSITY OF MICHIGAN PRESS

First paperback edition 2004
Copyright © by the University of Michigan 2001
All rights reserved
Published in the United States of America by
The University of Michigan Press
Manufactured in the United States of America
⊗ Printed on acid-free paper

2007   2006   2005   2004   4   3   2

A CIP catalog record for this book is available from the British Library.

Library of Congress Cataloging-in-Publication Data

Hay, M. Cameron, 1965–
Remembering to live : illness at the intersection of anxiety and
knowledge in rural Indonesia / M. Cameron Hay.
p.   cm.
Includes bibliographical references and index.
ISBN 0-472-09785-7 (cloth : alk. paper)
1. Sasak (Indonesian people)—Health and hygiene.   2. Sasak
(Indonesian people)—Attitudes.   3. Sasak (Indonesian people)—
Medical care.   4. Traditional medicine—Indonesia—Pelocok.
5. Sick—Indonesia—Pelocok—Psychology.   6. Pelocok (Indonesia)—
Social life and customs.   I. Title.

DS632.S38 H38   2001
610'.9598'6—dc21   2001002486

ISBN 0-472-06785-0 (pbk. : alk. paper)

To Rob, with love

Contents

Illustrations

Maps

Figures

Acknowledgments

Sasaks frequently asked me, "Are you alone?" finding it difficult to believe that anyone would actually travel alone to live among strangers. What they could not see was that I was not alone. I carried the encouragement, support, and wisdom of others with me into the field. Nor was I alone during the long months at my computer, for the Sasak strangers had become friends, and their laughter and wisdom kept me company as I wrote about their lives. Only my name appears as author because I alone am responsible for this work's shortcomings. But for its successes, I thank those people who have kept me company throughout the years, making this project possible.

First and foremost, I am indebted to the people of Pelocok. From them, I learned more about being alive than could ever fit between the covers of a book. I have chosen to identify these people and their hamlet with pseudonyms and thus shall not list them otherwise here.

Outside Pelocok, there were a number of people in Indonesia who offered indispensable assistance, friendship, and encouragement. These people were Andrew Toth, Masnin, Made Mastika, Iwan Mucipto, Edi Ardius, Prima, Parsa and Yadek, Suwenno Sudjono and his family, and especially Suwetomo Sudjono, Zahrah, Purnawati, and their families. I also would like to thank those people who assisted me in preparing to go to Indonesia, including Judith Ecklund, Beth Povinelli, Mary Steedly, Susan Turner, Achmad Budiman, Maria Sumintatmadja, and the teachers of the Southeast Asian Studies Summer Institute (SEASSI) in 1992 and 1993. The fieldwork would not have been possible without the financial support of the National Science Foundation (grant number SBR-93139), the Southeast Asia Council of the Association for Asian Studies, and Emory University. I am grateful for a Citation of Merit Award from the Association for Women in Science, as well as for fellowships to study Indonesian from SEASSI.

I thank Lembaga Ilmu Pengetahuan Indonesia for its support, particularly Dewi Soenarijadi, E. K. M. Masinambouw, and Kalam Sebayang. I. Gusti Ngurah Bagus of Udayana University gave me support for the required visas and freedom to do the work. Setyoko, Director of Rumah Sakit Umum in Mataram, willingly came to my aid to solve a bureaucratic dead end. Others who facilitated my work in Lombok include N. Nursamsi, V. J. Hermann, Sabar, Habib, and the Department of Health in Mataram.

The lively intellectual atmosphere of the department of anthropology at Emory University has been instrumental in this project from the beginning. Bradd Shore, Peter Brown, Fredrik Barth, Charles Nuckolls, and Karl Heider at the University of South Carolina each went above and beyond duty, reading multiple drafts, motivating my exploration into different theoretical approaches, and maintaining that essential balance between healthy criticism and encouragement. Others were helpful resources and perceptive commentators; they include George Armelagos, Peggy Barlett, Don Donham, Marcia Inhorn, Bruce Knauft, Mel Konner, Robert Paul, Debra Spitulnik, Carol Worthman, and Pat Whitten. Throughout the early struggles with writing, Don Donham as well as Alexander Hinton, Wynne Maggi, Matsheliso Molapo, Theodore Shurr, John Wood, and Mari Yerger were willing readers and encouraging friends.

Many others have listened patiently to field stories and writing dilemmas, suggesting variant interpretations, including Cristine Gardner, Mary Kroeger, Bart Ryan, Gregg Starrett, and Roger Paget. The writing of this ethnography has drawn on the works of countless others, but Unni Wikan and Carol Laderman deserve special mention. Their writings about everyday concerns and medicine in Southeast Asia influenced both the conception of the project and its resulting ethnography.

I want to thank my editor, Ingrid Erickson, and the series editors, Rita Kipp and David Chandler, for their enthusiasm and their aid in bringing this book quickly to fruition. For detailed comments on the entire text, I thank David Hay, David Chandler, and an anonymous reviewer. My thanks also go to Janice Brill for carefully copyediting the manuscript.

There are others who gave me ways of seeing and understanding the world that have impacted my life and therefore my work profoundly. Jon Andelson at Grinnell College introduced me to an anthropology that did not lose its humanity in its quest for knowledge. I thank Cam and Margaret Carmichael for their hospitality at critical academic junctures, and Michael Malchow-Hay for teaching me how to be easy with strangers. Hugh and Carol Hunt taught me the joy of philosophy and the dignity of poverty. My parents, Mary and David Hay, instilled in me the desire to travel alone to corners of the earth regardless of the worry it cost them. I doubt my father's visit to Lombok lessened their worry, but my work certainly benefited from his curiosity about Indonesia and insight into people's lives there. During the final stages of writing, my children, Turner and Sydney Rollins, provided joyful distractions to contemplating the often painful details of my fieldwork. My deepest thanks go to my husband, Rob Rollins, who uplifted me with his visits to the field and patiently nursed me back to health when I finally came home. His belief in me, dedication to my career (at considerable personal cost), and down-to-earth criticisms of "this rhetoric is all nonsense" have made my work far better than it otherwise could have been.

Introduction

A certain degree of abstraction is of course required,
otherwise we would get nowhere, but is it really necessary
to just make a book out of human beings?
　　　　　　　　—E. E. EVANS-PRITCHARD

Laughter rings throughout Sasak compounds even though illness and death knock constantly at their door. Sasaks live on Lombok, the island immediately east of Bali in the Indonesian archipelago. Of Indonesia's thousands of islands, Lombok consistently has one of the country's worst health records. How do people cope with the fragility of their lives so that they can return to laughter? This ethnography, about Sasak ethnomedicine in a pluralistic medical setting, argues that the organization of medical knowledge that enables people to cope has profound consequences for their health.

In order not to "just make a book out of human beings," I will tack between descriptions of cultural knowledge and personal knowledge, processes of maintenance and processes of change. While clarifying theoretical positions on the relationships between culture and people, our focus must be on what matters, namely, on people's lives and the concerns that compel them. The following pages are filled with the serious, sometimes tragic side of Sasak life, but we must begin by getting the ethos right. We begin with laughter.

LIVING LIFE WITH LAUGHTER

Laughter rang throughout the compound. It was my last night in the hamlet of Pelocok, the place I had called home for nearly two years. As a parting gift, I entertained a gathering of about 75 people with video-tapes of themselves. As I played the tapes, people jammed together to see their images dancing across a makeshift screen. They laughed uproariously, pointing at themselves. Everything was hilarious. Children running off to school. Men playing dominoes. It all made them laugh with delight.

I had chosen the films with care, putting aside films of private or semiprivate events: cosmological discussions, births, and the like.[1] But tacked onto one film labeled "Everyday life—children playing" was the acute illness episode of Inaq Nori. Not exactly a private event, for at least 50 people had witnessed her convulsions and confused speech; nonetheless, I had not wanted to show anything that might remind friends of difficult events. I tried to turn it off, but Inaq Nori herself stopped me. I need not have worried. The group just continued to laugh. Inaq Nori laughed loudest of all and pointed at the screen, bursting out with "Look at me!" "What am I doing?" "Look, my stomach hurt!" I changed the film to one of dancing, and the laughter continued.

Inaq Nori's laughter was, perhaps, as much with embarrassment and self-consciousness, as with delight. But it was not laughter to mask distress or unhappiness. When she had cares, anyone who knew her knew it instantly. Her normally jovial disposition became quiet, her eyes lost their sparkle, and she would answer questions of everyday politeness with words that gave voice to her cares. For example, one morning she answered my inquiry if she wanted to go visiting with me with "No, I'm not going anywhere. My son ran away yesterday and my heart it goes . . ." and she made a jerky up-and-down movement with her fist in front of her heart. Later that night, after her son had returned, I met her again. This time the smile was again evident in her eyes, as she said that her son had just gone visiting and hadn't told anyone. The disappearance of her son obviously had troubled her, but with his return, she too returned to laughter.[2]

Inaq Nori was not unique in this respect. Every Sasak person with whom I had even a passing acquaintance readily communicated current worries, anxieties, griefs, and ills. Yet, with few exceptions, once these cares were past—for better or worse—people seemed to accept

---

1. Cosmological knowledge is considered potent, secret knowledge, and therefore the discussions I had been permitted to videotape were inappropriate for public viewing.
2. A phrase borrowed from Laura Bohannan's classic work *Return to Laughter* (1964).

the emotional and physical scars they made and turned their attention to the business of living another day.

In the pages that follow, the fragility of Sasak lives is palpable. Their world is riddled with dangers seen and unseen, spoken and unspoken. Illness is an everyday event. Death, in people's perceptions and in reality, is often lurking just out of sight, ready to pounce on the most unlikely person. The goal of this ethnography is to explore how people cope with such fragility.

The Sasaks of Lombok

Of Indonesia's thousands of islands, Lombok consistently has among the worst health records in the country. Moreover, statistics have shown that in spite of increases in biomedical infrastructure the overall health of the population has not significantly improved. This suggests that the problems of health care in Lombok lay beyond simple availability of biomedical facilities (Corner 1989). This ethnography explores those problems by focusing on the population for whom health is the gravest concern, the rural Sasaks.

Sasaks constitute approximately 2 million of the island's population of 2.5 million, with Balinese, Chinese, Javanese, and Buginese making up the remainder. As with any people, it is difficult to generalize about Sasaks. Roughly 20 percent of them live in urban settings, and the rest live in rural areas.[3] All Sasaks are Muslims, but some are more orthodox and others more syncretistic.[4] Almost all can communicate in the Sasak language, but only some have the formal education to be fluent in Indonesian. Some Sasaks are capitalists and some are peasants. Some have satellite dishes and computers, others have neither electricity nor running water. Some have traveled to distant islands while others have never gone beyond the closest market town. These are the primary variables that differentiate Sasak ways of life. This ethnography is about those Sasaks described by the latter characteristics, that is, the rural, syncretistic Muslim peasants with little formal education, minimal experience with the wider world, and almost no access to technological conveniences. Specifically, this ethnography is about the Sasaks who

---

3. This figure is an approximation based on overall population statistics; see Mboi 1995, 178.
4. A minority of Sasaks have converted to Christianity or Hinduism. Gerdin (1982) argues that Sasaks who marry Balinese and convert are no longer truly Sasaks, because by definition to be Sasak is to be Muslim.

live in the hamlet of Pelocok, but its arguments could have been drawn from countless Sasak communities where these characteristics hold true.

It is among these rural Sasaks that life is most fragile.[5] That is not to say that those Sasaks with wealth and formal education are free of illness, but their wealth and knowledge make these dangers less imminent and provide better resources for managing them. In contrast, for the rural poor illness and death are a daily reality not easily coped with.

Many Indonesian peoples are conscious of social, political, and physical dangers continually surrounding them. Various ethnographies speak of an Indonesian tendency for perpetual vigilance to avoid these dangers by maintaining emotional harmony and equilibrium. It is this desire for harmony and equilibrium that seems to be the root of the proclivity toward performance suggested in many descriptions of Indonesians.[6] Indonesians are expected to perform in everyday life, showing contented faces to cope with their concerns.

In Lombok, the concerns of Sasak people are much the same, yet, surprisingly, masks do not usually slide into place to cover strong emotions such as anxiety, grief, and anger. Sasaks do not struggle to keep a bright face when confronted with health concerns and death, even though they do have an ideal of maintaining personal equilibrium. With few exceptions, Sasaks cope *without* putting on bright faces. They genuinely live their fragile lives with laughter.

HISTORICAL AND ECONOMIC
BACKGROUND INFORMATION

Lombok is in eastern Indonesia, but its history and resulting cultural patterns tie it more closely to its western neighbors of Bali and Java. Lit-

---

5. This study does not address the concerns of the urban poor. The majority of Sasaks living in cities and towns are, in comparison to rural peasants, financially well-off. For heuristic reasons, throughout this text I make a simplistic distinction between rural and urban Sasaks. Urban Sasaks and their ideologies, practices, and economic well-being are more diverse than I imply. The simplistic characterization of urban Sasaks does, however, reflect the perception of them from the standpoint of rural peasants.
6. For more detailed accounts of this vigilance against danger, the tendency toward maintaining equilibrium, and performance, see, e.g., Bateson 1982; Siegal 1986; Errington 1989; Heider 1991; Wikan 1990; Barth 1993; Geertz 1973; Peacock 1987; Hobart 1985; Keeler 1987. Note that Wikan (1990) argues persuasively that, for the Balinese at least, the concern is less with external performance (cf. Geertz 1973) than with maintaining inner equilibrium.

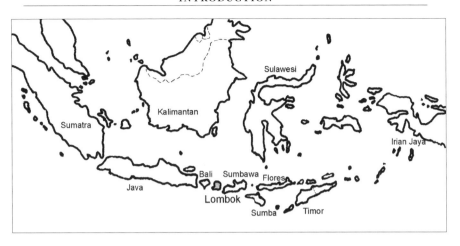

MAP 1. Indonesia

tle is known of Lombok's early history excepting the introduction of Islam by Makassar traders and widespread conversion in approximately 1600. At the beginning of the seventeenth century, the Makassarese gained influence over the aristocracy of eastern Lombok, while the Balinese arrived and established themselves in the western half of the island. From 1740 until 1894, the Balinese dynasty of Klungkung ruled all of Lombok. In 1894 the Dutch ousted the Balinese and took over ruling Lombok until 1942.[7] From 1943 to 1945 the Japanese occupied the island. Then the Dutch returned until 1949, when Indonesia gained its independence and Lombok became, with the neighboring island of Sumbawa, the province of West Nusatenggara.

In historical records from the early 1800s, we know that Lombok used to be agriculturally rich, exporting substantial surpluses of rice and tobacco. By the late 1800s, there is evidence of occasional famines caused by drought. In addition, the land taxes and corvée labor required by the Balinese kings were an increasing burden to Sasak peasants. The Dutch years were no blessing economically because the peasants were taxed on everything from owning or leasing land to slaughtering animals to selling produce to any side income a peasant might have. On top of this, there began a cycle of drought and famine,

---

7. For limited historical accounts of Lombok, see Bosworth et al. 1986; Vlekke 1943; van Leur 1976. For a fuller account of Lombok's recent history see van der Kraan 1980.

striking every seven to nine years (Williamson 1984): "While there is no evidence of the existence of a class of paupers under Balinese rule, towards the end of the colonial era it was common knowledge among Dutch officials that about one-third of Lombok's population was destitute" (van der Kraan 1980, 169). During Japanese occupation, things only got worse. It was only after Indonesian independence that the livelihood of Sasak people began to improve, and famines became less regular. Although much of the rural population still lives with hunger tapping at the door, Lombok now has an urban middle class.[8]

LANGUAGE

The official language of Lombok is the national language, Indonesian. But most everyday interactions outside of businesses and government offices are conducted in Sasak. The Sasak language is an Austronesian language with strong grammatical and lexical similarities to the languages of Javanese and Balinese, including speech levels with distinct lexicons and speech inflections.

Yet, unlike Javanese and Balinese, the lower Sasak language levels do not retain the softness of tone or the gentle inflections of the highest level. As used among commoners, Sasak takes on abrupt and staccato sounds, with a majority of words ending in sharp *k*s and glottal stops. In addition to the levels of the language, different areas have different dialects. People living in hamlets only an hour's walk in distance can have distinct dialects, different in tone and word choices. Sasaks did not have trouble communicating in different dialects, although they often poked fun at the dialects used in different places. In contrast, when codes were switched from Sasak to Indonesian, many rural Sasaks were no longer able to understand everything or to contribute actively to an interaction.

---

8. With the dramatic drop in Indonesia's currency value in late 1997 that continues into the present, the economic boom of the 1980s and the early 1990s has slowed dramatically. The rural dwellers who are tied to the land are and will continue to be less affected by the financial crisis than urban dwellers, but cycles of poor crops do send rural Sasaks to the marketplace for rice and other essentials. With considerably higher food prices, Sasak peasants are hungrier than in years past, but, with the forests to gather from and their social system of sharing any surplus on a daily basis, the economic crisis should have little impact on their lives overall unless it leads to widespread violence.

FIELDWORK

This ethnography is based on 22 months on the island of Lombok. I was there for two months of preliminary work in 1990, then carried out fieldwork from November 1993 through September 1994, and again from February 1995 through October 1995. The vast majority of this time was spent in the hamlet I call Pelocok (phonetically, Pe-low-choke, accented on the second syllable and ending with a glottal stop).

Pelocok is a pseudonym, as are the place-names of surrounding small hamlets, although the rest of the place-names are real. Similarly, the personal names of people in Pelocok are pseudonyms. The decision whether to use actual names or pseudonyms is difficult. When I asked Sasaks, they always wished their names to be used. But I was thoroughly unable to make clear to them the possible risks of using correct names. Those risks include the possibility that my writings could be used to forward biomedical and political agendas that singled out "Pelocok" as a target for potentially aggressive intervention. Also there loomed the possibility that tourist promoters would find my writings and make "Pelocok" into a tourist attraction—a sort of human zoo—as has been done elsewhere on Lombok. My purpose for using pseudonyms is to shelter the privacy of those who befriended me. I have otherwise not altered their circumstances, personalities, or histories in any way.

I was introduced into Pelocok by Raden Suwetomo. His inherited title of Raden, nobleman, would have made him second only to kings in the hierarchical system that reigned on Lombok until the Dutch occupation. Today the title still commands the highest levels of respect, but it is through his willingness to help peasants in financial and political difficulties that Suwetomo has earned the unquestioned loyalty of a large number of villages and hamlets in Lombok. During pilot work in 1990, Suwetomo suggested various hamlets that might be suitable for the kind of research I had described to him. I visited each, and when I returned in 1993, Suwetomo offered to use his influence to get me established in the hamlet of my choice. I chose Pelocok for its relative creature comforts: situated in the foothills, the air was cooler and water more plentiful. The choice made, Suwetomo arranged for me to live with the "Mol" family. The people of Pelocok would never have tolerated my presence long term—even with my stack of official Indonesian permits and letters of introduction—if I had not been introduced by someone trusted and respected like Raden Suwetomo.

People in Pelocok almost exclusively speak a low-level dialect of Sasak. During the first six months of fieldwork, I concentrated on learning their dialect. Indeed, so few villagers spoke Indonesian that there was no alternative. I eventually mastered the language to approximately 70 percent fluency and only had trouble following conversations when people talked swiftly. With people outside Pelocok, I almost always spoke Indonesian. Although Sasaks have no trouble understanding various Sasak dialects, my language skills were not so versatile.

Although I made my share of social blunders, I became generally well liked and trusted in Pelocok. Throughout the fieldwork, I lived and worked as a villager—excepting my odd habits of retiring to "study" (write my field notes) and of carrying around a tape recorder and sometimes a camera or video camera when visiting. Although I developed a circle of friends who would explain things in context for me, I never had any assistants or informants. My status as an educated outsider made me a favorite ritual and drinking companion of older men in the community, with whom I would sit and talk for hours on end. My gender invited the companionship of women with whom I went about the everyday tasks of cleaning, washing, cooking, caring for children, and working in the fields. During the last five months of the fieldwork, I apprenticed myself to an old midwife and healer (Papuq Isa), and from her—in the wee hours of the night so no one could overhear—I learned secret knowledge to treat illness.

In the course of my research, I collected over a hundred illness case studies. These case studies include direct observation of treatments as well as attention to how patients and others talked about the particular illness. The majority of cases involved relatively minor illnesses such as colds and stomachaches. About 20 cases were of serious illnesses that prompted more conversations and more treatments. I spoke with all the healers in Pelocok and observed the healing treatments of two shamans (*dukun*s) on numerous occasions, but my closest contacts with ethnomedical specialists were two healer-midwives (*belian*s). In addition, I spoke with and observed the preventions and treatments of a large number of Sasak laypersons, mostly people from Pelocok, but also some from surrounding hamlets as well as a handful from urban areas. My interactions with biomedical personnel were less numerous. I spent a considerable amount of time with the local biomedical midwife (Indon., *bidan*),[9] and, to a lesser extent, with a clinician in a distant

---

9. Throughout the text, the language of foreign words is designated with "Sas." for Sasak, "Indon." for Indonesian, "Bal." for Balinese, or "Ar." for Arabic. If no language is specified, it is Sasak.

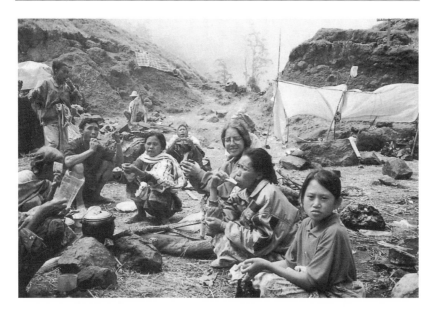

FIG. 1. Anthropologist and Pelocok villagers having coffee in the volcano basin (1995). (Photo by Rob Rollins.)

hamlet. I also spoke with four doctors on the island at length and observed how doctors interacted with rural Sasaks on two occasions. It should be noted that most of the illness episodes discussed in this ethnography were from the more serious case studies because these were the ones that prompted more conversations and through which the relationship between personal and cultural knowledge through the medium of social interaction was made clear.

Studying social interactions made it necessary to capture people's words, to understand not only what was said but also how and in what contexts it was said. Toward this end, I used a tape recorder and to a lesser extent a video camera, always with participants' permission. The longer conversations in this ethnography are transcriptions of interactions taped in Sasak and translated into English. Some of the shorter interactions are also transcribed and translated from recordings. I indicated these recorded data by providing both the English translations and the Sasak transcriptions. When recordings were not possible, interactions were written from memory as soon as possible. I wrote my notes in English but tried to capture people's turn of phrase and often noted the Sasak words they used. With practice, I became good at committing conversations and people's particular statements to memory. Nonetheless, those conversations not accompanied by Sasak transcriptions are not as accurate as those recorded with audio equipment.

AMBIVALENCE AND SETBACKS

Fieldwork is inherently problematic because the anthropologist must be a participant observer: both a sympathetic and active member of a community and an objective outsider. In the spaces where these contradictory roles clashed most strongly, I experienced difficulties. One was a personal ambivalence regarding health care; another was a clash with villagers who would not permit me to be both a member of their community and collect statistical data.

While in the field, I constantly struggled with ambivalence regarding Sasak health care. I highly respected Sasak ethnomedical practices; indeed, I was impressed by treatments that healed sicknesses in ways that I still can not explain. Nonetheless, I personally believed that for many conditions biomedical treatment could be more efficacious (cf. Hahn 1995). When I was sick in the field, I put little faith in the ethnomedical treatments I submitted to and, more often than not, sought biomedical care at the first opportunity. On the other hand, although I put greater stock in the efficacy of biomedicine in general, I did not particularly trust the knowledge, skills, and technologies of biomedical personnel on Lombok (see chap. 7). Moreover, I was frequently angered by the way rural Sasaks, their knowledge, and their skills were dismissed as inconsequential by more elite members of society, especially biomedical personnel. I appreciated the struggles of rural Sasaks to maintain dignity and pride in a larger society that marginalizes them. My ambivalence regarding biomedicine and ethnomedicine on Lombok colored the fieldwork.

While my ambivalence was an internal struggle, my efforts to collect statistical data in Pelocok prompted an external one. The most comprehensive statistics are the official ones collected for governmental purposes and gathered with some degree of conscientiousness by Amaq Her, the head of Pelocok's Islamic school (*pesantren*).[10] Officially, "Pelocok" encompasses a geographic region significantly larger than

---

10. The education at Pelocok's *pesantran* consisted of learning basic Arabic and learning to recite passages from the Qur'an. Attendance cost a nominal fee usually paid in rice or produce. Most elementary school-age children attended it sporadically—particularly in the holy months of Ramadan and the prophet Mohammed's birthday—whether or not they attended the regular elementary school.

the one in which I worked. Locals identify two hamlets within this region: Lakongak and Pelocok. There is no significant social, religious, or economic difference between the two that would skew these statistics. When I refer to the population of Pelocok as hovering around 800 persons, I am referring to the hamlet called Pelocok within the governmental region of the same name. In chapter 1, I primarily use these official statistics because I was unable to complete any kind of systematic and detailed census of the area where I immediately worked. When I attempted to do a census after I had established fairly good rapport with the people, I used the word *sensus,* which is an Indonesianized version of the English word, thinking that using this word would make my activities more clear to them. This was an error. *Sensus* is associated with an activity government officials complete before each national election. When I attempted to do my census, the hamlet mayor, neighbors, friends, and even my "family" reacted strongly and suspiciously, destroying what census data I had collected. My attempts to correct my blunder and explain why I wanted the data were futile. I was told in no uncertain terms: "You may study our language, our ways, and our traditions. But you may not make a *sensus.* You may not count. You do not need to know that. That is the business of the government. You are not government. If you want to count, you must leave Pelocok." From that day forward, I never tried to do anything that remotely could be considered counting nor did I ever collect data with notebook in hand; all details I tucked away in memory and wrote into field notes later. I tried to gather the same data by asking questions about property and income, genealogy, marriage, and children when appropriate within normal conversations, and then people were not at all hesitant to share this information. It was, after all, information available to anyone. The problem was not the content of the information but the manner in which I had attempted to collect it. Unless designated as official, the statistics I cite occasionally throughout this ethnography on the hamlet of Pelocok are from the data I was able to collect in this unsystematic manner. Much of the data are from the 33 households I knew best, with patchier data from some 50 others out of a total of about 135 households in the hamlet.

My Sasak "Family"

The family that adopted me deserves particular mention, for their influence over my life and work was considerable. The father, Amaq

Mol, is a prominent religious leader whose laughter and quiet companionship I treasured. It is through him that I gained semiandrogynous status: I was able to sit with the male religious leaders at rituals and with men gossiping over palm wine. His wife, Inaq Mol, is the mother of his children (then 10, now 11; only 7 are still living). Inaq Mol is a part-time or lay healer. She enjoyed answering my questions, and I learned much from her; but because she controlled the family finances, contention between us arose whenever she discovered I had given gifts to people outside her family.[11] Her daughter, La Nan, did the majority of the domestic chores. She was my earliest companion, and, although our relationship changed after her marriage—as much from my decision to disengage myself from a sole companion as from her enchantment with marriage—she remained a friend, telling me her cares, answering my questions, laughing with me at my blunders, and sharing any current gossip. Her husband, Amaq Sunin, was from a distant town and spoke a different dialect that was difficult for me to understand in the beginning. In addition, I resented his tendency to cut off informative conversations I was having with others by saying "She doesn't need to know that" (see chap. 4). But by the end of the fieldwork, our relationship was friendly. Then there were the small children, who made me laugh, taught me much, and were the heart and joy of the household. Amaq and Inaq Mol had 5 sons in 1994 ranging from about 2 to 13 years old. Amaq Sunin and La Nan (who became Inaq Rhea) had a little girl late in 1994, bringing to 11 the total number of persons living in the 18-by-15-foot house. It is through their

---

11. Negotiating finances in the field was never easy. On the one hand, I needed to pay for my room and board; on the other hand, I did not want to give the Mol family so much money that others became envious. Moreover, my funds were quite limited, there were others to whom I was also indebted (primarily Papuq Isa and Papuq Alus), and periodically I gave small gifts of clothing or money to others in the community. With the Mol family, I never set up an exact amount that I would pay them. Instead, whenever I went to town, I came back with grocery bags full of foodstuffs and gave Inaq or Amaq Mol cash in varying amounts but averaging 10,000 to 15,000 rupiah a week ($5–$7 or just above what a person in Pelocok could earn in cash during a week). In addition, I funded all of the life-cycle and religious rituals the Mol family hosted (14 in number), provided capital for their cash crops, and twice gave them cash gifts amounting to over two times their annual agricultural income. I did not demand any special food and insisted that I enjoyed vegetables as much as meat so that they would not spend extra money on my food. Nonetheless, Inaq Mol often lied to me to get more money (e.g., by telling me that something cost more than it did), and she became angry each time she heard that I had given gifts to others in the community. Asking for money from others and using lies in such manipulation occurs among Sasaks themselves, and, gradually, I learned to sidestep those demands I could not afford to give in to.

social ties and relatives that I initially made my way into the community; throughout the fieldwork my position as a "child" of Inaq and Amaq Mol colored how I was perceived and what I was told.

It is difficult to speculate on how the fieldwork would have differed in a different living situation. Living by myself was not an option because Sasaks' distrust of strangers, particularly ones that have no family or friends to live with, would have made fieldwork very difficult. Moreover, by living with a family I could more quickly learn Sasak, become involved in everyday life, and generally find my feet. By living with the Mol family rather than with the hamlet's mayor's, I unwittingly insulted the latter, who never took me into his confidence. Had I lived with a family with stronger ties to the surrounding communities, I might have gained a more objective understanding of how typical Pelocok was in the region.

A DEGREE OF ABSTRACTION

In seeking to understand the lives of these people, we begin with what seems a simple question: how do Sasaks cope with the fragility of their lives? Its simplicity is deceptive. In seeking an answer, we shall have to delve into the central theoretical problem of anthropology, namely, how can we conceptualize the dynamic relationship between culture and individuals?[12]

One of the most promising answers has come in the form of cultural models or schemas through which culture provides individuals with shortcuts for interpreting events and situations.[13] The notion of models or schemas changes the concept of culture from an object into loosely shared perimeters and guidelines for interpretation that are built up through lifetimes of shared experiences and shared social environments. Internalization is the process by which widely held schemas of interpretation are accepted by an individual, even though each schema is not internalized to the same degree (Spiro 1987). Some schemas are rejected, some are accepted only superficially, and some

---

12. These next pages ground the theoretical discussions found throughout the book in the wider anthropological and ethnographic literature and set the stage for the theoretical approach I take. However, those readers eager to engage Sasak lives and concerns may prefer to skip to chapter 1 and return to these pages as they read the discussions of theory in later chapters.

13. The cultural models literature referred to here is Holland and Quinn 1987; D'Andrade 1992; D'Andrade and Strauss 1992; and, especially, Strauss and Quinn 1997.

become deeply motivated filters for making meaning. Schemas are distributed unevenly among those within a social milieu. This allows for any given individual to have particular ways of interpreting the world (intrapersonal schemas) that are related to widely distributed cultural ideas (extrapersonal schemas). Schemas can thus be studied as patterns for interpretation that allow for human action to rest upon "networks of often highly stable, pervasive, and motivating assumptions that can be widely shared within social groups while variable between them" without reducing cultures to bounded, coherent, and timeless systems of meaning (Strauss and Quinn 1997, 4).

In this ethnography, I am concerned with many of these same issues and draw heavily upon this literature. Yet in two particulars, I find this approach limiting. Like psychologist F. C. Bartlett (1995), I find the terms *models* and *schemas* problematic.[14] These terms imply stable patterns. They are further complicated with the adjective *cultural,* which implies that all persons within a social milieu, like automatons, will have and use the same schemas . This is *not* what the cultural models literature argues, but these terms get in the way of the theoretical concepts. In this manuscript I use *cultural knowledge* to refer to those ways of perceiving and interpreting the world that are widely distributed within a social community. The term *knowledge* is more conducive a concept for understandings that people can value, use, transform, or reject as fits their particular motivations. Moreover, while *schemas* require processes of internalization with their corresponding implication of long-term indoctrination into a shared way of living, *knowledge* is batted about in everyday life. Knowledge can be garnered in casual social interaction as well as built up over a lifetime of learning. It has a flexibility about it that the term *schemas* lacks. Knowledge, while it can be deeply motivated and tenaciously held, is constantly subject to social critique and revaluation in interaction. The ontological reality of people's lives is one that revolves around not abstract schemas but everyday knowledge. In our terminology as well as our descriptions, we must strive to "*get our ontological assumptions right*" (Barth 1987, 8, emphasis in original).

My other concern with the cultural models literature is that it does not provide a framework for studying large processes as well as the smaller ones. In laudably emphasizing how particular cultural models are internalized within persons who then interpret and act upon their worlds based on those schemas, it neglects providing any tools for

---

14. See also Wood 1999.

examining those cultural processes whose structures may affect the content of the schemas. How people interpret the world is not just a matter of what schemas they have and how motivated those schemas are, it is also a matter of *how* they have access to the world. For these reasons, I find it useful to take the insights of the cultural models literature and develop them within the anthropology of knowledge approach.

The anthropology of knowledge is the examination of how knowledge is gained, distributed, and organized within a society (its sociology) as well as what characteristics, qualities, motivations, and meanings knowledge is understood to have by people within that society (its culture).[15] I understand knowledge to be a discrete and distinct entity—any particular idea, notion, expression, or interpretation, both verbal and nonverbal—that can be traced intersubjectively, within interactions and over time. This definition incorporates everything anyone does or says, and at first appears impossibly unwieldy. But by attending to the actions and words surrounding particular topics or incidences, the study of knowledge becomes more manageable. For example, one can study what is done or said in the room of a woman in labor or what is done in efforts to treat a man's broken hand. This approach simultaneously takes into consideration the constraints society puts on individual actors as they get and express knowledge, yet allows room for personal interests to transform received knowledge. Most works using the anthropology of knowledge approach look at large-scale processes of knowledge within communities, particularly at how knowledge is organized and distributed within communities.[16] The anthropology of knowledge literature thus far lacks ethnographies that expand the approach to look at microprocesses of how, in a particular instance, any bit of knowledge is put forward by someone and then received, interpreted, or rejected by others.

In what follows, I attempt to do both. I move back and forth from descriptions of cultural knowledge and the social organization of that knowledge to descriptions of idiosyncratic, personal knowledge and specific health concerns. Thus in asking the question how rural Sasaks cope with illness, we look simultaneously at how specific Sasaks cope with specific concerns as well as how rural Sasaks as a people are con-

15. For studies and commentaries on the anthropology of knowledge see, e.g., Barth 1987, 1990, 1993; Borofsky 1987; Crick 1982; Keesing 1982; Latour and Woolgar 1986; Lindstrom 1990; Taussig 1987; Nuckolls 1996.
16. Barth's work in New Guinea (1975, 1987) and Bali (1990, 1993) are examples of ethnographic writings that examine the overall social organization of knowledge and the cultural ramifications of those particular organizations (see also Latour and Woolgar 1986).

fronted with and have cultural resources to resolve problems of health. In so doing, this book develops the anthropology of knowledge approach into a theory bridging personal and cultural knowledge through small and large social processes.

This theory is founded on basic assumptions about knowledge, interpretation, and communication. Knowledge must be known or held by some person; it does not reside in things or in some nebulous region between people. That said, the degrees of variation among people's knowledge can be conceptualized as falling on a continuum with idiosyncratic understandings at one end and synonymous understandings at the other. Knowledge that falls at the more idiosyncratic end of the continuum is referred to here as idiosyncratic or personal knowledge. Knowledge that approaches the other end of the continuum is referred to as cultural knowledge.

A person's knowledge is formed and transformed through the mechanism and context of its transmission.[17] These transformations require that the theory incorporate an understanding of creativity. Creativity is the process of interpretation through which knowledge is transformed in keeping with the motivations of the knower, her understanding of the context, and her own constellation of prior knowledge. Thus creativity is what happens when a person uses what she knows of her social and cultural world to interpret events, to transform received information into meaningful knowledge. Interpretation, the individual act of making meaning, is simultaneously personal and cultural, individual and social.[18] Because all interpretation is personal and individual, it is to some extent creative. Yet, because we are necessarily cultural and social beings, the tools we use to generate creative interpretations are as much tools of cultural knowledge as they are idiosyncratic perspectives.

The success of these interpretations or creative constructions of knowledge is determined when it is expressed in social interactions. Others' reactions either legitimate or constrain knowledge production. Legitimacy depends on the degree to which the knowledge expressed

17. For different philosophical, sociolinguistic, or psychological perspectives on how the processes of gaining knowledge transform its content, see, e.g., Bateson 1979; Duranti and Goodwin 1992; Peirce 1955; Polanyi and Prosch 1975; Tedlock and Mannheim 1995; Volosinov 1973; Bartlett 1995.

18. How the personal and cultural are related remains a theoretical problem. In addition to the cultural models literature, for writings focusing on symbolism as the mediator between the two, see, e.g., Obeyesekere 1983, 1990; Shore 1991, 1996, 1997; Munn 1986. For writings focusing on social processes as the mediator between the two, see, e.g., Berger and Luckmann 1966; Willis 1977; Luhrmann 1989.

by a given person fits with the recipients' expectations, motivations, and prior understandings of the topic. I assume that persons desire to have their knowledge legitimated, and therefore they reformulate and/or constrain their expression of knowledge in accordance with their perceptions of the context and their social relationships with the recipients.[19]

Three signs that knowledge has been legitimated within a particular context are that other persons will defend it from criticism, they will further distribute that knowledge, or they will enact the knowledge in their behavior. Knowledge is thus more than the verbalization of concepts, ideas, and beliefs. Knowledge is also embodied. Gestures, facial expressions, and ways of physically interacting with other beings and objects are all expressions, albeit nonverbal, of knowledge.[20] Embodied knowledge is also legitimated by others' reactions to one's behavior. Legitimated verbal or nonverbal knowledge is deemed socially acceptable and thus more likely to be widely distributed. Only widely distributed knowledge can become cultural knowledge that people use to further interpret their world and judge others' interpretations. By systematically tracing the patterns of creativity and legitimation of verbal and nonverbal knowledge in the processes of everyday health care, I develop a theory that inherently connects personal knowledge with cultural knowledge while remaining grounded in the dynamic and contingent processes of everyday life.

STUDYING MEDICAL KNOWLEDGE

> All knowledge is the product of a natural process, social
> and cognitive in character rather than logical and
> axiomatic, through which human beings and groups of
> human beings struggle to make sense of their world.
> —CHARLES LESLIE AND ALLAN YOUNG

Medical knowledge, be it part of a global medical tradition or an individual person's own understandings, is subject to these processes of

---

19. See Bourdieu 1977a, 1991 and Goffman 1973.
20. The theoretical position here, informed by work on embodiment (see, e.g., Bourdieu 1977b; Csordas 1994; Foucault 1977, 1978; Lock and Kaufert 1998), draws largely on ethnographic work on kinesthetics and nonverbal knowledge, detailing behavior in social interaction; see, e.g., Hall 1973; Birdwhistell 1970; and Kendon 1990.

individual and social interpretation and is geared toward coping with health concerns. It is surprising then that medical anthropologists have not examined these processes in an integrated way. Many have studied either cultural identifications and interpretations of physiological characteristics or the personal knowledge of medical specialists. And recently, critical medical anthropologists have focused on the social dynamics and power inequalities between those who experience illness and those who control the knowledge and healing of illness.[21] This book does all three, linking them in the processes through which people gain, distribute, and legitimate knowledge.

Moreover, as Leslie and Young note in the quotation above, these processes are motivated by the struggle to make sense of a world of illness, pain, and death. The pain and anxiety of sickness drive behavior and motivate understandings in deeply salient ways.[22] Purely cognitive examinations of knowledge are inadequate to the study of knowledge when lives hang in the balance. The processes through which people gain, distribute, and legitimate knowledge about medicine are emotionally charged. They are motivated by anxiety about health. This ethnography explores personal knowledge about medicine, analyzes how it is emotionally motivated as it gains or loses authority in the details of social interactions, and shows overall patterns of interaction among different medical traditions that affect people's health.

Furthermore, in studying realms of sickness, works in medical anthropology tend to focus exclusively on when people are sick. For our purposes, *sickness* is the umbrella term for both disease and illness, with *disease* defined as pathological states and *illness* defined as interpretations and experiences of abnormality (Young 1982, 264–65).[23] Examining sickness can answer many important questions in medical anthropology, but not all of them. Anxiety about health shapes peo-

---

21. For works in medical anthropology on cultural interpretations of illness, see, e.g., Turner 1967; Nuckolls 1991; Brodwin 1996. For works on the knowledge of health specialists, see, e.g., Kleinman 1980; Fraser 1998. For studies on the politics of medical care, see, e.g., Singer 1990; Vaughan 1991; Farmer 1992; Taussig 1992; Lock and Scheper-Hughes 1996.

22. See, e.g., Good et al. 1992; Good 1994; Kleinman 1980; Desjarlais 1992; Finkler 1994a.

23. Later, Young defines sickness as "a process for socializing disease and illness" (1982, 270–71). In some ways my project of looking at the processes of coping with illness could be defined as a study of sickness using this latter definition. I have nonetheless avoided this terminology because *sickness,* as a noun, somehow does not fit with the notion of process. To my way of thinking, process requires verbs such as *coping* that do not necessarily have an end point, unlike *socializing,* which implies that an illness will eventually become socialized, and process will end in routine.

ple's lives and actions even in the absence of actual sickness. Indeed, how people experience their bodies and understand their selves while healthy influences whether sickness episodes are recognized and how they are diagnosed and treated.

Finally, medical anthropological studies tend to describe consistent medical systems reflecting specialist knowledge.[24] This is problematic because the vast majority of health care occurs at the popular level, in which laypersons rely on their own knowledge rather than consulting health specialists (Kleinman 1980). Moreover, as Dentan (1988) argues, such consistent systems are anthropologists' models that do not accurately describe the "hodge-podge flavor" of the popular sphere of health care. His data show a "welter of mutually contradictory diagnoses, etiologies and cures" (857). In other words, there is a need for studies in medical anthropology that focus on popular rather than specialist health care and that seek to understand the ontological processes whereby illness is actually managed. The approach used here shows how it is possible to study the relative coherence of specialist health traditions side-by-side with the disorderly nature of popular health care.

STUDYING MEDICAL KNOWLEDGE ON LOMBOK

Lombok is a place of multiple medical traditions. These medical traditions emerge out of particular cultural values and practices, or ethnographic environments, and thus are all *ethno*medical traditions. Here, I adopt a commonly used shorthand for distinguishing among them. *Biomedicine* refers to medical knowledge that is based on Western biological and chemical science. I reserve the term *ethnomedicine* for those traditions whose knowledge emerges out of other notions of medicine and healing (Brown 1998).

Lombok has one biomedical tradition and multiple other ethnomedical traditions (although the latter have family resemblances). Among those resemblances is a tendency to emphasize personalistic causes of illness, as opposed to biomedicine, which exclusively recognizes naturalistic causes (Foster 1976). But the most distinctive characteristic of Sasak ethnomedicine is that everyone is a potential healer. This characteristic complicates how people resort to health care. Rural

---

24. While this remains largely true, there are some notable exceptions; see, e.g., Price 1987; Olesen et al. 1990; Romanucci-Ross 1986; van der Geest 1991; Pool 1994; Farmer 1992.

Sasaks do not have a clear hierarchy of resort, jumping among different traditions, medical experts, and laypersons opportunistically. Medical care on Lombok falls along a continuum with biomedical care in a hospital at one extreme and the exclusive resort to spells at the other. Generally speaking, rural Sasaks tend to utilize the biomedical end of the spectrum far less frequently than urban Sasaks.

When I entered the field I had no intention to become a medical anthropologist. Yet, the longer I remained in Pelocok, gathering ethnographic materials on every imaginable topic, the more I came to recognize illness and death as central, everyday experiences. People lost beloved spouses, parents, and children regularly, yet people somehow went on with life, laughing along the way. Health is, I suggest, a continual, daily concern that shifts in and out of focus as other subjects take precedence. Jean Comaroff (1981) cautions medical anthropologists against doing themselves and theory a disservice by prematurely factoring out aspects of life not directly related to disease and healing. So we follow the trails and loops, finding connections among subjects like peasantry and relations with biomedicine, anxiety and remembering, vulnerability and personhood, illness and secret knowledge. Among Sasaks, health concerns are never out of sight. Our interest is to understand how they cope with them in the midst of everyday life.

How Do Sasaks Cope?

Barth (1987) admonishes anthropologists to stay carefully grounded in the materials, not attributing anything to them that we do not have reasonable evidence to show them to possess. With this in mind, we must ask whether the theoretical assumptions of the anthropology of knowledge approach fit with how Sasaks conceptualize their ability to cope with their health concerns.

Sasaks use the word *tauq* in ways English speakers use the word *cope*. *Tauq* means to be capable of doing something (similar to Indon. *bisa*). It involves agency. The Sasak word *bauq* appears similar to *tauq* but has distinct connotations. *Bauq* means for something to be possible, but it lacks agency. For example, if one's sandals are broken, one can say, "*Ndeqku bauq begawa leq bangket*" (I am not able to—it is not possible for me to—work in the paddy field), but if someone says, "I am not capable [*tauq*] of working in the paddy field" the implication is that, whether or not it is physically possible, the person does not have any motivation, any agency to work. This distinction is important in understanding coping with health concerns. When *bauq* is used, an ill person is not perceived to have any agency in managing the illness. When *tauq* is used, a patient is an active agent in managing the illness.

The agency connoted in the word *tauq* is shaded by the definition of "to know," like the Indonesian word *tahu*.[25] Thus, when answering a question like "Do you already have this spell?" a Sasak person would respond with "I already know" (*Tauq aku wah*). Knowing something is conceptually the same thing as being capable of doing something or having the will to do it. Knowledge is equated with capability. For example, when one man was so grieved at the death of his son that he retired from the community to live in a mountain hut for over a year, people said that he was not capable (*tauq*) of living in Pelocok, because he still saw his dead son everywhere he went. He had not yet *coped* with and did not *know how to deal* with his son's death.

For Sasaks, living is a matter of *tauq*—a matter of being capable and knowing to live. More than once, sitting apart with an old midwife I would ask what were an ill person's chances, and she would answer in low tones, "He doesn't know—isn't capable of living" (*Ndeqne tauq idup*).

The title of this ethnography comes from the most heart-wrenching moments of fieldwork, when I heard a spouse, a parent, or a child at once commanding and begging a dying loved one to "Remember! Remember!" (*Ingat! Ingat!*) To stay alive, one must be capable (*tauq*) of remembering. Understanding how remembering keeps death at bay is the essential key to understanding how Sasaks cope with illness and its anxieties.

Because Sasaks themselves recognize knowing as the key component to coping with illness, our own examination, foregrounding the sociology and culture of their medical knowledge, fits well with the materials. It fits so well, in fact, that confusion can arise between the knowledge that Sasaks use and knowledge as a theoretical concept. For that reason, throughout the text, I use the Sasak terms *ilmu* (knowledge) and *puji* (small words) to refer to the specific emic knowledge that Sasaks use to cope with their health concerns. I reserve the word *knowledge* for broader, more etic descriptions, analyses of medical systems, and

---

25. *Tauq* has another meaning distinct from the "being capable, to know" constellation of meanings, namely, the word also means "to occupy a space, to be in a space." For example, *"Wah iye tauq keteq"* means "He has already come here once." The distinction in meanings is made contextually in conversations. For our purposes, this second meaning of the word *tauq* is irrelevant, and for simplicity's sake, I omit this definition throughout the ethnography.

processes of individual creativity and social legitimation involving interpretation and action.

VENTURING OUTSIDE THE TENT,
OUTSIDE THE GATE

After returning from the field, I reread Indonesian ethnographies and
was inspired by some, humbled by others, but always had the vague
sense that, regardless of the cultural similarities, historical overlaps,
and evocative anecdotes, the lives of these Javanese, Sumatran,
Sulawesi, Sumbanese, and Balinese peoples did not seem, well, familiar.
This was even more disconcerting when I reread earlier dissertations
written about Sasak people. I recognized the Sasak words, as well as the
customs, politics, economics, social organizations, and histories. But I
didn't recognize the people.[26] Then I read Dettwyler's *Dancing Skeletons*
on her research in Mali, West Africa. I read smiling at the coincidences
between the images she wrote and my own experiences on the opposite
side of the world. These coincidences catapulted me back to Pelocok to
the extent that I finally scrawled in the margin, "This could be Lombok!" In the dirt and the rain, in the overcrowded trucks and the over-
worked mothers, in the swollen stomachs and the demands for medicine to cure malnutrition, I recognized my Sasak friends.[27]

When Westerners think of Indonesia, images of beautiful green rice
fields and elegant artistry come to mind. Even anthropologists, well
versed in this darling of a field-locale, know Indonesia for political
intrigues, social grace, elegant theatrics, complex emotion work, peasant economies, elaborate discourses, rituals and myths, and captivating
"webs of significance."[28] Indonesia is perceived and valued—and

---

26. Clifford criticizes the "consistent tendency among fieldworkers to hide, discredit,
or marginalize prior written accounts" (1986, 117). While I accept this critique, it is
important to note that this corpus of ethnographic data is not lacking in what it
does—indeed, materials and interpretations are often astonishingly rich and insightful—but that these writings about Sasaks, in topic as well as writing style, largely do
not resonate with me personally.
27. Bart Ryan, an anthropological colleague whose fieldwork overlapped my own, did
work with urban Sasaks. The Lombok he knew, rich in politics, rituals, and religious
negotiations, I glimpsed in visits to the cities. The Lombok I knew he glimpsed in travels through the countryside. But I doubt he would recognize his Sasak friends in the
pages of a book on hunger in Mali. What is interesting is how well the desperate realities of rural peasants are hidden or beyond the realms of relevance for those in urban
settings.
28. See, e.g., Geertz 1960, 1963, 1973, 1980, 1983; Anderson 1990; Pemberton
1994; Heider 1991; Kipp 1993; Bateson 1982; Siegal 1986; Steedly 1993; Peacock
1987; Atkinson 1989; Errington 1989; Sears 1996.

rightly so—as a place of immense beauty. In contrast, when the world thinks of Africa, at least one of our stereotypical mental images is of starving children. We expect death to be brutal and ugly in Africa. In contrast, in Indonesia death is an opportunity for splendid rituals: the magnificent Balinese cremations, the exotic Torajan effigies. But that is not the Indonesia I know. My images are of splendid vistas with caskets carried through them, of elaborate rituals and everyday hunger and illness. For Indonesia's poorest citizens, death is as much hovering over their compounds as it hovers over compounds in Mali.

Appadurai has said that gatekeeping concepts "define the quintessential and dominate questions of interest in the region . . . [thus] the over-all nature of the anthropological interpretation of [a] society runs the risk of serious distortion" (1986, 357). The major gatekeeping concepts of Indonesia emphasizing cultural elegance and intrigue neglect the brutality of everyday life in places like Pelocok. In the field, I did not venture outside of the anthropologists' gate until I sat in a pool of blood at the feet of a woman hemorrhaging to death with a retained placenta and then watched as her infant died 24 days later of starvation and neglect. This was an Indonesia beyond all my expectations. And this was everyday reality in Pelocok.

This ethnography strives to make our images of Indonesians more complex. They are not as bad off as many people in the world, and there is no widespread hunger or starvation now (although there is in recent memory for rural Sasaks), but in some areas, everyday hunger and undernutrition are the norm among the poor. For these poor, everyday life is closer to that found in our images of African dancing skeletons than of Balinese Barong dancers. International aid organizations and the Indonesian government know that poverty and health are critical concerns in some regions, but this has not penetrated our gatekeeping concepts. In reading this ethnography, I ask you to suspend disbelief and venture outside the gate with me, for this too is Indonesia.

—●—

PART I

Less than Healthy

This ethnography is written in two parts. It begins by guiding the reader into thoughtful acquaintance with rural Sasak people. Chapter 1 explores maps: the map of Lombok within which Sasak people live, the map leading geographically to the field site, and the maps written on people's bodies pointing to realities defining their lives and health. Chapter 2 abandons maps and surface writings on bodies in order to explore the various ways in which rural Sasak laypersons and health specialists *understand* their bodies.

Those understandings shape people's anxieties about their health that surface daily *in the absence of illness*. A typical work of medical anthropology probably would start with Part II, in which I examine how people cope with illness episodes. Instead, by exploring how people communicated and acted upon knowledge that had any remote connections with health, well-being, or illness, I learned that how Sasaks cope with illness in its absence has a profound impact on how they cope with it in its presence. Chapter 3 explores Sasaks' sense of vulnerability toward illness, their anxieties about it in its absence, and chapter 4 examines Sasaks' capabilities or agencies to act upon their anxieties and prevent illness.

~ 1 ~

Written on the Body

It was late afternoon on my third day in the field. I was sitting on a mat just inside the doorway, a glass of too-sweet coffee in my hands. Two men, Amaq Mol and a neighbor, were drilling my limited Sasak vocabulary. Inaq Mol and her daughter were shelling beans and laughing at my errors.

A man I did not recognize crept silently into the house and sat leaning against the open door. The others apparently took no notice of him. The language lesson continued for perhaps 10 minutes. Then the conversation shifted to include the quiet stranger. Their conversation, like all conversations within the hamlet, was in a local dialect of Sasak. Only with non-Sasaks or government officials do they speak Indonesian, and then clumsily at best. At this point I understood only Indonesian, so all their conversations, including this one, were incomprehensible. Then the quiet man said *sakit,* a word meaning "sick" or "hurt" in Indonesian as well as Sasak. Inaq Mol got up and, weaving her way around our legs, her upper body bent down looking at the floor, she went out of the house.[1] Their conversation continued. A few minutes later she came back with a cracked saucer holding about a tablespoon of cooking oil. She knelt behind the quiet man. He took off a shirt that was more holes than fabric. Inaq Mol blew her breath on his back, moving her lips as she did so. Evidently the light was too dim, and they repositioned themselves so that the man's back was turned toward the open doorway and in my line of vision.

Then it was obvious to me what was *sakit,* sick. There was an angry red welt, the size of an egg, at the base of the back of the visitor's neck.

The title of this chapter is taken from Jeanette Winterson's *Written on the Body* (1993).

1. Such bent posturing is an action of respect and politeness common in many areas of Indonesia.

I initially thought it was perhaps an ulcer of some kind or the result of an injury not yet healed. Inaq Mol began giving him a back massage, dipping her hands in the oil so that they would work the muscles rather than tug at the skin. Of course, I thought, it is just an enormous knot in his neck muscles. And I waited for Inaq Mol to begin massaging it, to begin smoothing out the muscles of the knot. But she never did. She completely ignored the spot. Stopping the massage, she chewed a quid of betel, spat its red juice all over the man's back, and asked if he wanted a cup of coffee.

Her response to the word *sakit*, the massage, was over, with nothing done to resolve that enormous welt. I was baffled. But over the next few days, I noticed that the man's welt was not unique. In fact, every man beyond puberty in the entire hamlet had such a welt! In retrospect the massage had probably been for sore back muscles from working in the fields too hard that day. The welt was not *sakit*. It was an enormous callous developed over years of carrying produce and wood balanced on a beam over the shoulders and the back of the neck.

Whereas women *beson*, carry things on their heads, men *mikul*, carry things on their shoulders. Everything that must be moved either rides on women's heads or on men's shoulders. Heads can carry as much as 20 kilograms, but shoulders can easily double that. Thus it is primarily men's shoulders that carry crops home from the fields, wood down from the forest, and houses from one compound to another. To carry most loads, men tie them to wooden poles, perhaps one and a half meters in length and eight centimeters in diameter. The poles are worn glossy and dark with years of rubbing on sweating skin. The poles and their loads are balanced over the back of the neck and steadied by the man's hand holding it in front. Boys will begin by carrying light loads on narrow poles. Gradually, as they become stronger, their loads become heavier, and the calluses rubbed onto the back of the base of their necks grow larger. In towns, people rent horse carts to move heavy objects. Even if there were horse carts as far north as Pelocok, they couldn't make it along the narrow dikes of the paddy fields or up the steep paths to the forest. In Pelocok, a man's ability to move things on his shoulder is essential to his livelihood. The resulting welt is a mark of peasantry.

— • —

This ethnography is about bodies. These bodies are blemished and scarred, scratched and broken, quick and dead. Bodies are written on by life, but how does that writing take place? Following the signatures on the body, we trace the loops of who or what does the writing, how and why.

I will argue that the writings are the results of dialectic and dialogic processes, uncountable and contingent, through which people reshape their worlds and, along with them, their bodies. In essence, dialectic processes are direct interactions between two objects—in this case the body and the environment—that mutually react to and affect one another.[2] Blisters and calluses form in direct response to the rubbing of the carrying pole. They are physical manifestations resulting from actions Sasak people take to make a living in the environs of Pelocok. Over time a callus develops into a welt making a man capable of carrying much heavier loads, thereby enabling him to transcend his earlier limitations and act with greater effect on the land. Most physical manifestations on the body are the result of similar dialectic processes. On the other hand, dialogic processes are the mutual, sequential relations of *interpretation* among communicating subjects (Bakhtin 1986, 117). If one takes the abstract structured relationships of dialectics and adds motivated, personal voices intent on understanding, judging, and communicating with other people, one gets dialogic processes (147). It is in dialogue that people perceive and make sense of the physical manifestations on and pains in their bodies. Illness is defined in terms of individual and cultural constructions of physical, physiological, and psychological states. I will argue that it is through dialogue that people construct illness. But we cannot lose sight of the physical manifestations on the body that stimulate those dialogues. Thus we begin by examining bodies. The goal of this chapter is to let the reader see the normal writings on rural Sasak bodies, understand the direct interactions between their bodies and their environment, and touch the surface of the interpretations those writings stimulate.

— • —

Lombok has 4,738.7 square kilometers of land to host its population of 2.5 million. The island is economically poor with an optimistic domestic product of 194,853 rupiah (approx. $100) per capita[3] and is, as I was frequently told by other Indonesians and some Sasaks as well,

---

2. "He sets in motion the natural forces which belong to his own body, his arms, legs, head and hands, in order to appropriate the materials of nature in a form adapted to his own needs. Through the movement he acts upon external nature and changes it, and in this way he simultaneously changes his own nature" (Marx 1977, 283).

3. The currency of Indonesia is the rupiah with an average exchange rate of U.S.$1.00 = 2,210 Rp in 1995 (throughout this book, rupiah equivalents are in U.S.

totally lacking in culture (Indon., *kebudayaan*). Perhaps for this latter reason, Lombok has not drawn many anthropologists. Of the hundreds of anthropologists who have worked in Indonesia, only six have written ethnographies on Sasaks, discussing cultural change (Krulfeld 1974), marriage customs (Ecklund 1977), religion and politics (Polak 1978; Cederroth 1981), poverty (Judd 1980), and a history of Lombok's colonial era (van der Kraan 1980). There are also a handful of anthropological writings on Sasak customs (Hidajat 1972), music (Toth 1978, 1979), poverty (Williamson 1984), and maternal health (Grace 1996; Hay 1999; Hunter 1996). Works on the Balinese people of Lombok (Harnish 1985; Gerdin 1982) and travel journals and colonial accounts round out the literature.[4] Of varying quality, these texts succeeded in putting Lombok on the anthropological map although they did not ignite the anthropological imagination.

To sketch the portrait that emerges out of these ethnographies: Sasaks prefer to hide behind the swords of others rather than fight themselves; their customs are symbolically interesting but not elaborate in comparison to their Balinese neighbors; their poor are skillful manipulators of social hierarchies and ideologies; they accept economic development and accompanying social changes with little fuss; and there remains a bitter and political tension between two Islamic groups on the island, the "traditional" Wetu Telu and the "orthodox" Wetu Lima. If anything, it is this last that kindles the imagination, but not enough to attract more than the passing tourist. Indeed, those tourists are generally disappointed, for the mythic Wetu Telu are always said to be living in the next village over.[5] In short, Lombok has failed to ignite imaginations and is considered an unimportant island that one

dollars). The per capita amount was for 1987 and is the combined figure for Lombok as well as the neighboring island of Sumbawa. Sumbawa, with only half Lombok's population and a much larger land area, is likely to inflate the regional domestic product per capita (Kantor Statistic 1988, 284).

4. See, e.g., Wallace 1922; Vogelsang 1922; Cool 1896; Goris 1936; Graaf 1941; Hooykaas 1941; Liefrinck 1927; Zollinger 1847. For a thorough listing, see van der Kraan 1980.

5. Islam is indeed very interesting on the island, because it has many divergent forms. Islam as practiced and believed in one hamlet can be remarkably different from that practiced and believed in the hamlet less than a kilometer away. But whereas the designation of Wetu Lima and Wetu Telu makes some sense in the Bayan region of North Lombok, elsewhere it makes no sense at all. At most the distinction is one used by orthodox Muslims to deride Muslims with different practices, or it is used by educated, self-designated Sasak philanthropists and NGO workers who wish to "protect" a nostalgic image. Even though outsiders told me I was living in a Wetu Telu area, I never met anyone that others designated Wetu Telu who recognized it as an appropriate designation for her- or himself. See Hay 1997.

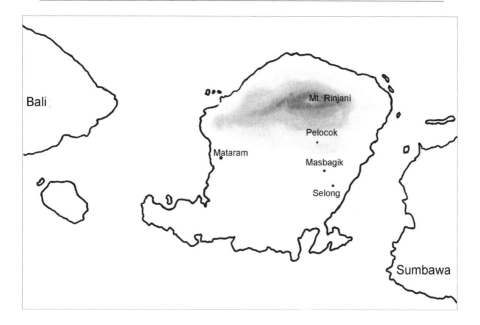

MAP 2. Lombok

passes through going east to Komodo and Sumba or west to Bali and Java.[6]

Geographically too, Lombok is a transitional island, straddling Wallace's line that divides the western, lush islands of Indonesia from the dryer, eastern ones. In its western half Lombok receives much the same precipitation as Bali, but as one travels east, Lombok increasingly resembles its more arid eastern neighbor, Sumbawa. The northern half of the island is dominated by mountains topped off by the volcano Rinjani, rising 3,775 meters, the third highest in the archipelago. Rinjani is active; during the summer of 1994 it burst forth with rains of volcanic

---

6. Aggressive advertising to tourists beginning in the early 1990s hoped to change all of this with the slogan "Lombok Primitive." Between 1993 and 1995 tourism at a place called Singgigi, a resortlike area of hotels and restaurants on the western coast, indeed attracted a good number of tourists, some of whom ventured out to smaller tourist attractions like the islands on the northwest coast, a beach area called Kuta Beach on the southern coast, the "traditional" Sasak village of Sade (a place that the government designated as a living museum similar to Williamsburg in Virginia), and sometimes the village of Tete Batu lying in the middle of the island. Tourism is growing, but Lombok remains a place tourists visit between Bali and Komodo; tourists don't come to Indonesia to see Lombok.

ash, killing much of the vegetation throughout the entire mountainous region in the east.

Between the arid south and the mountains lies a belt approximately 10 kilometers wide, where most of Lombok's people live and most of its produce is raised. The main road on the island cuts west-east across this belt, connecting the tri-city urban area of Mataram, Ampenon, and Cakranegara with Masbagik (an hour's ride away) and extending east to the coast.[7] Masbagik is a dusty, crowded town, attracting people from all around for its market. Twenty minutes by *bemo* (minivan) to the southeast of Masbagik is the town of Selong boasting a hospital. A distance to the north of Masbagik is the place I call Pelocok.

GOING TO PELOCOK

There are no minivans going up to Pelocok. Depending on road conditions, the time of day, and one's financial situation, one must walk, ride the back of a motorcycle-taxi (*ojek*), or climb onto the open bed of a large truck. The walk is uphill taking about an hour and a half and is pleasant if it is not raining. Riding the *ojek,* if one has 1,500 Rp ($0.75)[8] to spare, is the quickest mode of transport, but it only works if one is not carrying much baggage, and one still must walk through the muddy spots and up the steeper hills. I, like most people in Pelocok, usually rode in the back of the trucks. The trucks are inexpensive at 400 Rp ($0.20), and run every couple of hours in the morning, carrying people and their produce to and from the marketplace.

If one is lucky, the truck waiting to go up the road is already fairly full before one climbs on. Otherwise one could have a long wait sitting in the heat on the dirty truck bed and talking to the women there. While men will go to market to sell off entire crops or to buy their own clothing, it is the women who usually go to market, selling a basket of produce and buying food and goods unavailable in the *gawa* (forest), which is what people on the plains call the upland region bordering the foothills of the volcano. Tired from their morning of bartering, these women quietly discuss prices and gossip while waiting on the truck. A truck will not leave before it is jammed with people standing sardine-style along the perimeter of the truck bed with baskets of goods

---

7. This tri-city area had a total population of 300,500 people in 1994.
8. This is equal to or greater than the average day's wages per household for rural Sasaks.

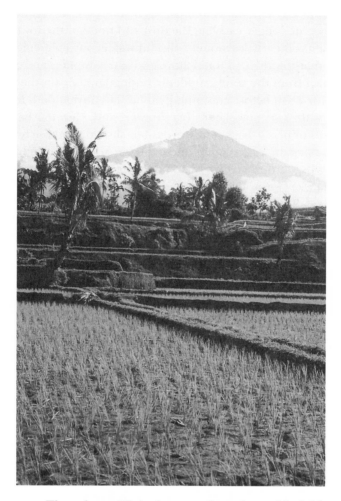

FIG. 2. The volcano Rinjani as seen from the paddy fields
of Pelocok (1995)

stacked waist-high in the middle. After it is full, if one is lucky, the truck
will actually start when it is cranked, and off it goes, with riders ducking
to avoid hitting branches of trees along the road.

As one travels up the winding road to Pelocok one can feel the winds
change. In Masbagik and everywhere on Lombok's plains, the air is
stiflingly humid and warm, usually hovering around 32°C (90°F). As
the truck turns off the paved road north of Masbagik, the landscape
changes from the brownish cream of towns to the emerald green of

fields and forest. The winds blowing against one's face become cooler and crisper, no longer carrying the dust and noise of the towns. Every few moments, the truck's money collector will let out a piercing whistle, the sign that the driver should stop, and a few women and men will climb down from the truck, suddenly urging another on the truck to come in for a visit before continuing home. This invitation is invariably rejected with "not now, later" (*bareh wah*), and, carrying baskets on their heads or plastic bags swung over their shoulders, those few will go off down a path or into a compound of brown houses. The lighter truck continues its journey northward and upward. About an hour after leaving the market town, the road bends and suddenly there is a breathtaking view. Brilliant emerald terraced paddy fields stretch from the road to distant rolling hills and above them in purple splendor rises Rinjani, the sacred volcano. The air is cooler here, ranging between 18°C (65°F) at night and only about 24°C (75°F) at *zuhurr*, the time of the midday prayer. The road bends and the view is again that of a tunnel cut out of green trees and brown compounds. Here, almost at the end of the road, one climbs off the now nearly empty truck and enters the life of Pelocok.

Written on the Body by Peasantry

The longer I stayed in Pelocok, the more I saw persons with distinctive personalities and characteristics. But as a new field-worker, unfamiliar with the local language, surrounded by swarms of people curious to watch the stranger, and not yet able to distinguish one from another, what I noticed first was bodies—warm skin tones, dark hair and eyes, and petite stature—which left me at five and half feet towering over all but the tallest of the men. These features are common to many Indonesian ethnic groups and in no way surprised me. But the longer I watched Pelocok bodies, the more I noticed other markings, common among them but different from the bodies of town dwellers. Watching these closely, I learned to read their bodies for what the markings could tell me about their everyday lives.

In Lombok what is written on bodies is economic situation. A peasant life-style writes a set of markings easily distinguishable from the markings of any other life-style. Once the markings are learned, one can distinguish at a glance a peasant in a crowd of merchants, housewives, teachers, and truck drivers. Because economic activity is so variable among townspeople and so limited among rural Sasak, I draw a dichotomy between townspeople's bodies and peasant bodies. This dichotomy oversimplifies townspeople and, to a lesser extent, rural people. However, it reflects the line represented by the distinguishing marks on their bodies. It also reflects rural people's perceptions of the distinction between themselves and outsiders. Understanding these writings on bodies allows us to comprehend the threats rural Sasak bodies are exposed to, the illnesses they develop, and the conditions that influence how they seek treatment.

To begin at the bottom, we look at feet. Feet in Pelocok are not soft or pretty like town feet. Young feet run bare and are marred by cuts, bruises, and wounds. As feet age, the heels become worn, hard, and cracked with dirt wedged deeply in the crevices. The balls of the feet are thick and callused. Old feet do not wound or cut. They can walk over and through anything—from freezing streams and muddy paths to sizzling dry compounds and sharp rocky roads. They do not bleed. Frequently the toes are splayed, particularly in feet over fifty years old. Those splayed feet, more resembling the triangular feet of ducks than the oblong feet accustomed to shoes, have amazing balance and agility. Having good feet is exceedingly important because walking is the only way to move about in the rural environment. Pelocok is spread out helter-skelter across a landscape of paddy fields and overgrown gardens. Extremely narrow footpaths jog around fields and gardens, connecting lone homesteads with small compounds, and smaller compounds with larger ones. The paths disappear and new ones appear as people move their homes, or they wall off paths with a new corral or garden. Feet must be sturdy to traverse this maze many times daily. Feet must be able to climb uphill for two hours into the mountain fields and trot back down carrying the extra weight of firewood or bundles of corn. Pelocok feet are ugly and unstoppable.

Very young and very old feet go bare: young feet, because sandals are inconvenient to the hurried carelessness of play; old feet, because there is no need for cushioning—the feet are sandals enough. But those feet in-between, of people from the mid-teens to the mid-forties, wear sandals, rubber flip-flops. A few feet wear nicer shoes, particularly right after Lebaran (*id 'al fitri*) when new shoes complete one's new wardrobe for that holiday which ends the fasting month. These nicer shoes, made of plastic, fall apart within a month. Rubber sandals are the norm, and the most practical. They offer a slight cushion from rocks and underbrush. They can be quickly removed and put on again at thresholds to homes. Moreover, they are affordable at 800 Rp ($0.35) for a pair that will last two or more months. After some weeks of wear, the slight ridging of the sandals is rubbed away by the imprint of the foot, and the sandals become slippery. Sandals that do not break will be used until they do, regardless of how slippery and worn they become. Not infrequently a hole the size of one's heel is worn completely through, and still the sandal is worn because it is better to have such a sandal than none at all. Aside from the embarrassment one would feel at not being able to afford sandals, not wearing sandals is treacherous because one's feet are directly exposed to the dangers that lurk unseen on the earth. As we shall see, feet are often the first entry point of an illness.

Pain in one's feet is tragic. I met a man in the spring of 1994 who had just lost his big toe in a machete accident. He and his wife were filled with concern. How would they eat? How would they feed their children? He was landless and had earned their daily bowl of rice by going up to the rain forest and carrying down two bundles of wood and selling them for 500 Rp each. A thousand rupiah is enough for a kilo of rice, spices, and perhaps a vegetable from the market or a piece of candy for his children. But how would they eat without his being able to walk? As it turned out, he stayed home with the youngest children until his wound healed, and his wife went out and worked in other people's fields or asked for food (*ngendeng*) from relatives and neighbors. They got by, as one does. As Amaq Wis once put it, "Here it is not like in America. There if someone is hungry, if you do not know them, you will not ask them in and give them rice. Here, it is not like that. It is not allowed. We must give food to everyone who comes. It is Islam to do so. If we do not have anything, all we have to do is ask for it [*ngendeng*]. If they have it, they will give it to us." No one is allowed to starve in Pelo-cok, but, as no one has very much, there is not a lot to share. A person with bad feet, unable to walk for whatever reason, is completely dependent upon others.

The other body part essential to daily livelihood is the hand. On most hands the nails are cut to the quick. Only a few people who no longer work in the fields—the hamlet mayor and three relatively wealthy men—can let their nails grow fashionably long. The fashion of long nails in men and women is set by town dwellers who do not have to work the land to eat.[9] Working hands do not have the luxury of

---

9. The fashion of long nails on men is widespread in Southeast Asia and may originate in mythical characters. The swordlike fingernail of Bima, one of the Pendawa brothers in the Hindu Mahabharata saga, as it is depicted in Javanese wayang, is a well-known symbol of Bima's strength and power. In Balinese mythology many powerful figures boast long fingernails, again symbolic of their power (e.g., Rangda, the witch

being fashionable. Most hands in Pelocok are strong and leatherlike. They don't tire when pulling sheaves off rice or holding the wooden pole used to pound rice into flour. Hands do not seem to grow stiff and painful washing clothes against rocks in freezing streams. Hands do not shy away from holding a glass of steaming coffee or moving a red coal from a fire into an incense bowl. Hands can plant, weed, and harvest fields from dawn to dusk and spend the evening delicately weaving palm fronds into tiny rice containers. Even young hands in Pelocok, hands of six-year-olds, are tough. They can use a hand knife to cut rice stalks one at a time for days on end, whereas my hands became bloody with cuts and broken blisters within an hour. The tops of Sasak hands are dry, with a sheen of skin pulled in creases across the bones. The undersides are padded with thick calluses. Their hands are not the smooth, soft, moisturized hands of townspeople. Their hands are all bones and pads.

There is little to ease the struggles of hands to extract food from the landscape. Tools in Pelocok are few and simple. The most widely used tool is a machete, a blade about a foot in length usually with a curved tip. Most men wear a machete at all times, the handle thrusting out from the top of their sarongs, the blade in its wooden sheath lifting the fabric of their sarongs at their backs as if a strange tail.[10] The machete is used for everything from chopping wood to cleaning fingernails. Some households also have a smaller knife for cooking, but because these tend to be lost, stolen, or broken, women frequently send children out to go get their father's machete so that dinner can be made. The thin white scars one often sees on hands and legs are the careless inscriptions of these knives.

---

of the barong dance). On Lombok today many if not most businessmen, students, and officials wear long nails, meticulously manicured even if on only one finger (à la Bima). These are taken by others as signs of a man's power/potency and status; thus fingernails are a cultural symbol easily "worked" if one's economic situation does not require hands to do hard labor (Obeyesekere 1990).

10. These knives seem to be a symbolic replacement for *kris*es. The *kris* is much discussed in the literature as *pusaka,* objects of spiritual power, which are never work knives (i.e., Geertz 1973; Anderson 1990). *Kris*es are still worn by some men in an area of South Lombok. In Pelocok, even if a man owns a *kris*, it is considered too powerful to be worn and is kept hidden in his house. Machetes are not considered spiritually powerful, but they are regarded in ways similar to how Balinese men regard their cocks (Geertz 1973). In Pelocok men go nowhere without their machete tucked in their sarongs, lifting it up in back. They take pains to sharpen the blade regularly and to make a wooden scabbard painted in bright colors. They pass machetes around for other men's examination and praise of the blade's length and sharpness. They tell stories of a blade's strength by citing how many strokes it takes to chop down a tree. The machete is a symbol of masculinity and power.

Other than the machete, there are few cooking tools. A mortar and pestle are used to grind spices for meals as well as ingredients for medicines. Metal or coconut-shell stirring spoons and plastic ladles are used to stir boiling vegetables, fry *jeje* (sweets), and scoop out steaming rice. These tools protect hands somewhat, but water, oil, and steam often scald, leaving hands marred with burns. In August women's palms are red-black from shelling coffee by using a scored board and mallet, although, since there are only a few such tools, many people shell coffee with their teeth. A final hand tool, a *pelocok*, is actually a tool replacing teeth.[11] A *pelocok* is a cylinder of metal no larger than the size of a long, thin finger, which has a metal plunger just fitting it. Sometimes food but more often betel is mashed by the thrusting and twisting of the hand-held poker in its sheath. The contents become a mush that old people who have lost their teeth can suck on or eat. These then are the only common hand tools in Pelocok. Their hands remain unsoftened by the luxury of work gloves (there were only three pair in Pelocok at the time of fieldwork), unmarked by pen's ink, and uneased by machines.

As with feet, the loss of one's hands renders a person helpless. On the last day of July 1995, Amaq Urin, a man in his early forties, had a bad fall in the rain forest leaving his right hand swollen and probably broken. The local understanding of his hand injury was that it was *polak*, a diagnosis used for any interior injury involving bones that leaves that body part painful, swollen, and hot to the touch. It was wrapped in leaves and treated daily with secret spells. While it mended, his grown, divorced daughter worked his fields and his sister made his meals, so he got by as one does, but their crops suffered substantially because his daughter was unable to care for them all by herself. Amaq Urin's hand improved, but even after three months he still did not have full use of his fingers. If feet are the key to motion in Pelocok, hands are the key to work. Both must be strong to do the normal tasks essential to living.

More subtle is the writing on the muscles of rural Sasak bodies. There are eight adults in Pelocok who have excess flesh. These people all have wealth and position, allowing them to choose not to work but

---

11. I chose the word *pelocok* as a pseudonym for the hamlet because of my personal association of the hamlet with betel chewing and the widespread use of *pelocoks* among the elderly.

to spend most of their days visiting and relaxing.[12] For the rest, muscles are chiseled out, jumping on the bones underneath a film of skin. One can watch the ripples of jaw muscles as people talk. The neck and back muscles of men and women carrying produce, honing logs into house posts, or washing clothing would put most American bodybuilders to shame. Adults typically weigh between 30 and 45 kilograms (that is, between 66 and 99 pounds, as the government midwife's scale showed when people would step on it out of curiosity). In contrast, the muscles of town bodies are usually masked under layers of flesh, giving townspeople a softer and rounder appearance.

Sasaks do not have many tools to ease the labor of their muscles. A wooden pole is the primary tool of back and arm muscles. As mentioned at the beginning of this chapter, this is the tool men use to carry things on their shoulders, which, in addition to causing a welt on the backs of their necks, builds bulging muscles. Women use this same pole to grind husks from paddy, and flour from rice. They stand above a wooden trough, a hollowed-out wooden stump, or even a mat on the earth and throw the pole vertically down on the rice with one hand, catching and raising it deftly with the other. It is a rhythmic movement of resounding tempo, beautiful to behold but incredibly taxing on arm and back muscles. Another such tool is a long, thin stick sharpened at one end that men use to make holes in a garden field, thrusting it down into earth. Women then drop seeds into these holes and, with their dirty feet, cover them with earth again. Special tools, such as hoes, cattle-drawn plows, hammers, and woodworking tools, are also used, borrowed from their owners once or twice a year.

Although not a tool, there is yet one piece of equipment that sharpens arm and neck muscles and is essential to everyday life: the container. Whether a clay water jug, a plastic bucket, a basket, or a painted metal basin, women are constantly lifting and carrying (*beson*) containers on their heads bringing water home, taking food and dishes out to workers in the fields, carrying laundry and dishes down to the stream, and carrying produce home from the fields. Containers, like wooden poles, pointed sticks, and other tools, encourage muscles to grow in strength and definition.

Creviced and splayed feet, leathery hands, the welts on the backs of men's necks, and incredible muscle tone all physically distinguish peo-

---

12. They are the mayor of the hamlet and his wife, an old man of wealth and high prestige, and the five women who manage food kiosks (Indon., *warung*s).

ple in Pelocok from their counterparts living in Sasak towns. These are the writings of peasantry.

Written on the Body by Poverty

Just as their peasant life-style leaves marks on their bodies, their economic poverty is written on their skin, their children's stomachs, their teeth, and their eyes. Poverty writes on the skin in black ink: in dirt and in black, scabby crusts. Dirt is everywhere inside and outside. In 1995 only a fourth of homes boasted cement floors. The rest, as well as all of the kitchen huts, had floors of packed earth. Nine in every ten houses had mat walls of woven bamboo, with cracks and notches through which the dust-bearing wind blows. Dirt is wedged in the crevices of people's feet and in the cracks of their hands. Perhaps a third of the total time spent bathing, for women at least, is dedicated to cleaning one's feet, scrubbing them with soap, if there is soap. But soap is a luxury most people can not afford. So they scrub themselves with sand, using rough weeds or stones to rub heels and hands in a vain effort to clean the dirt out of the cracks. If one's feet are dirty, others may comment *Tekill nainde* (Your feet are dirty). Despite all the work they do, feet should not be dirty. This is a comment that makes one ashamed (Indon., *malu*). One should never relax at home or go visiting before washing off any dirt. It is shameful not to be clean, so adults usually bathe two or three times daily. In towns, where people walk on paved paths and roads, and work in offices or shops, it is easy to keep one's body clean. Town dwellers bathe in bathrooms; people in Pelocok bathe in the open. Men most often bathe in the green, algae water of the mosque pool. Women and children bathed in streams running between irrigated fields until mid-1994; thereafter they switched to a new cement water tower surrounded by mud. Regardless of how well one scrubs one's body, the walk home from the bathing spot is enough to splash feet and calves with mud and dust. Then one hears again the gentle criticism *Tekill nainde*.

Dirt on children is tolerated. Toddlers are cared for primarily by older siblings who splash water on them once a day, but don't bother to scrub the little ones who leave their baths only to play in the dust and the mud again. Black lines of dirt encircle their necks, cross behind their ears and knees, and run underneath their arms. Often, on the heads of toddlers, what appears to be dirt encrusts a part of the scalp. It is not dirt but an infection that will gradually cover much of the head if an adult does not take over the chore of bathing the child. This crust is identified as an illness, but because it is seen as something normal, something that simply happens to children, it is not considered worth the expense and trouble of seeking treatment. Regardless of vigilant attempts at cleanliness, black dirt and scabs mark their bodies with poverty.

Whereas rural Sasaks condemn dirt, they do not recognize swollen stomachs as problematic. In fact, large stomachs in children are considered a sign of health. Thin children are considered ill, whereas children with bloated stomachs, even when suffering dysentery and bloody discharge, are considered relatively healthy. From an outsider's point of view, peasant children's stomachs also bear the writing of poverty. Hard and swollen, the bellies of young children host worms and other parasites. Worms can enter bodies in any number of places in a poor setting like Pelocok. The streams in which women and children bathe and from which they draw water are the same streams people use to defecate.[13] Babies and young children defecate in and around their house, and the discharge is either eaten by a dog or merely wiped up with a piece of clothing. Women do not wash their hands prior to preparing food. Meals are eaten with the right hand, not washed but only dunked in a finger bowl of water. I know that pinworms, giardia, and schistosomes abounded in the area. Bloody diarrhea, mucous discharge, nausea, wheezy breathing, and lethargy were common in young children, leading me to believe that roundworm, whipworm, and amoebas were also common. The protruding stomachs of children bear witness to poverty.

Sasak teeth are also written on by poverty. I never saw anyone under 15 or over 30 in Pelocok using a toothbrush. Toothbrushes are cosmetic items for young adults, important during the years of courtship when white teeth are considered attractive. But otherwise people do not use toothbrushes. There is no money for them, let alone for toothpaste or dentists. Yet Sasaks have a passion for sugar. Sugar in sweets and overly sweetened coffee takes its toll in painful cavities, abscesses, and pulled-out teeth. In addition, the teeth of people in their mid-thirties and older are mostly red-black, covered by layers of buildup from

---

13. In September 1994, pipes running mountain spring water to a cement reservoir in Pelocok were completed. After this time, except when the pipes were broken, women and children bathed and drew water from this cleaner and much more convenient source. It is difficult to say how this change affected health in Pelocok. Until I left the field in November 1995, I did not notice any marked changes in the sizes of children's protruding stomachs nor in the overall rate or variety of people's ailments.

mamaq (chewing betel). *Mamaq* is a combination of areca nut, lime chalk, and betel leaves all chewed together into a red mass and then held between one's teeth and cheeks, so that its juices can be sucked on. Adding a bit of tobacco to the red mass strengthens the effects of the juices and also provides a web to hold the mass as one talks. Betel chewing is said to confer many advantages, including healing powers and strong teeth. As a narcotic, betel also numbs the mind and quiets a hungry stomach. When rice was scarce, it was not uncommon to see parents rejecting their meals and chewing betel instead, leaving the available rice for their children. For many reasons, including cosmological beliefs, healing practices, and addiction, as well as hunger, betel chewing is essential to the adults of Pelocok. One young man joked as we sat with a group of habitual betel chewers, "If a baby dies, it dies. But if there is no betel leaf, they will send people running in all directions to find it." Chewing betel also distinguishes peasants from townspeople who generally shun the practice, neither needing betel's soothing effects nor wanting its urban connotations as a primitive practice.

No one in Pelocok wears glasses regularly. Glasses are a sign of poor eyesight, worn because one values seeing clearly. On Lombok, glasses are also a sign of wealth and education. The minimum cost of prescription glasses was 200,000 Rp ($91) in 1994. Among the middle classes in urban areas, many people wear glasses. I doubt that people's eyesight in Pelocok was better than elsewhere. Pelocok residents often asked why I wore glasses all the time, and I answered that without glasses everything was blurred (*keliru*). Invariably, people would then ask to borrow my glasses so that they too could see clearly. They would put them on and take them off immediately, saying that the glasses made them *pinung* (dizzy). This was understandable given the level of my prescription, but these conversations about my glasses suggested that many people felt their own vision was blurred. I did see some older men wearing drugstore-quality reading glasses while reading the Qur'an or a *lontar* (palm leaf book).[14] Amaq Mol and Papuq Junin both had such glasses, which they stored in the bulk of sarong at their stomachs whenever they attended rituals. Glasses, usually bent and bandaged at the rims, were prized possessions. But even with his glasses, Amaq Mol could not read very well. He would adjust the glasses and move the *lontar* closer or further from his face. If there was anyone who could take his place at the readings, he would say, "*Ndeqku tahu tegit-*

---

14. Lontars, written in ancient Sasak script, are said to contain the wisdom of the ancestors that is usually expressed in myths, stories, and histories.

aqne" (I can't see it) and pass the reading, along with the glasses, to that person.

Seeing clearly is desired, but it is not a necessity. Only local leaders and some people under 25 are literate. Most children, boys and girls alike, are now sent off down the road to begin first grade. Their parents save or borrow the money necessary to buy at least one of the two required school uniforms of white and red, and gold and brown. The children skip off to school, wet from frigid baths, at about seven in the morning, playing until the teachers arrive at nine. Around noon, after one or two hours of class and many moments of recess, the children come home and diligently take off their uniforms, draping a sarong over the shoulders of their otherwise naked bodies. When school becomes more work than play, or when their parents give them more farming responsibilities, most children quit. Those who actually finish the first year (about half) have begun to learn to read. According to school rosters, of the four hundred plus students who begin first grade each year, only about 30 remain by fourth grade. After all, what in their lives requires literacy? There are no books except a few *lontar*s and the Qur'an—none of which are in Latin script. There are no newspapers. There is no need for anyone but *kiayi*s (religious leaders) and the *kepala dusun* (hamlet mayor) to know how to write.[15] Any official document that needs signatures is "signed" with a thumbprint. The only people who ever leave Pelocok are some young girls marrying out and a handful of young men who go off to seek their fortune working in the rubber fields of Malaysia. For what, then, would one need to see clearly? Eyes are not important enough to pay a year's wages for glasses or surgery. Those with poor eyesight just live with poor eyesight.[16] Those with glaucoma, cataracts, xerophthalmia, or other eye problems simply go blind.

In Pelocok, the poverty people live with blackens their skin and teeth, swells children's bellies, and threatens their eyesight. Embedded in peasantry and poverty, rural Sasak bodies—normal bodies—bear the writings of their lives.

---

15. *Kiayi*s must know how to write "letters" to Allah, to be buried with old people who may forget that they are Muslims. *Kiayi* can also be spelled *kyai* or *kijaji* (e.g., Anderson 1990; Geertz 1960). The spelling chosen here of *kiayi* (key-ae-yee) most closely represents Sasak pronunciation.

16. Inaq Mol, the daughter of the most renowned *belian* (female healer), once told me, *"Ndeqne are owat care Sasak si kuat gen mata"* (There is no strong medicine in the Sasak way for eyes).

The Peasant Economy

The peasant economy and life-style set the stage where bodies and land mutually mark one another. Thus we draw back from the body momentarily to view the stage, to see the limited props available for people in Pelocok to use. Welts, splayed feet, hard hands, and black teeth arising out of daily activities are not considered problematic. But related writings on the body such as cuts, burns, sore muscles, scabby heads, and eye problems are considered ills. Peasantry figures directly and indirectly in making bodies ill. More than that, peasantry colors their world; it shapes how they perceive their bodies, understand their illnesses, and seek health care.

Recently, the concept of the peasant has been criticized as a stereotype that masks internal diversity, implies dualistic categories, and reflects a historical period when anthropology scrambled to come to terms with the end of colonialism (Kearney 1996). Moreover, the negative connotations of the word *peasant* call forth images of backwardness and static traditionalism that can have important political consequences (171). All of these criticisms are important, yet the term *peasant* still seems to me useful to introduce people in Pelocok. Later in the ethnography, as persons in Pelocok become differentiated, the term *peasantry* loses its descriptive power. But the connotations of backwardness and the stereotypes of poor people who work the land without expensive technologies remain constitutive of interactions between people of Pelocok and those with fancier clothes, cleaner bodies, and urban life-styles. Thus, while not a justifiable term with which to end an exploration into Sasak lives, *peasantry* is a good one to use at the outset.

Definitions of peasant economy have stressed different things. Peasants have been defined as those who have the "rudiments of capitalist (i.e., market) economy," simple technology, subsistence production, high population density, and production intensification (Dalton 1961, 209–10; Firth 1956, 87; Johnson and Earle 1987, 271). Fundamental to all of these definitions is that the "peasantry always exists within a larger system" that the peasant feeds and ideologically supports (Wolf 1966, 8, 48ff.). Paradoxically, then, peasants uphold social systems—even in moments of resistance—that marginalize and denigrate them (107–9; see also Scott 1976, 1985). By any of these standards, Pelocok has a peasant economy.[17]

These Sasaks are poor peasants. They engage in the market econ-

---

17. For a more general analysis of Lombok's peasant economy see Krulfeld 1974.

omy and depend upon cash to purchase necessary items ranging from salt to sandals, from ceramic dishes to clothing. Yet their technologies remain simple, using half a dozen tools to meet all of their needs. Land is scarce. Every available corner is used. Even so, only a handful of people produce more than subsistence quantities.

In October 1995 the population of the Pelocok area stood at 1,918 persons, divided among 395 households.[18] Young households may have as few as two or three persons. Birth control is something people know about and could use, but children are a prime source of pleasure and pride as well as help, therefore a typical couple has between five and eight children. Thus a household at its peak may have ten or more persons, often including ailing parents and married children. Eventually a household will wane, as widowers are taken in by daughters and widows head small households of one to three people. This growth and waning of household size corresponds loosely to the growth and waning of land ownership.

There are three kinds of land available. The most valuable are the irrigated paddy fields (*bangket*), followed by the unirrigated garden fields (*kebun*), then the unirrigated mountain fields (*kontak*). Irrigated fields cost as much as 2,000,000 Rp ($905; over 10 times the average annual income per household) per *arah*. Fields are measured in *arah* (Indon., are) and *hektar* (Indon., hectare).[19] Unirrigated garden lands are much less expensive, priced as little as 100,000 Rp ($45) per *arah*. The combined hamlets of Pelocok and Lakongak owned 22 hectares of irrigated fields and 160.7 hectares of garden fields in 1995. Approximately one in five households owns any of the valued irrigated fields. Irrigated fields tend to have better luck than other fields with cash crops, and one can depend on them for a good annual rice harvest.

---

18. As discussed in the introduction, I did not complete a census. These official census figures are for the region designated as Pelocok, although locals identify two hamlets within it: Lakongak and Pelocok.

19. According to the metric system, one are is the equivalent of 100 square meters and one hectare the equivalent of 100 are or 10,000 square meters. Repeatedly, I was told by men in Pelocok that an are was equal to 10 square meters and a hectare equal to 100 square meters. While the official records given might use the correct metric equivalents, the sizes of the holdings I saw were more in keeping with the equivalents given to me in Pelocok. In other words, their actual landholdings were much smaller than the official metric equivalents imply. Were the official estimates of arable land correct, landholdings in Pelocok would include 220 square kilometers (86 square miles) of irrigated lands, and Pelocok's population density would be 1 person per square kilometer of arable land—figures that are untenable considering the area's constant land shortage, poverty, and the sizes of landholdings. Unfortunately, I was unable to do any exact calculations of landholdings because people perceived any counting or censusing on my part as threatening (see Introduction).

Most households own only unirrigated garden fields. The poorest households, those headed by women or by young men, own as little as one small garden in which to grow vegetables, or they own nothing at all.

In addition, every male-headed household has rights to an unirrigated mountain field (*kontak*). The mountain fields are government lands that villagers are allowed to use on the condition that they plant trees on their plots to reforest the foothills. Annually government officials come and lecture the village men that they must plant more trees. And annually the villagers of the area nod in agreement, with no intention whatsoever of planting more trees. Trees take away from the usable size of their assigned plots. Access to these plots is inheritable and also can be leased out to others, should the "owner" not have the time or resources to plant it himself.

Land is most easily acquired through inheritance. Inheritance rules require that sons be given two-thirds and daughters one-third of parental property. In actuality, usually more than two-thirds is handed over to sons, which is justified as Islamic *rukun* (Sas., religious obligation) for land inheritance.[20] A 20-year-old married son will live with his parents and work their land until they die or agree to give him his inheritance. Then he will set up his own household. If his crops are successful, he will buy more land. As he ages, his sons and daughters will gradually take over the work of his lands. Eventually he will give them his lands, trusting them to care for him until his death. This is an ideal scenario. It often happens that parents are so poor there is next to nothing to bequeath. Even if the parents are well-off, there are often so many children that the children do not inherit enough to make a living.

Subsistence and Land Usage

One has the impression that every square inch of land is used. Like those in Bali or Java, the irrigated lands in Pelocok and throughout Lombok are terraced and worked intensively to maximize their size and produce (e.g., Lansing 1991). Less obvious is the intensive use of land surrounding compounds. At first glance these areas of dense overgrowth seem to be a mass of weeds; actually they are horticultural gardens filled haphazardly with tubers, beans, chayote, squash, chilies,

---

20. Islamic law follows al Qur'an, Surah 4:11, which states: "Allah (thus) directs you as regards your children's (inheritance): to the male a portion equal to that of two females" (Ali 1989). In Pelocok, inheritance to daughters is not strictly apportioned, but if there is anything to inherit all daughters must receive something.

cloves, bamboo, chocolate, coffee, banana, and durian. Planted and ignored until ripe, this produce was then gathered for the next meal. If no vegetable was ripe, a few leaves off of a squash vine (*walu*), the tender new shoots of a certain kind of fern (*baku*), a wild mushroom—all can be used for a meal. People in Pelocok are fond of saying, "Here we are rich in food. In towns they have to use money to eat. Here we only have to go out and find it." Even so, food is not abundant, and there are often periods of meager meals resulting from crop failure, the dry season, and, occasionally, volcanic ash that coats vegetation.

On their lands people plant three times annually at most. The crop rotations correspond to the seasons. Pelocok's rainy season begins in December and lasts through April. The rest of the year is dry, with water truly scarce in August and September. The first crop, planted in December and harvested in February, is rice. The second crop, usually a cash crop, is planted in April and harvested in the dry months of June and July. The third crop is usually vegetables or a second rice crop, planted and harvested in the fall. This schedule of planting must be adjusted to allow for different growing seasons, land differences, climatic variations, and the industriousness of the workers. The only certainty is that everyone with access to land will plant a rice crop at least once a year. A good crop on an irrigated field will sustain a large household for six to eight months. Dry field rice crops yield less, usually only enough to support a household for two or three months.

The shortage of irrigated fields means that many households in Pelocok can not subsist on their land holdings. Land shortages are common throughout Lombok, which had a population density of 540 persons per square kilometer in 1994.[21] Lombok participates in Indonesia's transmigration program (Indon., *transmigrasi*) in which the government pays for persons willing to relocate from islands of high population density to islands of low population density. In 1995, a group of households from the hamlet north of Pelocok chose to transmigrate to Maluku. Their transmigration caused a stir in Pelocok. Some young men spoke of wanting to transmigrate because it was too difficult to make ends meet in Pelocok (literally, too difficult to get enough to eat, *sekat ite mangan*). But they were silenced by their elders and their wives who stressed that no matter how difficult, Pelocok was home. Transmigration was not considered an acceptable option; instead, people sought subsistence in other ways.

---

21. The population density was calculated by using the population estimates from Dinas Kesehatan 1994 and geographic figures from Kantor Statistic 1988.

Sources of Cash

For those with access to at least some capital, the second growing season is when hopes are planted for financial gain. Garlic (*kesunah*) has the potential for the most rewards, but the starting bulbs are the most costly, 300,000 Rp[22] per *quintal* (100 kilograms), which is enough to plant 3 or 4 *arah*. Moreover, the crop is delicate. In 1994, the garlic crops were successful. Many people tripled or quadrupled their investment leaving them with enough to invest in a cow, chickens, clothing, and the like. In 1995, everyone planting garlic lost the entire crop because of too much rain.

The second favorite cash crop is shallots (*bawang abang*). Not as expensive an investment at 135,000 Rp ($61) per quintal, its potential is also not as great. Shallots are equally fragile. The 1994 crops failed because of lack of rain. In 1995 the crops fared better, but did not double investments as they are fabled to do. Many families suffered consecutive years of failed crops, planting shallots in 1994 and garlic in 1995.

Garlic and shallots are both high-risk, high-return crops that are labor-intensive and occupy a field for a relatively short period out of the year. The other common cash crops have long growing seasons; therefore, while low risk, they have the drawback of occupying precious farmland for long periods. Pineapple is one such crop, requiring only 12,000 Rp ($6) per quintal of seedling (*bibit*). It is a hearty plant that generally triples the investment, but it has an 18-month growing season. Another crop is sugarcane. Its growing season is a full year, but it regenerates itself after a harvest. In 1994, a crop on 10 *arah* sold for 180,000 Rp ($81) but in 1995 the season was poor and the same field's crop sold for only 63,000 Rp ($29).

There are other crop options that can produce marketable surplus, but the investments and the surpluses are so minimal that to call them cash crops exaggerates their significance. Moreover, these hearty plants are mingled together in a field or garden, emphasizing their main purpose of providing food for the household rather than surplus to be sold. These plants include corn, tubers, various beans, chilies, cherry tomatoes, cloves, squash, cabbage, coffee, coconuts, bananas, and durian.

---

22. This equals $136 or the income an average Pelocok household could expect to earn over a year and a half.

Any significant amount of cash gained in selling produce is usually invested in a cow. Cows are the savings accounts of peasants. There were 135 cows in Pelocok in 1995, about one in every four households. Cows are not milked and are used only in plowing irrigated fields and breeding. They are owned, petted, prayed over, and cared for rather as one would an antique car one is afraid to drive too much. Families will buy and keep as many cows as possible as security against hard times. Occasionally cows are sold for rice to feed a family. Most often, cows are sold or killed for ritual obligations. Grown cows cost between 150,000 ($68) and 600,000 ($272) Rp, whereas bulls can be as much as 1,500,000 Rp ($680). If one owns cows, one's economic situation is not so precarious; one has a walking safety net.

Even so, life in Pelocok is tenuous: one completely ruined crop, and food becomes scarce. In 1994 one family borrowed 4,000,000 Rp ($1,800) to buy seed for a shallot crop. But that year all the shallot crops failed. The family had no means of paying off the debt and no relative who could afford to lend them so much. They sold their land, their cow, their home, and all their belongings and moved with the clothes on their backs to Sumbawa where the father hoped to get work as a day laborer. They went from peasants to homeless poor in a few short months.

Approximately a quarter of the households in Pelocok own no more than a small garden or no land at all.[23] These people largely live in female-headed households or young, impoverished, male-headed households. These people rely on day labor (*beboreh*) and their own ingenuity. Day laborers working in others' fields are fed breakfast, coffee, and lunch and given a portion of the produce collectable at harvest.

Other than day labor, landless peasants rely on their own ingenuity to feed their families. One physically difficult but common path of young men is to gather bundles of wood in the rain forest, a two hour hike into the mountains, and carry them back on a wooden pole balanced on the welt at the base of their necks. Two bundles, all a man can reasonably cut and carry in one day, can be sold for 1,000 Rp ($0.45). The most common way for women to bring in money is to act as a middleman: buying produce in one place, transporting it, and selling it again. Pelocok women would buy surplus vegetables, transport them

---

23. Estimates suggest that the number of landless peasants in the province of Nusa Tenggara Barat (incorporating Lombok and Sumbawa) amounted to 38 percent of the rural population in 1973 (Kano 1994).

down to the market, and resell them there, often profiting only 500 Rp. Larger profits could be had if a woman, or more likely a group of women, could buy an entire crop, such as a coffee crop. They would work together to harvest the beans, then shell and resell them. If the crop was good, each woman in the group could earn as much as 20,000 Rp ($9) for her labors. Regular marginal profits could be had for those few women with a little capital who bought produce, candy, and other small goods at the market, then sold them at a marginal profit either in their own food kiosks (Indon., *warung*)[24] or out of baskets they carried on their heads as they walked from compound to compound.

One final way for the landless poor to make ends meet is to scavenge on the harvested lands of others. It is the right of the poor that after a rice harvest they can go onto others' fields and pluck up fallen rice kernels and unharvested stalks. Many a day I helped an old woman, Papuq Alus, pick up kernels in a field strewn with emptied rice stalks, only gathering enough rice for her evening meal.

Another potential source of cash is engaging in illegal activities.[25] The favorite among older men was gambling at cockfights. Winnings were relatively rare, and the losses sometimes went as high as 100,000 Rp ($45). Winnings were taken as windfalls and immediately spent on alcohol and clothing. Among young men *maling* (Indon., theft) was a favored source of income.[26] Cows were the preferred prizes of theft, but thieves did not shy away from stealing an entire cash crop, harvesting it by moonlight. Both kinds of theft are dangerous.[27] If caught by villagers, the thief is often beaten to death; if caught by police, the thief is usually imprisoned. More common than *maling* is *nyalet* (Sas.), the

---

24. Unlike *warung* in towns of Lombok and elsewhere in Indonesia, these *warung* were simple affairs. Sitting or sleeping on a bamboo bench, a woman would sell her wares from a thatch-covered bamboo table. The smaller *warung* just carried teaspoon-sized packets of sugar, cigarettes, matches, and sweets (*jeje*) for children. The three larger *warung* also carried dried fish, tofu, chilies, eggplant, tomatoes, cabbage, beans, cucumbers, eggs, *piksin* (MSG packets), salt, *terasi* (shrimp paste), plastic tubes of cooking oil, kerosene, soap, shampoo packets, and sandals.

25. Gambling and large-scale theft were *not* engaged in by many men in Pelocok. It is difficult to estimate numbers because people were fairly secretive about participating in illegal activities, particularly large-scale theft (*maling*). Perhaps four out of five household heads gambled two or three times a week during periods when farm work was minimal. I would estimate that only one out of every five households had a man who engaged in *maling* once every few months.

26. Sasaks have a reputation for being thieves, particularly among the Balinese (i.e., Wikan 1990).

27. The victims of cow and crop theft suffer, particularly victims of crop theft. While cattle are usually equivalent to a savings account, cash crops, often planted with borrowed capital, are the primary source of annual income for land-owning peasants.

stealing of small, inexpensive things.[28] This is a regular and daily occurrence among men, women, and children of all ages in Pelocok. Although I heard some people vehemently condemn the practice, I also saw community religious leaders laugh about how they had stolen an egg from underneath a neighbor's chicken. A few rupiah, foodstuffs, and cooking utensils are most commonly taken. I leave cockfight winnings and gains from theft aside in the figures on income given below because, being illegal activities, people were extremely hesitant to speak about them.

The final source of cash available to only some people some of the time is payment for special services: providing alcohol, conducting rituals, or treating illness. This income is nominal. Alcohol in Pelocok is *tuaq* (palm wine), tapped directly from the *now* tree. A one-gallon plastic gasoline jug of good *tuaq* costs 1,000 Rp ($0.45). The owners of these trees could sell their *tuaq* to neighbors putting on rituals or to outsiders from towns coming to Pelocok for *tuaq*. But this lucrative if seasonal income was drastically curtailed by friends and neighbors coming over and urging the owner to sit and drink the *tuaq* together. Thus the income gained from selling *tuaq* is sporadic at best. Another kind of service, that provided by a religious leader (a *kiayi*), is essential to every ritual. There were eight *kiayis* in Pelocok in 1995, although only four of them were regularly invited to pray at rituals. A *kiayi* earns between 100 and 200 Rp per prayer session in addition to ritual food, varying from one rib of bananas to two or more baskets of ritual food. While this is a substantial supplement to the average household income, it is sporadic and insufficient to be a household's sole support. The third special service is that of a healer. Local healers are generally paid in kind with a small basket containing a cup of uncooked rice, an areca nut, a pinch of lime chalk, betel leaves, a little tobacco, a circle of cotton string, and 100 to 200 Rp for treatment of minor ills.[29] Payment increases if the required treatment is for a more serious illness. For example, a person with a broken hand might pay 500 Rp ($0.23). Childbirth earns the midwife approximately 1,000 Rp. Someone ill

---

28. Small, inexpensive items and small amounts of cash were taken from me rather regularly. This was bothersome, but even worse was my fear (shared by my "family") that thieves (*maling*) would come in to steal my camera and tape recorder. This prompted me to ask that a wall and door be built in my corner of the house. It was, and thereafter I kept the door locked. The wall was a flimsy mat wall, like the exterior house walls, affording little privacy or much security against a very determined thief. But my room was never broken into.
29. These baskets are both payment and gifts to the healer's spirits and gods that aid in the healing.

because of a black magic attack could pay 10,000 Rp. Nearly every adult in Pelocok has healing knowledge for some kind of illness, but only three have enough patients to substantially contribute to their income.

Household Economics

In total, the average daily income for a household where one person sought cash income hovered between 500 and 1,000 Rp ($0.25–0.46).[30] For those who did not seek daily cash incomes, namely, the landowning peasants who counted on harvests to feed the family, the average annual income *per household* hovered around 200,000 Rp ($91) in 1994 and 1995. This can be compared with the average *per capita* income in Lombok of 200,000 Rp in 1988 and the average in Indonesia of over 2,200,000 Rp ($1,000) cited by then-president Suharto in his state-of-the-nation address in 1996. Even taking the different years of these statistics into account, the income of Pelocok peasants is low indeed. These statistics measure only cash income. Nonetheless, they give some indication of Pelocok's poverty, a poverty all the more profound when compared to the costs of living.

There are a few things for which cash is used. The most essential item is rice, usually costing 650 to 750 Rp ($0.29–$0.34) per kilogram. For a two-month period in spring of 1995, prices skyrocketed to 1,200 Rp ($0.50) per kilo, leaving many villagers hungry. For a small household, one kilo can last two days. For a larger one, two kilos a day were necessary. Note that the cost of rice is equal to or higher than the highest possible daily cash income, and not surprisingly, when households are reduced to buying their rice, they quickly run out of resources and sometimes sell livestock and belongings to continue to eat. Houses cost anywhere from 100,000 Rp for the smallest hut to 2,500,000 Rp ($1,131) for a house with a cement floor, stucco walls, and glass windows. Most houses in Pelocok cost between 300,000 and 800,000 Rp ($136–392). Clothing and household costs are between 20,000 and 50,000 Rp ($9–23) per adult annually. Annual land taxes for average households are between 8,000 and 20,000 Rp ($3.50–9). Livestock taxes are about 5,000 Rp per cow. Then there are collections for community projects, such as building a new mosque, that total between 20,000 and 50,000 Rp depending on a household's means. If one lives sparsely and works hard, one can make ends meet. The problem is that

---

30. In theory, if a person worked 300 days a year, this would work out to an annual income of between 150,000 and 300,000 Rp, which would be about equal to the incomes of landed peasants.

unexpected and costly events, such as total crop failure, theft, severe illness, or (most frequently) life-cycle rituals, affect each household at least once a year.

The Economic Requirements of Ritual

There are five life-cycle rituals (*begawai*): marriage, *besumbut* (a first pregnancy ritual), *molang-malik* (a name-giving ceremony), circumcision (full entry into Muslim community), and *bekuris* (a rite signifying full entry into the cosmological and cultural community). While these last two can await the parents' financial capabilities, the first three ceremonies cannot be delayed. The most embarrassingly spartan marriage ceremony costs about 50,000 Rp ($23). A *besumbut*, the least expensive ritual, only costs about 10,000 Rp ($4.50). One can scrape by with 35,000 Rp ($16) for a *molang-malik*. Circumcisions and *bekuris* rituals cost at least 85,000 Rp ($38).

In addition to life-cycle *begawai*, there are seven *begawai* that must be given at each death, on the first, third, fifth, ninth, forty-fourth, hundredth, and thousandth day after death. One of these seven, preferably the one on the ninth day after death, must be a large ceremony where a goat or a cow is sacrificed, many baskets of goods and belongings are given to community leaders, and all surrounding neighbors are fed. This one ceremony costs at least 150,000 Rp ($68 or almost the entire annual income of a typical household). The minimal cost for each of the other death ceremonies is 10,000 Rp. Thus every household is responsible for giving every member twelve *begawai*s throughout their lives at a bare-essentials cost of at least 475,000 Rp ($215).

The households of community religious leaders, *kiayis*, have the additional responsibility of hosting five ceremonial meals (Indon., *selamatan*)[31] at a cost of 10,000 to 30,000 Rp ($4.50–14) each on the holy dates of the Islamic calendar: *Nisbu* (the night of Ascension), *Malaman* (the 29th day of Ramadan), *Bubur Putih* (the month of white porridge),

---

31. Geertz (1960) discusses the ceremony of *selamatan* or *slametan* in detail, describing it as a communal feast. Remarkably similar to the *selamatan* as described by Geertz for the rural Javanese, among Sasaks the *selamatan* is different only in the food that is served, the easygoing, casual manner, and the role of the host. Among Sasaks, although the host will welcome guests and chat with them beforehand, he sits apart from the actual ceremony, leaving all prayers to the invited *kiayis*. Moreover, no speech is made to explain the general reason for the rite; it is assumed all the guests already know, but those who don't can figure it out from the words of the prayers. As for the Javanese, the *selamatan* is a core or basic ceremony fundamental to all formal Sasak rituals.

Bubur Abang (the month of red porridge), and *Maulid* (Mohammed's birthday).[32] Each of these life-cycle, death, and Islamic rituals is considered *rukun*, unquestioned obligations of intertwined Islam and *adat* (Indon., custom).[33] It should be noted that the people of Pelocok are unusually devoted to *rukun*. Surrounding hamlets to the north, east, and west, and the towns of the south and elsewhere on Lombok do not celebrate all of these events. People from Pelocok speak with derision of these others who do not follow the words of their ancestors and who care more about money than about *rukun*. Regardless of the economic straits that one of the larger *begawai*s can put on a household, people in Pelocok rigorously adhere to their *rukun*.

Part of that obligation is in preparing elaborate ritual foods that make up the primary cost of rituals. In contrast, everyday food is very simple and nutritionally bare. Rice is the only daily standby, with every person having at least one bowl of rice per day, even if they have to eat at a relative's or beg from a neighbor. Rice is essential for eating. Indeed, unlike in Indonesian, in Sasak there are two words for "eating": *mangan* and *naken*. *Mangan* is eating rice. *Naken* is eating anything else, comparable to snacking in English. Rice is essential, everything else is just snacking. Thus, while people recognize that eggs and meat are desirable if unaffordable, Sasaks do not see their economic situation as causing malnutrition as long as they have rice. In addition to rice, there is nearly always a boiled vegetable seasoned with non-iodized salt and a spicy paste (Indon., *sambal*) of chilies, onions or garlic, and shrimp paste. Protein sources such as eggs, dried fish, bamboo worms, tofu, or tempeh are rarities gracing a meal maybe twice monthly. Surprisingly, fruits are also rarely eaten: instead, durian, bananas, and pineapple are sold as cash crops. Thus the nutritional value of daily foods was largely limited to starchy grains and green vegetables.

Life in Pelocok is the life of poor peasants who are tied to the land for their daily sustenance, supplementing their household incomes with cash-earning ventures. Between covering their minimal living costs

---

32. To my knowledge, Bubur Putih and Bubur Abang are unique to Islam as it is practiced among some communities of Sasaks. The *selamatan* and related taboos of these two months are not practiced among the majority of Sasaks on Lombok, although they too call them the months of Bubur Putih and Bubur Abang. In East Lombok, I was aware of fewer than two dozen communities, all of rural peasants, that upheld some version of the *selamatan* and taboos.

33. The word *rukun* in Indonesian is used to mean the pillars or basic principles of Islam. The usage of this word in Pelocok has Islamic connotations while closely resembling the Indonesian *rukun syarat* meaning "customary, minimally obligatory rules" (Echols and Shadily 1989).

and their ritual obligations, rural Sasaks remain in a precarious economic situation. There is little money to spend on soap, vitamin-rich food, or other niceties. Their peasantry and their poverty write on their bodies and make them particularly susceptible to various illness. At the same time, financial concerns are omnipresent, coloring their decisions, including how they react to concerns of the body.

READING THE WRITINGS ON THE BODY

As we have seen, living in peasantry and poverty leaves writings on normal bodies. Peasantry inscribes itself on bodies by building welts on the backs of men's necks, by making feet hard and splayed, by adding leathery pads to hands, and by shaping muscles so that they are efficient and strong. Poverty inscribes itself on bodies by blackening skin and teeth, swelling children's stomachs, and denying treatment to those with poor eyesight. These writings give evidence of some of the challenges their bodies must face.

Nonetheless, in themselves these writings do not mean much. In my opinion, when at their best, bodies in Pelocok are active, quick, and strong. Even though inscriptions of peasantry and poverty can be spotted instantly in a crowd of townspeople, rural Sasaks always looked healthier and stronger to me than the rounder and softer townspeople. Yet Pelocok women and men would regularly describe their own bodies as *lenge* (ugly, bad) in comparison to the bodies of their urban-dwelling counterparts. They idealized white or paler skin, skin not tanned by working long hours in the sun. They idealized the soft, plump (*mokoh*) bodies that do no hard physical labor and have plenty to eat. They idealized the black shiny hair, which many think comes from the luxury of shampoo rather than a well-balanced diet. They idealized the soft, clean hands with long nails of those who work in offices. They idealized the feet that rarely walk far and are hidden within shoes. They expressed these ideals often, particularly in words either praising or criticizing me.

Indeed, while I was consciously working to mark my body somewhat like theirs, they strove to keep my body like those of townspeople. My pale skin was admired, but as it tanned, women would scold me for not staying out of the sun. They worried about my weight loss, pushing more food in my direction. Older people would forbid me to work beside them in the fields because, they said, I would hurt or tire myself. Then, after I stubbornly worked anyway, they would look at my dirty body and blistered hands and feet, telling me that I should have listened to them, and that now I looked bad/ugly (*ide gitaqne lenge*). Where were my real shoes, my skirts and dresses? Why didn't I use *smir* (hair dye) so that my hair would be good (*sola*), meaning black, rather than brown? Why didn't I pay for a motorcycle-taxi to ride everywhere rather than walking or riding the dirty trucks? Eventually I succeeded— against all their efforts—in marking my body with something of the peasantry and poverty of their lives. I sensed they took it as a compliment even as they could not understand why I would want a body like theirs. After all, as they told me, their bodies were *lenge*.

In the same breath, they would say things like "Even though we Sasak are ugly, we are strong" (*Dengan Sasak lenge laguq kuat*) or "We are ugly, but we know the ways of finding food" (*Ita lenge laguq tahu ita carenya mete nasiq*). There is a pride in the ugliness and hardness of their bodies even though they denigrate their bodies and idealize the bodies of those who do not work the land or live in poverty. It would be misleading to leave out this complexity, this contradiction in the *meanings* Pelocok people give to their marked bodies. The marks on the body draw us in because they are also signs pointing toward myriad meanings.

Charles Sanders Peirce (1955) argues that interpretation is inherent in all perception. That is, as soon as something is perceived by a mind, the mind must make sense of it. A mark once perceived becomes a sign, something that is meaningful. Peirce discusses this in terms of indexicality[34]—the intermediary connecting one sign with another. Each such connection in turn indexes another sign. Meaning arises in the endless indexing of one sign with another, what he calls *semiosis*. Through repetition of connecting signs with particular perceptions, in this case of writings on bodies, habits of interpretation are formed (358–59). People develop habits of interpreting the same or similar perceptions in a particular way or ways. For our purposes here, we look in passing at the habits of interpretation I made and other Indonesians made, but concentrate on the interpretations rural Sasaks themselves tended to make when perceiving the marks on their bodies.

The everyday writings of everyday activities I habitually interpreted as signs of peasantry and poverty. Indonesian officials, urban dwellers, and others with different agendas habitually interpreted these marks as signs of backwardness, laziness, and stupidity. In the Indonesian pecking order of occupations, peasantry is rock-bottom. Because of a deeply embedded national ideal of *maju* (Indon., progress, development,

---

34. Which Peirce also calls the interpretant or thirdness.

modernity), being poor can seem almost treasonous. There are, of course, many things that index a person as a poor peasant: ignorance of the national language, worn and shabby sarongs and shirts, a humble and creeping demeanor. But it is the roughness of their written-on bodies that, even when dressed in borrowed clothes and talking out of earshot, identifies them as poor peasants who can and should be treated with condescension. Thus, one habitual pair of interpretations rural Sasaks make regarding the writings on their bodies includes denigration—calling them *lenge*—mixed contradictingly with pride in their bodily strength, both of which arise in comparison with the idealized bodies of the nonpoor nonpeasants. The other habitual way rural Sasak tend to read the writings on their own bodies is in terms of health.

THE UNHEALTHY NORMAL BODY

In Pelocok I never met one person who, if asked, described herself as healthy. If a person had just recovered from an illness, I might ask if she was now healthy (*Wah sehat ide?*). Often the answer would be "Yes." Yet when fellow household members, neighbors, or strangers in apparently perfect health requested medicine from me, and I responded "What medicine? You are healthy, right?" each of them invariably answered, "I am not healthy" (*Ndeqku sehat*) or, less frequently, "I am sick" (*ku sakit*). This would then be followed with a litany of complaints and another plea for my medicines.[35] I was bewildered by their common complaints of being too small, not strong enough, or not fat. I had never seen such muscle definition, such strength and activity as displayed by these peasants. After repeatedly and vainly seeking biomedical answers in *Where*

---

35. Like any anthropologist, I had a small bag of medicines with me: bandages, antibiotic ointment, aspirin, chloroquine, a bottle of hydrogen peroxide, Fansidar, Pepto-Bismal tablets, and assorted cold medicines. I struggled ethically about how to share these meager supplies. I did not want to become a local pharmacy, first because I was there to study their ways of managing illness, second because I could not afford to supply the entire hamlet, and third because I am not qualified to give out more than the most basic first aid. On the other hand, if I could help ease pain, I felt an obligation to do so. Throughout the whole two years, I maintained an uneasy balance between interfering and not. The bandages, antibiotic ointment, and cold medicine I gave out regularly. A handful of times I offered people chloroquine or a pain reliever when I was certain the drugs would be of help. I sometimes took people to a clinic and paid for their medicine there. At other times, I did not have or know of any medicine for a particular illness. Mostly I sat with the ill and their caregivers, offering sympathy and any knowledge I might have about the symptoms, but not posing as a healer myself.

There Is No Doctor (Werner 1992) for these complaints that I wrongly took as based on physiological symptoms, I realized that they were sick because they were not *sehat* (Indon., healthy). That is, they have a commonly assumed interpretation of what health should be that is built upon their perceptions of others' bodies. As Saltonstall reminds us, "health is . . . a constituted social reality" (1993, 12).

Rural Sasaks define health through how they perceive others, whether real or mythical people. The tall and apparently strong European or Australian tourists that they occasionally see are said to be so healthy because of secret medicine (*owat*) that they are unwilling to share. Indeed, more than a dozen times, people became angry with me for not sharing this secret medicine so that they and their children could become tall and strong too.[36] Stories of Sasak grandparents who could pound rice for hours without tiring, or make two trips daily into the forest for wood, or bear eighteen children without difficulty, kindled complaints of weakness. "The ancestors were strong, what had been their medicine?" they would ask rhetorically, bemoaning the knowledge that had been forgotten. Then too, contemporary Sasak men have reputations of mythical sexual strength.[37] Pelocok men complained that they should be able to make love twelve or more times a day. They would say, Sasaks can not be without a wife even for a week, and if they could afford it, they would have two, three, or four wives. They pointed to the crowds of naked children always underfoot as proof of their virility. Then in the same breath, they would tell of so-and-so from Masbagik or Timbanuh or Selong who had sex from dusk until dawn without stopping. They complained that they would always get too tired.

Finally, to fit their ideal of health, one should be fat. This is an ideal common among poor around the world (Brown and Konner 1987). People in Pelocok acknowledge that fatness comes from having enough to eat, particularly plenty of meat and eggs. Yet fatness must also come from some kind of medicine, because the only really necessary food is rice. As an older man once said to me, "I eat a lot. Two plates of rice I can finish. But I don't become fat. What is the medicine?" Fatness is the equivalent of health according to a commonly

---

36. I was considered large but neither huge nor strong. Apparently, it was thought that I must possess the secret Western medicine, but that for some reason it didn't work as well on me as on the gigantic *dengan turis* (tourists).

37. This ideal of virility is popular throughout much of Indonesia. Anderson (1990) persuasively argues that for Javanese virility is linked with and a sign of power—political, social, and cosmological. His argument could equally be made for Sasaks. See also Hay 1998a.

cited proverb, *Lamun ie mokoh, sehat ie* (If you are fat, you are healthy). Not being fat is a symptom of illness, as well as an illness in itself. Fatness, unlimited virility, untiring physical strength, and tallness, these are the signs of health. With health defined in such terms, it is not surprising that apparently healthy people were always seeking medicine.

Some of the stories supporting the ideals of health were told by the traveling medicine man. With stories to convince people that they were not up to par, an extremely worried look upon hearing each complaint, and a pill to cure every ill, the traveling medicine man reinforced insecurities about one's health. During the first year of my fieldwork, before there was a government midwife in Pelocok, once every three weeks or so, Amaq Jumi would come walking up the dusty road carrying a worn black vinyl briefcase. He was from Masbagik and would walk from hamlet to hamlet selling his wares. Amaq Jumi would stop at the largest *barugah* (covered platform) in every courtyard and sit down talking about the weather or the crops. The wife or daughter of the household who owned the *barugah* would scurry into the kitchen hut to boil water. She would send one child to a neighbor's to ask for some coffee grounds and another child to a small food stall to buy a tablespoon of white sugar wrapped in plastic for 25 Rp. Men and women would gather on the *barugah* talking with Amaq Jumi, finding out the news of his family and of Masbagik. Children would stare at him silently, sitting in their parents' laps. The glass of coffee would appear. Then one of two things would happen. In the first scenario, the household head or the person with the highest social status on the *barugah* would say, "There is no money." If no one else said anything, Amaq Jumi would drink a sip of his coffee and gather his things to move on. The assembled women and men would urge him to not rush off, but this would really mean that they were ready for him to go.

In the second scenario, an adult would interrupt the small talk with, "I am not healthy." She or he would go on to say she didn't feel strong, or he coughed all the time, or she couldn't work long hours without tiring. Amaq Jumi would pull out his blood pressure cuff and take the person's blood pressure. Never in all of Amaq Jumi's peddling visits did I ever hear that a blood pressure was normal. It was usually too low, occasionally too high. Luckily, he had just the thing. The briefcase held a wide assortment of different colored vitamins and pills. During my first encounter with Amaq Jumi, my neighbors introduced him with praise, boasting that he even had a government certificate. Amaq Jumi proudly pulled it out for me. Indeed it did certify that he was allowed to be a traveling salesperson selling *obat* (Indon., medicine). Of course, it had expired two years previously. Amaq Jumi would open an array of bottles, saying that this pill would cure insomnia, this pill would make a person strong, this pill would make men virile (sexually), this pill would make a person fat, and so on. He sold the pills at 500 to 1,000 Rp per tablet, the equivalent of a day's labor. Multivitamins that sold in town for 50 Rp apiece he sold as pills to make one strong at 1,000 Rp apiece. Insomnia pills, fat pills, and the like were marked up as much as 800 percent.[38] Yet people were willing to buy them, perhaps because they did not know the retail prices or perhaps because they did not recognize the packaging as I did.

In almost everything else, rural Sasaks impressed me as very shrewd: women would haggle over the price of a bag of sugar for five minutes. Why could a traveling medicine man with an expired license convince them to spend a day's wages on a pill? Why did apparently healthy people believe they were less than healthy?

The answers can be partially found in their notion of health. Health is what townspeople are thought to have. The picture of health is seen daily on the ragged posters people have tacked to their mat walls. There are posters of plump girls in tight black leather straddling motorcycles and of soft, round-faced Javanese actors in beautiful modern clothes with their chubby, smiling children. To be healthy means to be fat, tall, strong, virile, and also *wealthy*. Poor people's definition of health stems partially from envy of the wealthy: envy of their soft bodies, easy jobs, nice clothing, and expensive commodities. Hand in hand with envy of the wealthy is being *malu* (Indon.), embarrassed by the stigmata of peasantry and poverty. While many of my Pelocok friends have staunch pride in their *adat,* these same friends borrowed my clothes when going to the hospital in Selong or visiting distant hamlets, so that they would not be *malu.* They would buy a little soap so that they could scrub themselves really clean. Dressed up and clean, they were still country mice—too thin and rough and angular, too cowed by traffic and uniforms, too talkative to strangers, too awkward sitting on chairs and eating with utensils. Townspeople would ignore them or answer them too briskly. My friends recognized the rudeness with which they were treated, yet they came back to Pelocok often raving enthusiastically about the courtesies they had encountered and how *kurang sehat* (Indon., less than healthy) they were. Didn't I have some medicine for them? The rudeness of the townspeople was too embar-

---

38. This is in comparison with the prices of medicines sold in town that had the same wrappings.

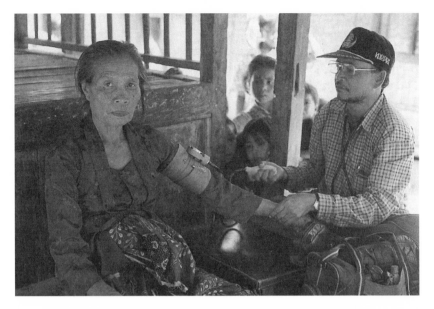

FIG. 3.   The traveling medicine man taking a woman's
blood pressure (1994)

rassing to admit to and, instead, seemed to be taken as a reminder of
the inferiority of their less than healthy bodies.

Health perceived from the perspective of a biomedical paradigm is
generally understood as an objective state identified as the absence of
distinct physical and physiological diseases. For rural Sasaks, health is
the green grass on the other side of the fence. They can never be as fat,
as pale-skinned, as tall, as strong, as virile, as wealthy as their ideal, and
thus they always perceive themselves as *kurang sehat,* less than healthy.
Another reason they believe they are not healthy is that they see themselves as vulnerable to sudden illness and death.

"IF I LIVE LONG ENOUGH,
WE WILL MEET AGAIN"

The first time I heard this sentence it was spoken by an elderly mother
to her son who was leaving to find work in Bali. These words of parting
gave me pause, but because she was old and because I suspected that
she had an advanced case of tuberculosis, I was not particularly sur-

prised. I was very much surprised when these words of parting were used when I was leaving for a four-month return to the States. I thought that maybe people in Pelocok did not believe that I would return. So I tried to convince people, giving them the approximate date in their calendar and showing them all the equipment I was not taking with me. But even so old people, middle-aged people, and even an extremely healthy woman in her teens responded, "Yes. It is good and right that you come back home in time for Puasa [Ramadan, the Islamic fasting month]. Hopefully I will live long enough to see you again."

Was this simply a social convention for saying good-bye? Surely, I thought, they were not serious. Surely it was just a form of politeness, not wanting to insult Allah by assuming control over one's fate. Yes, it is a social convention for saying good-bye. But it also reflects a perception of the tenuousness of life and the imminence of death. I can not imagine such a parting in America where denial of mortality is the norm. In Pelocok healthy people spoke often of their potential deaths. After a few months of attending funeral ceremonies and discovering that I could hardly leave the hamlet without someone dying in my absence, this conventional sentence of parting took on more significance for me.

People in Pelocok worry about their health with reason. Illness and death can and do strike with amazing swiftness. The provincial Department of Health Statistics indicate a number of diseases particularly prevalent on Lombok; among the more deadly are diarrhea, pneumonia, malaria, hepatitis, tuberculosis, typhoid, typhus, meningitis, cholera, and tetanus (Dinas Kesehatan 1993, 1994). Because most people in Pelocok do not seek biomedical care, these diseases may have had a more profound impact in Pelocok than I am aware. Among people in Pelocok, I recognized water-borne diseases (stomach ailments, diarrhea), parasites, diseases from poor nutrition (kwashiorkor, anemia, xerophthalmia), respiratory diseases (tuberculosis, pneumonia), and tetanus—most of which can be linked to their poverty and peasant adaptations to their environment (Brown et al. 1996).[39] Its high elevation protects Pelocok from malaria and dengue fever, but three times during my tenure there men returned from working on Sumbawa with all the symptoms of malaria (*P. falciparum*), although in each case villagers diagnosed it as Sumbawa illness (*penyakit Sumbawa*) rather than as malaria.

---

39. In 1992, a reported 71 percent of pregnant women in the province had anemia (Mboi 1995, 186).

During my time in the hamlet of Pelocok, out of a population of about 800 people, 42 persons died; of these 40 percent were under 1 year of age. This translates into a crude death rate of 26.3 per 1,000 persons, which is over twice the official crude death rate for the province of 11 per 1,000 persons in 1993 (Dinas Kesehatan 1993).[40] Other statistics further show the tenuousness of life in Pelocok. During my fieldwork, of the 36 infants born, 16 died, which translates into an infant mortality rate of 444 per 1,000 births.[41] In comparison, the official statistics for the province list the infant mortality rate at 93 per 1,000 births in 1993, reputedly the worst in all of Indonesia (see also Corner 1989, 191, 196).[42] The national infant mortality rate was 65 per 1,000 births in 1993,[43] and the comparable rate in the United States was 8.4 deaths per 1,000 births (U.S. Department of Statistics 1993). Reproductive histories that I gathered in Pelocok show that a woman can expect approximately *half* of her children to live. Maternal mortality ratios are another indicator of overall health. Lombok is esti-

---

40. I have some evidence that the published official health statistics tell a more positive story than their raw data supports. The best such evidence is the statement of an Indonesian doctor who had worked for 14 years on Lombok: "Did you know that NTB (Nusa Tenggara Baret, the province of Lombok and Sumbawa) has the worst health record of all of the 23 provinces in Indonesia? Actually my specialty is in education and I used to work and do research in the health department. Six months ago they transferred me to the hospital. I don't know why. Maybe I caused too much trouble for them. In the statistics, in the research, I always insisted on reporting the truth, the truth about the health conditions here. But the directors of the health department did not like that; they have to make the statistics better for the government. I made things difficult for them so they transferred me here. If you want my opinion, the reason health conditions are so bad in the villages is an administrative problem between the officials in the health department and local leaders. They do not share information. Officials do not tell local leaders why or the reasons for doing things like keeping wells clean."

41. The infant mortality rate includes all infants who die within their first year. Of the 16 infant deaths, 10 were within the first two weeks of life.

42. This is half the official infant mortality rate for the province in 1979, which was 182 deaths per 1,000 live births (Williamson 1984, 94). Figures this widely divergent over a time span of fourteen years suggest either dramatic improvements in health care, a different censusing method, or problematic reporting of statistics. The latter explanation is suggested by the discrepancy of the 1993 figure above (cited from Lombok's department of health statistics) with an infant mortality rate of 110 for the province in 1993 cited from an Indonesian national health statistic report (Mboi 1995, 184). The late 1980s and early 1990s did have an increase in the number of rural clinics, which might account for some of the reported drop in infant mortality.

43. Indonesia's reported infant mortality rate dropped to 57 in 1994 (United Nations 1994), suggesting that the country is making annual incremental improvements in infant health care.

mated to have the highest maternal mortality ratio in all of Indonesia,[44] where national estimates range from 390 to 647 deaths per 100,000 births (Iskander et al. 1996, 10, 12; Mboi 1995, 183). Of the 36 births in Pelocok, there were 3 maternal mortalities. These numbers imply that a woman's chance of dying in childbirth are 1 in 12. A final indicator of overall health is life expectancy. In 1995, the national average life expectancy was 65 years. In Lombok it was 53 years according to the head of the largest hospital on the island. Because age is not something people keep track of in Pelocok, it is impossible for me to calculate their life expectancy, but probably it is well below the Lombok average because of their general living conditions, poor diet, and health-care choices. These statistics show the fragile reality reflected in the words, "If I live long enough, we will meet again."

Life in Pelocok is precarious. Thus even when all the writings on their bodies are normal for their peasant and impoverished life-style, rural Sasaks understandably see themselves as less than healthy and continually vulnerable to illness and death.

---

44. Although officials at the provincial Department of Health, the former director of that department and current director of Lombok's largest public hospital, and Grace (1996) all maintained that Lombok's maternal mortality ratio was the highest in the archipelago, the precise figures remained elusive.

Learning Sasak Anatomy

In late February 1995, nearly every household in Pelocok had at least one person ill. In my household three of us were ill; I was one of them. The illness usually lasted more than a week and seemed flulike: fevers, loss of appetite, fatigue, and stomach pains. Everyone, I was told, was sick with the same thing: "*Enyakitne pede doang*" (The illness is just the same). Everyone said it was a *penyakit biese*—a usual illness.[1] Nonetheless, people admitted that it was not normal for illness to be epidemic (*te'rinduqan*). I tried a number of times to get at a theory for the spreading of disease, but to no avail. Sitting one morning with Amaq Mol, both of us feeling under the weather, I tried one last time:

> *Cameron:* Why is everyone sick these days? Everyone is sick with the same thing.
> *Amaq Mol:* Yes. Everyone is sick now. It's the same sickness everywhere.
> *Cameron:* Yes. It is the same sickness everywhere. How does the sickness go from one person to another?
> *Amaq Mol:* Yes. Everyone is sick now. It's the same thing.
> *Cameron:* Yes. But how does it happen that illness goes from one body to another?
> *Amaq Mol:* Yes.
> *Cameron:* Everyone is sick with the same thing?
> *Amaq Mol:* Yes. Everyone is sick with the same thing now. It is the same sickness for everyone. Everyone is sick.
> *Cameron:* Does the illness walk from one body to another?
> *Amaq Mol:* Yes.

---

1. Sasaks distinguish between usual and unusual illness. I discuss this distinction further in chapter 5.

Cameron: How does it?

Amaq Mol: It goes from one body to the next. It is the same thing.

Cameron: Yes. What is the path the illness uses to go from one body to another?

Amaq Mol: It walks from one body to another.

Cameron: Yes, but how? How does illness go from one body to another?

Amaq Mol: Yes. It is given by Allah. Do you want some more tea?

This interaction reminds me of Evans-Pritchard's frustration in trying to learn a person's name among the Nuer (1969, 12–13). But whereas in Evans-Pritchard's case, the Nuer deliberately kept knowledge deemed valuable from him, here I was asking the wrong questions based on my agenda, not theirs. Understandings of bodies and their susceptibilities to illness emerge in context based on perceptions of relevance; they do not fit neatly into a description of "Sasak ethnomedicine" or even a description of medical pluralism in Pelocok.

— • —

There is no Sasak version of *Grey's Anatomy* lying around Pelocok. Nor is there a single widespread version of cultural knowledge about anatomy. People's interest is not with anatomy, an intellectual understanding of the physical body and its operations. Rather, they are concerned with their own immediate physical state relative to their ideals of health. As we have seen, rural Sasaks generally ascribe "health" to the fat, tall, strong, virile, wealthy bodies of outsiders, mostly well-to-do townspeople. In comparison, they tend to consider their own bodies as *sakit* (Indon., ill) or at least *kurang sehat* (Indon., less than healthy). Sasaks are aware that their bodies are vulnerable. Their concern is pragmatic—they want to know what precautions and preventions they should take, not intellectualize about the mechanisms involved.

This pragmatic and contextual interest is also reflected in how they learn about anatomy. Like many people in the world, Sasaks learn anatomy by living, by listening to the admonishments of others, by engaging in conversations, and by watching the illnesses of others. To what extent does this manner of learning about the body yield a systematic, widely accepted understanding of what bodies consist of and how they operate? Persons' particular constellations of knowledge do have family resemblances, which is hardly surprising given that Sasak people tend to learn most within their family circles and most people in Pelocok are related in one way or another. Moreover, everyone in Pelocok has healing knowledge, and many are called regularly to identify or treat specific illnesses even though they are not considered health experts. In a society where everyone is a potential healer, family resemblances in no way predict or limit the possible understandings of the body in Pelocok.

Nonetheless, among the different types of experts, understandings differ in predictable ways. For example, a *dukun* (a man adept at healing problems through communicating with spirits and ancestors) emphasized a spiritual anatomy. A *belian* (a woman adept at massage, herbal medicines, and midwifery) most often described the body in humoral terms. A *bidan* (a biomedically trained midwife) tended to understand the body in terms of biomedical mechanisms. Each of these three experts represents a tradition of knowledge: a clearly demarcated understanding about the body that is recognized by the roles of *dukun, belian,* or *bidan.* These traditions of knowledge can loosely be understood as branches of the medical pluralism in Pelocok, although each branch is not equally different. The tradition represented by the *bidan* varies more substantially and is referred to here as biomedicine. In contrast the traditions of the *dukun* and *belian* have more blurred areas of overlap and are each referred to as ethnomedicine. But even experts were less than consistent, capable of changing views of the body at the drop of the proverbial hat.

Simply put, anatomy was considered important only insofar as it enabled one to recognize the difference between a healthy body and an ill body and to take the steps needed to prevent illness and make an ill body healthy again. Fabrega (1980, 9ff.) suggests that the understandings of bodies and their functioning are infrequently discussed by medical anthropologists.[2] This is unfortunate because anatomy is a topic that shapes and is shaped by understandings of illness and therapeutic technique. Assumptions about anatomy and the corresponding mechanisms of illness are found both in widely distributed cultural knowledge and in the idiosyncratic personal knowledge of individuals utilizing multiple medical alternatives (Garro 1982, 1451). These complex and often conflicting assumptions underlie the preventive practices and methods of treatment discussed in later chapters.

---

2. For exceptions, see Fabrega 1980; Good 1980; Helman 1994; Laughlin 1963.

ANATOMY IN METAPHOR

In examining illness in Pelocok, it became clear to me that the various diagnoses and treatments had family resemblances. That is, rural Sasaks work from a widely distributed set of assumptions—or cultural knowledge—about anatomy. Following Lakoff and Johnson (1980), we can examine the fundamental bodily ways in which Sasaks experience and conceptualize the world that are implicit in their everyday speech.[3]

Rural Sasaks speak of their bodies as something that illness and medicines go into (*tume*) and go out of (*sugul*). They use a body-as-container metaphor.[4] Culling through my notes, I frequently found sentences like these:[5]

Owat iye ndeqne tauq tume.
Her medicine doesn't know how to enter the body.

Lamun ndeq tebebubusanne, tauqne tume penyakit jemaq.
If [the infant] is not *bebubus*ed [a red dot of betel placed on its forehead] illness will be able to enter later.

Ndeqne meleq sugul penyakitne.
It doesn't want to go out, the illness.

Lamun wah tesugul, sehat iye.
Once it [the illness] has gone out, he will be well.

Dewa seket wah sugul iye. Masih are seket leq dalemne si harus teowatin.
One of the *dewa*s [spirits/gods] has already gone out. There is still one inside that has to be treated.

Ndeqne man sugul penyakitne?
It hasn't gone out yet, the illness?

---

3. See also Johnson 1987; Lakoff 1987; Sontag 1990; Kirmayer 1992.
4. This fits Lakoff and Johnson's prediction that people perceive their bodies as containers (Lakoff and Johnson 1980; Johnson 1987). However, the Sasaks' perception, well supported by their language use, should not be used to substantiate Lakoff and Johnson's prediction that this is a basic human metaphor; for example, the neighboring Balinese do not have such a metaphor or perception (Hay 1992).
5. These sentences serve the purpose not of proving my argument but of exemplifying the data I used in my interpretations.

Illness is something that goes into a body.[6] When it goes out of the body again, the person is well. Other than when speaking about bodies, the words *tume* and *sugul* are used most frequently to describe people's movements in and out of houses. Passersby are invited to *Tume wah!* (Come in already!), and at other times, people—mostly children—are ordered to *Sugul!* out of a house or kitchen hut. Their uses of the terms imply an analogy in thinking between a house and a body—both of which are containers with permeable boundaries other entities can enter and exit at will. It is worth noting that people used the word *tume* much more rarely when talking about bodies and illness than they did *sugul.* This hints that Sasaks are not as concerned with etiology, how one becomes ill, as with how, once ill, a person is made well again. People are concerned with how to make illness go out of a body. A body can't be cured of illness because illness can't be cured, in their terminology. At best, the illness can be made to go out of the body. Once outside the body, illness does not dissipate, but lurks out there, waiting to enter another body.

A related metaphor Sasaks use is enough/not enough (*cukup/ kurang*). The body is a container that has either enough of a substance or not enough. Enough (*cukup*) is synonymous with health; the container has an adequate supply. Not enough (*kurang*) has negative connotations; the body has less than an adequate supply and therefore is less than healthy.

Cukup kuat aku.
I am strong enough.

Ilmune wah cukup.
Her/his knowledge is already enough.

Kurang idapku.
I feel not enough [less than well].

Darehku kurang. Ape owatne?
My blood is not enough. What is the medicine?

Kurang sehat tian.
I am less than healthy.

---

6. Indeed, Sasaks even call an illness that resembles what Americans call colds "*masuk angin*" (Indon., entering wind). *Masuk angin,* a Malay-Indonesian phrase for cold, is used in many places throughout the archipelago.

Kurang, kurang tauq ku mangen.
I am not able to eat enough.

The examples using *cukup* in reference to oneself were rare, and when used they always occurred in conversations in which social status was questioned.[7] In contrast, people frequently used *kurang* in referring to how they felt physically, implying that they needed more of something (more blood, more food) in order to be healthy. The body as a well-filled container is healthy, physically and socially, whereas the body that is conceived as a container with less than enough is lacking physically and, by implication, socially.

A third metaphor Sasaks use is the opposition "up/down"(*taik/ turun*).[8] Things, usually fluids, are spoken of as rising or falling within a body. Rising is understood to be negative and dangerous. Going down is understood to be positive: the illness is on its way out of the body.

Sakit bahaya iniq. Taik wah tianne.
This is a dangerous illness. His stomach has risen.

Dareqne tiak. Atas gati. Bahaya si genone.
His blood has risen. It is very high. Such is dangerous.[9]

Lamun kadu iniq, turun jemat barakne.
If you use this, tomorrow the swelling will go down.

Ite urut ngeno serene aditne tauq turun penyakitne.
We massage in this way so that the illness will go down.

When Sasaks spoke of elements inside the body rising—blood, stomachs, livers, hearts—these were considered descriptions of particularly dangerous physiological situations. Recall that the traveling medicine

---

7. I use social status here as a shorthand for qualities of personhood that are negotiated in a social arena and determine the social respect one can command.

8. Up/down is also a metaphor that Lakoff and Johnson (1980) claim is a human universal.

9. *Dareq taik* is translated into Indonesian as *naik darah* (risen or rising blood), which in parts of Indonesia such as West Sumatra is used as a euphemism for anger (personal communication with Karl Heider). I never heard Sasaks use either the Indonesian *naik darah* or the Sasak *taik dareq* to refer to anger. Instead, Sasaks use the phrase to describe a perceived physiological increase in blood. This increase can be measured by biomedical blood pressure cuffs, as discussed in chapter 1 in the interactions with the traveling medicine salesman.

salesman made pill recommendations based on the results of a blood pressure test. High blood pressure was accepted as a sign of *sakit* (illness) because it fit Sasaks' assumption that things rising in the body are bad.[10] In contrast, *turun* (Indon., down) is considered a sign of impending health and is used more to describe a general state of the illness rather than the position of specific bodily elements. Specific concerns about the dangerous rising of bodily elements are replaced by more general ones when the treatment is proving successful and the initial diagnosis is no longer important. Illness must go down (*turun*) in order to go out (*sugul*) of the body. Indeed, all massages, all treatment motions, go from top to bottom, because it is assumed that illness only knows (*tauq*) to go out (*sugul*) through the feet or through the fingers.

In both the *sugul/tume* (go in/go out) and the *taik/turun* (up/down) pairs of metaphors there is an assumption of movement. Bodies, substances and organs inside bodies, and elements that affect bodies (such as illness) are all mobile. A metaphor commonly used, but only in its negative, is *lekaq* (to walk, flow, move), which explicitly marks the assumed importance of movement.[11]

Ndeqne lekaq aiq dareqne.
The blood is not walking.

Salah urat satikne ngeno. Ndeqne tauq lekaq aiqne.
Salah urat is the name of pain like that. The water isn't able to walk.

Movement, the fluidity of substances within the body, particularly water/blood, is considered essential to being healthy (e.g., Ferzacca 1996, 431ff). When fluidity is blocked or reduced (*kurang*), that blockage is considered an illness.

Another metaphor used when discussing the body is the contrast between pure (*suci*)[12] and dirty (*luge* or *kotor*). Only pure and clean bodies can be healthy. Dirty bodies and dirty bodily elements are conditions of illness. In this, Sasak understandings coincide with formal

---

10. Low blood pressure interestingly uses the metaphor of not enough (*kurang*), discussed above with its connotations of being less than healthy, rather than a metaphor of down (*turun*), which would be considered an indicator of impending health.

11. These metaphors—entering/exiting, rising/falling, and walking—are all consistent with Lakoff and Johnson's (1980) prediction of metaphors of movement, or a foundational schema of movement (Shore 1996).

12. The word *suci* is Arabic. Thus, the use of this word by Sasaks carries with it a plethora of religious meanings and indexes.

Islamic ones about purity and impurity. In essence, the Islamic view is that pure bodies reflect pure selves who would be blessed by Allah and therefore not become ill. Dirtiness, on or in the body, reflects spiritual imperfections. Sasaks also share the Islamic view that most bodily waste is dirty (*kotor*).

> *Lamun wah jok Gunung, suci jeri awakne. Ampokne tauq betian.*
> When she has already climbed the volcano, her body will be pure. Then she will be able to get pregnant.[13]

> *Wahan tebesunat iye, suci jerine. Sehat iye terus.*
> Once he [an ill child] has already been circumcised, he will be pure. Then he will be healthy.

> *Harus sugul seleput dareq si kotor. Wah ngeno baruq tauq iye sehat.*
> All of the dirty blood must go out. Only then will she be healthy [after childbirth].

For rural Sasaks purity can be ascribed to an entire person or body. *Suci* is almost an aura a person's body can have and is reflected in that person's overall health and virility. When using the word *kotor* (dirty), Sasaks always described a specific element in the body, most often blood, never the body or the person as a whole. In these metaphors, we see an assumed connection between the health of a body and the person's religious strength and faith.

The final common metaphor is hot/cold (*benung* or *panas/nyet*). This is a descriptive metaphor familiar in the literature on humoral medicine throughout much of the world.[14] A healthy body is *mul*—neither warm nor cold.[15] For the Sasaks both hotness (*panas*) and coldness (*nyet*) are signs of illness.

> *Mul idapku. Kenyang aku wah.*
> I feel neither warm nor cold. I am already well.

---

13. Gunung Rinjani, the active volcano on Lombok, is the most holy place in the world for rural Sasaks. It was frequently described to me as equal to or better than Mecca.

14. See Foster 1994; Tedlock 1987; Logan 1977; Fabrega 1980.

15. According to Laderman (1992), this varies somewhat from the Malay healthy body, which is slightly toward the cooler end of the hot–cold scale, and also from medieval Islamic thought, which maintained that healthy bodies should be toward the warmer end of the scale.

Panas dalam iye. Ngenone nyakitne.
He is hot inside. That is the illness.

Nyet gati naine. Ndeqne tauq lakaq dareqne.
Her feet are cold. The blood can't walk.

Bakat wah iye leq dalemne.
He is already burned inside.

Hotness can be both a symptom and an illness in itself. In contrast, coldness is never considered important unless the person is already ill. Although identified by touch, hot and cold are not merely descriptive of temperature. Often when people would ask for medicine or when I accompanied *belian*s on their calls, patients would say they were *benung* (hot) or were *sakit* (ill) with *benung*. Their skin temperature was usually what I considered normal; the hotness was on the inside (*benung dalam*). Hot and cold are used as metaphors to describe *qualities of illness*, not necessarily detectable through touch. The extreme of hot is *bakat* (burned) meaning that a body part became so hot that it was burned, a potentially life-threatening condition.

Moreover, as in humoral traditions elsewhere, bodies suffering from hot or cold are treated with foods also classified hot or cold. Rice, for example, the primary food and itself a symbol of human beings, is *mul* and therefore at the center of the continuum between really hot (Sas., *benung*, or Indon., *panas*) and really cold (Indon., *nyet*) foods. Foods classified as hot are those that taste spicy, salty, fatty: alcohol, peppers, spices, garlic, onion, and fried foods of any kind. Cold foods are those that taste sour, juicy, and bitter, particularly unboiled water, squash, edible tree and vine leaves, and spinach. In other places with humoral traditions, people seek food of the opposite temperature to balance out an illness; for example, a hot body is cooled by eating cold foods (see, e.g., Laderman 1992). In Pelocok, the opposite is true. When one is ill with a cold illness, one should avoid all hot foods that would be a shock to one's system. Cold foods might even be part of a healing treatment. But cold foods must be carefully avoided if one has a hot illness, again for fear of shock that could result from the sudden clashing of temperatures. Any kind of shock or surprise—including events like the trauma of birth or a sudden fall—precipitate an illness called *taget*.[16] If while ill

---

16. *Taget* is analogous to the Indonesian *kaget* (to be surprised, shocked). Like *taget*, *kaget* is also used as a noun to indicate the illness resulting from surprise or shock.

a person eats the wrong foods, he will acquire *taget* too. In short, the metaphors of hot and cold inherently incorporate assumptions of connectedness between foods and bodies and also humoral assumptions of balanced hotness and coldness in a healthy body.

From the frequent and common usage of these metaphors we can make general characterizations of how rural Sasaks understand bodies in relation to illness. They commonly assume that their bodies are containers that illnesses enter and rise in or go down and exit from. Bodies can repel illness by being *cukup* (enough) and *suci* (pure), but unfortunately bodies in Pelocok are more usually *kurang* (not enough) and *kotor* (dirty), as we saw in the first chapter. Finally, bodies and elements within bodies can heat up or cool off, both of which are signs of illness. Only these most general understandings are widely distributed among the people of Pelocok. Experts on the body have more specific ideas that are distributed piecemeal throughout the community.

THE *DUKUN*

*Dukun*s are healers who focus on those illnesses that have spiritual or supernatural causes. In this, Sasak *dukun*s vary from the description offered by Geertz (1960) of Javanese *dukun*s.[17] Geertz shows how Javanese *dukun*s have a range of understandings at their disposal, only some of which—the emphasis on souls (*dewa*s) and mystical connections for healing and sorcery—apply also to Sasak *dukun*s (86–111; see also Woodward 1985).

In Pelocok only three persons were called *dukun*s with any frequency. Only one, Amaq Deri, earned a considerable portion of his living from healing. Moreover, as he liked to say, he had been called to heal people in places as far away as the towns of Masbagik, Ampenon, and Sembalun. The spread of his healing fame beyond the borders of Pelocok to these faraway places gave him an authority that no other *dukun* could claim. Indeed, Amaq Deri was highly respected in the community because his *ilmu* (secret knowledge) was desired by people in faraway places. Because of the reputed strength of his *ilmu*, his circle of close friends in the community was limited to his immediate family; others feared the dangerous results of inadvertently insulting him dur-

---

17. The words *dukun* and *belian* or *balian* are used to designate healers in many places in Indonesia, but the activities of those healers vary substantially. For example, based on descriptions, Sasak *dukun*s resemble Javanese *dukun*s (see Geertz 1960), but are dissimilar to Balinese *dukun*s (see Wikan 1990, 230).

ing normal socializing. Unlike the other *dukun*s, Amaq Deri occupied an ambiguous position as a healer because the strength of his knowledge was said to be evidence of his dangerous knowledge of black magic. Amaq Deri was economically relatively well-off, able to support two wives and maintain their separate households. He had a distinguished bearing and was a compact and self-sufficient man; he was the only *dukun* to always wear a black cloth, folded and tied around his head, as a symbol of his expertise. The black cloth is significant in contrast to the white cloth *kiayi*s wear during rituals. *Kiayi*s' expertise is in matters of religion and purity; a *dukun*'s expertise is in matters of spirits and magic, the shadow side of the religious world.

For Amaq Deri, each person is born with an invisible *dewa*.[18] *Dewa*s vary in complexity, strength, and wisdom from person to person. *Dewa*s give energy, talents, and knowledge to people. The virtues of being virile, fat, strong, and wealthy are signs that that person's *dewa* is particularly strong, complex, and wise. Weaker *dewa*s are not strong enough to deflect even the weakest black magic. But even strong *dewa*s can be wounded if tested or tried (Indon., *coba*) by black magic, and they can be insulted by social slights or shocked by sudden occurrences. All the sufferings of the *dewa* are played out in the body. Persons become ill relative to the degree of insult, suffering, or shock their *dewa* has sustained. There are also disembodied *dewa*s, as well as other spirits (jinn, ghosts), who can invade or bump into the body, making it ill. For Amaq Deri, the physical body is the site on which unseen and potent agents act and struggle.

Other than this very general understanding of the body and a cryptic comment that "there are two hundred and fifty illnesses and only forty kinds of treatments, but those forty can heal all of the kinds of illness," Amaq Deri was extremely reticent about his knowledge. Part of his reticence was triggered by my being female. Indeed, once when I asked him why he had no one that he was training to become a *dukun*, he answered that all of his children were daughters. If he had had a son, he would have given him his *ilmu*. Amaq Deri himself had learned from his father. It was *ilmu* that must be passed down and kept secret. Thus, because he considered his *ilmu* a family secret only to be given from father to son, I doubt Amaq Deri's understanding of the body and its functioning was accessible to the wider Pelocok community in more than the general terms outlined.

---

18. *Dewa* in Indonesian means "god." In Pelocok, *dewa*s could inhabit streams, rice stalks, trees, mountains, and springs, and in all of these, "*dewa*s" refer to gods or spirits. But the word *dewa* was also used interchangeably with *bakat* (a kind of jinn or spirit), *nyiwa* (soul, spirit), or *epene* (twin, shadowy twin, soul).

THE *BELIAN*

Belian means "midwife" for Sasaks, but it also connotes a general healer.[19] A *belian* is distinct from a *dukun* because a *belian* is fundamentally a midwife, always female, and lacks the negative associations of dangerous knowledge (*ilmu* with the implications of black magic).[20] There were four *belian*s in the Pelocok area, all older women. Only two of these women, Inaq Hapim and Papuq Isa, were called upon frequently to assist women in labor, and only Papuq Isa, the oldest of the four, had daily clients seeking treatments for all sorts of illnesses. I developed a particularly close relationship with Papuq Isa. When she learned that America lacked *belian*s, she began to teach me much of her *ilmu* so that I would be able to treat myself when ill or giving birth. Papuq Isa's three grown daughters—one of whom was Inaq Mol—claimed to know only some of her secret *ilmu*, but none of them had been trained to become a *belian*, because they did not want to attend women giving birth. Papuq Isa was training a granddaughter, who was about 11 years old in 1995, to become a *belian*. This child's training was only haphazard; she went with Papuq Isa to see patients maybe once a week when she could get out of her chores. Generally, Papuq Isa was fairly open with her knowledge; much of it she tried to pass on to her clients, reserving only knowledge she thought would frighten them (such as knowledge of their imminent death) and the secret knowledge of *jampi* (spells) and medicine making.[21]

Part of this secret knowledge had been given to Papuq Isa by her elders when she was young, part she accumulated through experience,

---

19. A Sasak *belian* is not the same type of healer as a Balinese *balian*. Connor et al. (1986) describe a Balinese balian as a "traditional healer" with many possible specialties including reading archaic texts, divining, midwifery, spirit mediumship, providing massages, setting bones, selling charms and love magic, dispensing advice, and performing preventive rituals (22–23; see also Hobart et al. 1996). Among Sasaks, archaic texts on medicine and magic are read by *kiayi*s, *dukun*s, and various others in the community, but none of the *belian*s I know were literate in the languages of old (*bese laiq*), including archaic Sasak and Javanese-Balinese scripts. *Belian*s as well as others with healing knowledge in the community do divining, provide massages, set bones, and dispense advice. Sasaks to my knowledge do not have a tradition of spirit mediumship and trance so common in Bali, and Sasak *belian*s leave the selling of charms and love magic to *dukun*s, *kiayi*s, or other men.

20. *Ilmu* means potent or powerful knowledge. As such it can be both dangerous—as is the black magic form of *ilmu*—and healing. While *belian*s are reputed to have *ilmu* that is as potent as that of *dukun*s, their *ilmu* does not carry similar dangerous connotations.

21. A *jampi* is a healing spell mouthed during an illness treatment.

and part she gained from direct communication with the spirit world. Unlike the other three *belians* in Pelocok, Papuq Isa claims to have never undergone any sort of formal training or apprenticeship to become a midwife. After having 14 children of her own, she simply started assisting others. She credits much of her knowledge about how to conduct massages and how to make certain medicines to her experience of catching generations of babies. But Papuq Isa's most potent secret knowledge she gained directly from spirits, dead ancestors, or her own personal *dewa,* usually during dreams or divinations. Like Amaq Deri, for Papuq Isa, a person's *dewa* and relationship with the spiritual world directly impact that person's health.

Papuq Isa is also concerned with the body as a homeopathic and humoral system. In this, she is in keeping with a grand tradition of knowledge with probable medieval Islamic and regional roots (cf. Foster 1994). Homeopathic and humoral concepts of the body are widespread throughout Southeast Asia,[22] yet rather than describing Papuq Isa's knowledge as a variant of a larger theme, I prefer to keep our feet on the ground, understanding her own constellation of knowledge as she has made it.

According to Papuq Isa, the most vital element in the body is its fluids, what she referred to interchangeably as *aiq* (water) or *dareq* (blood), which flows through *urat* (fluid channels analogous to blood vessels but including muscles). Most illnesses, except those of skin abrasions and broken bones, are illnesses of the waters in the body. There are four kinds of waters—or waters of blood (*aiq dareq*)—in the body distinguished by their different colors: red, white, yellow, and black.[23] Menstruation, for example, is a surfeit of red blood/water. Urine is a surfeit of yellow blood/water. In healthy, pain-free bodies these waters are balanced and circulate without hindrance through the *urat.* Excessive amounts of any kind of blood are dangerous, and these buildups must be redispersed in the body through massages and spells. If there is not enough (*kurang*) of any of these types of blood, the lack can be made up by boiling teas out of a like color: a chip of a particular red wood to replenish red blood lost in hemorrhages and a chip of a particular white wood to replenish the lack of white blood signaled by fevers. The waters/bloods must all be *cukup* (enough) for a body to be healthy. Equally important, the waters must flow unhindered through

---

22. See, e.g., Laderman 1983, 1991; Geertz 1960; Endicott 1979; Kuipers 1990.
23. Among the Bugis of Sulawesi there is an association of white blood with high social rank (Errington 1989). To my knowledge, there is no similar association among Sasaks.

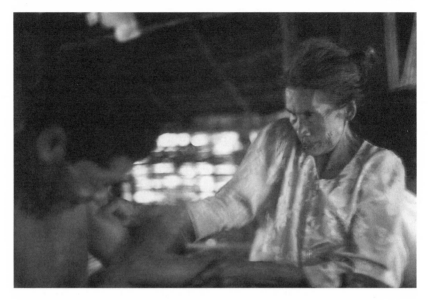

FIG. 4. Papuq Isa giving a massage (1994)

the *urat*. If *urats* are blocked, twisted, knotted, or their paths shift, the waters no longer *lekaq* (walk, go), and any number of illnesses can develop. Dearth of waters flowing in one body part is identified by the coldness (*nyet*) of that part; heat (*benung*) in the body is caused by a buildup of fluids usually caused by some blockage of flow in the *urat*. Such problems with *urats* can either be caused by overexertion or by other illnesses that enter through the feet and rise in the body. In either case, healing is a matter of smoothing out the *urat*, forcing the illness down and out through the feet. Furthermore the body is organized vertically, so that pain was experienced higher up in the body than the site of the actual source of the pain. For example, the source of a headache is in the lower front of the neck. Pain experienced in the abdominal region just under the rib cage is caused by twisted *urat* in the calves. Pain rises faster in the body than does its cause, the illness. Treatment entails pushing both pain and the illness down and ultimately out of the body.

All of Papuq Isa's homeopathic and humoral knowledge was available to everyone, whether they asked for her explanations or not. Unlike Amaq Deri, Papuq Isa was not feared. A warm, chipper, insightful woman with a self-confident demeanor, she had a way of putting patients at ease and engaging them in discussions. On August 16, 1995, a man and his teenage son arrived from a village to the south to seek treatment for the son's illness:

Amaq Jo [the father, indicating the son]:	This one is rather sick. He can only walk with my help these days.	*Iniq, iye semait sekitan angkak. Iye kan, doang barengku belembar wahan mesaqne.*
Papuq Isa: [She started examining the young man, concentrating on his stomach while his father continued.]	He is not able.	*Ndeqne bauq.*
Amaq Jo:	We even took him to Selong to be injected, but the sickness just stays.	*Kan ite leq Selong jauan iye ampokne tebesuntikan, laguq, anuq, tetap doang nyakitanne.*
Papuq Isa:	Of course. Injections are not able to heal something like this. Injections are dangerous. The injection reaches that which has nothing wrong. But this *urat* here is knotted. That is the illness.	*No. Ndeqne bauq suntikan si ngene. Behaya suntikan kan. Timaq ndeq te wah ngene wah ngumbe. Laguq mbelitik uratte sine. Nyo sakitne.*
[She pauses, during which Papuq Isa presses the young man's stomach, causing grimaces of sharp pain.]	[Pause]. See. See. There is the illness, this urat. The smallest *urat* is knotted; if it were a large *urat,* you would be quickly healthy.	[Pause]. *No. No sakitanne, urat sino. Urat paling kocet mbelitik, lamunne uratte si beleq jelap tauqmet sehat.*
Lo Jo [the young man]:	Yes. That is the place.	*Aoq. Ngeno ngena dengan.*
Papuq Isa:	Imagine as if it were a twisted *urat* in the mid-	*Cobaq malik lamun bongkorta bauq araq iye*

dle of your back, it is hard to find it. Just any healer will not know to find it and the treatment will not work tomorrow if the spell is not strong enough to meet it.

mbuteng urat kocet leq papah tengaq, sekat dengan daitne. Kurang-kurang sine pete si jejampi ndeqne bauq lamun ndeqne araq jejampine ndeqne dait iye jemat.

Lo Jo: It's as if it were an *urat* [the size] of a hair?

Sang munne urat bulu sino?

Papuq Isa: Like an *urat* of hair. Who can find it?

Maraq urat bulu, saiq ndait iye?

Lo Jo: If that is the case, what is the name of this large *urat?*

Wah no pe aranne urat belek sine?

Papuq Isa: Your large *urat* here is knotted, it is the one that makes you feel achy. Like the feeling of a needle is your small *urat*. This small *urat* feels achy like a needle. Then all you have to do is describe it thus, and I will know to look for it there. You would get tired waiting if I looked for it there where the pain is. It is lower. Ruined already is your *urat*. Only slowly will you recover.

Urat beleq meq sine je bengel iye, sino iye sineruk idapne. Maraq idap jarum urat meq si kodeq ino. Ka urat si kodeq ino sineruk maraq jarum idapne. Iye, ampok lamunne doang meq badak aku sakit ndeq soku pete iye tono. Lelah so anta munta pete iye tono lamunne ngene tonokne sakit. Bawaqan tauqne. Sede iye wah urat meq. Adeng-adeng doang tauq meq meleq malik.

Amaq Jo: Oh, so this is where it is?

O, mula sine wah taoqne?

Papuq Isa: [Reaching over and putting her right hand lower on the young man's abdomen]: Further down, there you seek it, and then from the top down massage so that again it is smoother, and then seek it further down.

Itehan bawaq ito pete amokq atas langan urutne maleq terus longgar iye bebawaq terus pete itu.

In this brief excerpt from the dialogue, we can see Papuq Isa's style of teaching. She does not examine a patient and jump immediately to the tasks of treatment. She explains, answers questions, and describes her understandings of how the body works. Here, we see her describing a difference in problems with large *urat*, which are signaled by dull pains, and knots in tiny, threadlike *urat*, which are signaled by sharp pains and are more difficult to treat. She tells how the pain is higher up in the body than the actual location of the knot. She also tells of treatment as a matter of easing the knot and pushing down the illness, working top–down in massage treatments. Finally, she hints at a theory of efficacy in treatment: medicine must fit the illness exactly in order to be able to find it. Only the best *jampi* (treatment spells) can meet and drive out illness.

Note also Papuq Isa's expression of animosity toward injections; the mildness of expression in this case was perhaps because these people were relative strangers. Given her central concern with promoting unhindered circulation of waters through *urat*, this is not surprising. According to her, injections break the skin and damage *urat*, causing blockages in water/blood flow. Thus, injections make people ill. Papuq Isa was adamant in denouncing the skills of clinicians and doctors generally and injection treatments in particular. At the same time, she never contradicted me whenever I consulted her about taking a particularly ill child to a clinic or hospital for medicines, usually given in the form of injections.

Lo Jo and his father returned to her house four times in the following two weeks, but otherwise, within the period of fieldwork, they never consulted Papuq Isa. Certainly some of what Papuq Isa told them was understood and remembered, and became part of their own constellations of knowledge. But they were not with her long enough for her to give them any thorough understanding of anatomy and the mechanisms of illness as she understood them. Even though most of her patients were from Pelocok and thus had more access to Papuq Isa, all of her knowledge about bodies and health she expressed in contextual, nonorderly conversations like the one above.

CHARACTERIZING PELOCOK'S
ETHNOMEDICAL TRADITIONS

Foster (1976) offers a useful model for characterizing medical traditions. He argues that the dominant concern when faced with illness is to identify its cause. Cross-culturally the recognized causes of illnesses fall into one of two camps: personalistic and naturalistic. Personalistic causes are those that are initiated by an agent; illness is the result of intentional action by a person, god, spirit, witch, or sorcerer. Naturalistic causes are those that are the unintentional consequences of biological, ecological, or environmental forces; illness is the unintended result of conditions and forces of nature. According to Foster, "in spite of obvious overlapping, the literature suggests that many, if not most, people are committed to one or the other of these explanatory principles to account for a majority of illness" (776). Furthermore, each of these explanatory principles is associated with a pattern of knowledge distribution. In personalistic systems magical and secretive knowledge are emphasized so that a healer's prestige increases if he guards his knowledge rather than distributes it. In naturalistic systems, the healer's prestige increases by teaching his knowledge to others (Brown 1998).

In looking at the traditions of the *dukun* and the *belian,* deciding which camp rural Sasaks fall into is difficult. On the one hand, the *belian*'s concern with humoralism and a bodily equilibrium (also found in cultural metaphors) as well as her willingness to share some of her knowledge bespeak a strong tendency for a naturalistic explanatory principle. On the other hand, the metaphors of purity and dirtiness, the concern with spirits and souls, as well as the *dukun*'s reluctance to distribute any of his knowledge bespeak a personalistic explanatory principle. In short, both explanatory principles are used in Pelocok. The *belians*' tradition of knowledge has a tendency to utilize naturalistic explanations a good proportion of the time, whereas the *dukuns*' tradition of knowledge is almost exclusively personalistic. Rural Sasaks find both types of explanations perfectly conceivable and use both.

The wider cultural environment tips the balance toward a more personalistic principle. Foster points out that in personalistic societies, religion, magic, and medicine are intertwined, whereas in naturalistic societies religion is largely irrelevant to how people understand illness (1976, 777ff.). Both the *dukun* and the *belian* rely on their relationships with spirits and dead ancestors to identify illnesses. Moreover, as we shall see, religious and life-cycle rituals are crucial to how Sasaks interpret their vulnerability to illness and are used to prevent illness. Rural Sasak ethnomedicine, then, is personalistic and, to a lesser extent, naturalistic. The third medical knowledge tradition found in Pelocok is unequivocally naturalistic.

THE *BIDAN*

The third expert with a specialist's understanding of anatomy as it relates to illness is a recent arrival to Pelocok. In April 1995, a government-sponsored PoLinDes (Indon., *Pos Salinan di Desa,* childbirth clinic) was opened and staffed by a 20-year-old urban Sasak girl named Rini as the *bidan* (Indon., biomedically trained midwife).[24] The Bidan ke Desa program is a recent attempt by the Indonesian government to combat high infant and maternal mortality rates by sending unmarried girls trained for one year in midwifery into villages for three-year terms. The *bidan's* position is a politically charged one in which she receives much pressure from above to persuade villagers to come to her for pre- and postnatal care, to deliver their children, and to start them on a government-controlled program of family planning (Indon., KB—*keluarga berencana*). She is expected to be an advocate of biomedicine and an intermediary between villagers and larger biomedical establishments (cf. Barbee 1986).

Rini, or Bu Bidan (Ms. Midwife) as villagers called her out of respect for her position, had delivered a total of 15 infants, all under supervision, before she came to Pelocok. Her formal knowledge of the body and its workings was restricted to what she had learned from a tattered book of photocopied pages, a course on midwifery, and three years of study in the medically oriented high school.[25] She is the only one of the three specialists discussed in this chapter whose knowledge was gained from a grand tradition of knowledge. Indeed, it is the global presence and scientific rationality of biomedicine that Rini thinks gives her knowledge its authority. Whereas the other specialists talk about their knowledge as *theirs,* given them by ancestors or spirits, Rini legitimates her knowledge by claiming that it is that of Science.

Rini's knowledge of anatomy was biomedically organized. The body was made of a number of interacting systems: respiratory, neural, circulatory, digestive, reproductive. For her, bodies were susceptible to germs, viruses, and bacteria infecting it by being ingested, physically contacted, or insufficiently prevented by artificial or natural immunities. She could list organs and their functions in a perfunctory way

---

24. In Java and in the Indonesian language, the word *bidan* does not distinguish between a biomedically trained midwife and a traditional birth attendant. On Lombok, the word *belian* is used for the latter, and *bidan* is reserved for the former.

25. It is like a trade school or prep school specializing in preparing students to go into health-oriented careers.

when I pressed her, but her concerns were primarily with childbirth and illness prevention and treatment. In this practical interest, she was much like others in Pelocok, and with practicality in mind, she emphasized actions that should or should not be done while communicating with villagers.

Her communications were always in the form of simple direct orders rather than explanations, more in keeping with Amaq Deri's style than Papuq Isa's. This mode of communication in itself was not problematic, except that it implied to rural Sasaks that Rini had *ilmu*. Yet Rini's therapies relied on pills and injections; they were technological treatments, rather like Papuq Isa's massages. For people in Pelocok, communications that are directive rather than explanatory imply the use of *ilmu;* this contradicted Rini's use of technological knowledge, which lacked any hint of *ilmu* in therapies.

Without explanations, Rini's communications did little to distribute biomedical understandings of the body throughout the community. She frequently ordered villagers to boil drinking water, wash their bodies and hair with soap daily, eat beans or meat and fruits daily, vaccinate their children, and come to her whenever they felt ill. While many of these things were either economically impossible or socially and ideologically uncomfortable to all but a handful of people in Pelocok, she did successfully communicate the importance of bodily cleanliness, reinforcing the negativity commonly associated with dirtiness as evidenced in metaphor use. Moreover, Rini's actions of giving injections and dispensing medications communicated some of the range of bodily ailments for which biomedicine has technological treatments. But she was unable to communicate how biomedicine understands normal body function, immunity, or susceptibility to bacteria and viruses.

Since Rini was an outsider, well-educated but with little practical or life experience, and in a position of government-sanctioned authority, the cards were stacked against her. People in Pelocok had seen biomedical clinicians, but only in other villages, towns, and cities. Pelocok had remained relatively isolated, a place where they could heed the advice of biomedical clinicians or not as they liked. Now, with a biomedical clinician in their midst, people in Pelocok were ambivalent. On the one hand, they appreciated the ease with which they could seek biomedical care whenever they wished. On the other hand, they did not appreciate their actions being supervised. Uninvited, Rini would show up at births or after births giving vaccinations and checking that all was going smoothly. Uninvited, Rini would lecture them for not boiling their drinking water or not taking the pills she had given them. In so doing, Rini was trying to do her job well and prevent future ills.

As an outsider, however, Rini did not understand many of the subtleties of how people in Pelocok approached health care or the social relationships that undergird resort patterns. While she seemed to understand the metaphors patients used when talking of their ills, she did not use them herself, nor did she ever refer to *dewa* or humoral imbalances. Instead she used scientific language in all consultations. As an orthodox Muslim raised in the most orthodox city of Lombok, Rini was unfamiliar with much of Pelocok's ritual life, which is derived from local rather than Islamic tradition, and she did not understand its importance in issues of health. She had her own maid and cook, a separate house and garden, a government salary, and no local relatives. This situation enabled her to keep herself apart from the life of the community; she never invited villagers into her home, served them coffee (except for me and the hamlet mayor), or reciprocated their gifts of food. In short, as an outsider, too young to have much experience to fall back on and in a position villagers were ambivalent about, Rini's ability to communicate her knowledge was curtailed by forces beyond her control. Even with the presence of a biomedical clinician, biomedical understandings of the body were not well distributed throughout the community.

ALL OVER THE MAP

Aside from these experts, people's understandings of anatomy and the mechanisms of illness were all over the map, even within a single household.

Inaq Mol, my "mother," is the daughter of Papuq Isa. She is fairly well-known for her abilities to heal two kinds of illness: broken bones and *sakit sedot* (illness located in the upper abdomen). Her patients, maybe two a month, are usually neighbors but sometimes come from the surrounding area. She claimed to have learned about healing from her own *dewa*, from her dreams, and from overhearing her mother when she was pretending to be asleep. While she shared her secret *ilmu* only with family members, she openly and authoritatively spoke of the workings of the body. For Inaq Mol, humoral considerations usually took precedence. The blood/waters of the body are always moving in the *urat* (fluid channels). When they do not move, one is very sick. Further, there are four different blood/waters: red, white, yellow, and blue (rather than Papuq Isa's black). The red waters in the body are given by the mother, the white waters are given by the father. Inaq Mol ties these waters to the annual ritual celebrations of Bubur Abang (Red Rice-Por-ridge) and Bubur Putiq (White Rice-Porridge), saying that they are rit-uals of thanks to the matriarchal and patriarchical ancestors respec-tively for giving the body these essential waters. Thus she saw blood as a gift of the ancestors, linking bodies ideologically to a mystical past. Inaq Mol also frequently spoke of *dewa*s and *nyawa*s in bodies. Once I asked if *nyawa* was the same thing as *dewa*. She answered, "Different. I also am confused about the difference. *Nyawa* is what leaves us when we die. When we meet someone who has died, it is their *nyawa* we meet. But *dewa*, when it comes, we get sick. There are many *dewa* that can come and make one sick. Or sometimes, a *dewa* makes us brave. It depends." In this overview of Inaq Mol's knowledge, we see strong elements from Papuq Isa's understanding of anatomy, as well as an emphasis on reli-gion and spiritual aspects of the body.

La Nan is Inaq Mol's only living daughter; she was about 19 years old in 1995. She claimed no healing knowledge of her own and was typi-cally quiet about matters of the body. Although she certainly put as much importance on the fluidity of waters in the *urat* as her mother and grandmother, La Nan spoke of the body more often in terms of hot and cold. She was particularly concerned with *bakat*—the burning that occurs within the body, as the result of illness, black magic, or ingesting extremely hot foods like alcohol. On the matters of *dewa*s, like Inaq Mol, she was unclear. At one time, she told me that each person has a *dewa* that varied only in its degree of complexity (*cecel*). Illness could be cured by sacrificing the number of chickens that correctly matches the level of complexity of one's personal and discrete *dewa*. Another time she told me that *dewa*s move between people, shifting from one to another and causing illness in whomever they inhabit. La Nan was the only member of the family who would occasionally seek pills and injec-tions from the Bu Bidan, although, just as frequently, I would overhear her deriding injections as dangerous to the integrity of one's bones. La Nan struck me as pragmatically oriented toward illness and its preven-tion.

Amaq Sunin is La Nan's husband. He claimed to have healing pow-ers of his own, although his patients in 1994 were few. As time went on, he became a popular source of love potions for amorous young men. Like Amaq Deri, he was reticent about telling his knowledge to anyone, saying to me more than once, "If you don't already know, you are not allowed to know." Nonetheless, I did learn some aspects of his under-standing of the body. For Amaq Sunin, there were five humors (*dareq,* lit., blood) in the body: white, red, yellow, black, and green. Like Papuq Isa, he believed that low amounts of a particular blood could be increased homeopathically by drinking medicines and teas made from like-colored leaves and barks. He emphasized humoral balance also in temperature moderation by seeking or avoiding foods based on their hotness or coldness. But unlike Papuq Isa, Amaq Sunin understood illness to be always localized where the pain was felt, he thought of fingertips as the point of illness entry and exit, and he believed illness could be moved out of the body not through massage but by the power of breath (Indon., *angin*). The most unusual aspect of Amaq Sunin's understanding of the body—although I know of two other men in Pelocok who had similar understandings—was his calendrical chart that enabled him to calculate on what days a person would feel relatively healthy versus those a person would feel ill, weak, or impotent.

In these three sketches, it should be clear that, aside from the cultural knowledge implied in their use of metaphor, there is no single understanding of the body that is *shared* among people of Pelocok. Instead, words and understandings about the body and the mechanisms of illness are distributed ad hoc, as needed, and with pragmatic goals in mind. There is no institution in which to study anatomy, no single expert from whom to learn. Moreover, all of these understandings, including those of the specialists, change over time, as they have different experiences and in interactions with other persons both inside and outside of Pelocok.

Yet people do communicate with each other and with all of the experts discussed here. How is this possible if their understandings are so different? Following the lead of others, I suggest that it is profitable to conceptualize the situation in terms of personal constellations of knowledge (Heider 1991). I assume that each person has a particular constellation of knowledge regularly drawn upon but constructed over many experiences within a social milieu and drawing upon commonly used metaphors, thus making communication within that milieu possible.

DISTRIBUTION OF MEDICAL KNOWLEDGE

This chapter began with metaphors used in everyday interactions that are so widely used throughout Pelocok as to constitute cultural knowledge about bodies. But the three traditions of expert knowledge are much less widely distributed; indeed, some specialists like the *dukun* are loath to give away any of their medical knowledge. When we stray from these experts to nonexperts of the same household—the persons most likely to distribute knowledge openly among themselves—their understandings of the body and how it operates vary significantly, even to the point of not having obvious similarities with any of the three "expert" traditions in the hamlet.

Others have noted the problem of variation in medical knowledge and the distribution of medical beliefs among healers and laypersons.[26] In her excellent study of variation in medical knowledge, Garro (1986) conducted interviews with 20 Tarascan Indian women in a rural Mexican community, half of whom were curers. She shows that there is a systematic variation in medical knowledge such that the bodies of knowledge of curer and noncurer older women were more similar than those of noncurer younger women who presumably had less experience with illness (366). This suggests that there is a "single system of beliefs common to both lay person and curer, with individuals varying according to their relative congruence with this standard" (357). Garro's model of systematic or patterned variation does not translate well onto the Sasak materials. Although metaphor analysis shows there is basic cultural knowledge about the body and its workings, there is not a single underlying system of beliefs among local healers, let alone among healers and laypersons. Garro mentions that the Mexican community has multiple medical alternatives (354); it would have been interesting to see what her results would have looked like if she had not restricted her research to a single belief system.

In Pelocok it makes more sense to examine the ways in which knowledge is distributed. The *dukun* who legitimated his knowledge through its secrecy, vowing that only a male heir could be given the secret knowledge, was very reticent about distributing anything more than the barest sketch of knowledge about the body. The *belian* was also extremely secretive about her healing knowledge, but would contextually give explanations of the body, thus distributing fairly widely through her clientele an understanding of spiritual, homeopathic, and humoral understandings of the body. Surprisingly, the one expert who legitimated her knowledge by referring to a larger body of knowledge, namely, biomedical science, which is supposedly open and public, did not attempt to distribute her knowledge. Perhaps the *bidan* was reticent because, as a well-educated and wealthy outsider to Pelocok, she lacked

---

26. See, e.g., Fabrega and Silver 1973; Kleinman 1980; Young 1980.

experience communicating scientific concepts and understandings to undereducated peasants. Thus secrecy and lack of experience combined with a lack of a contextual forum (a school, a village meeting) for systematically distributing knowledge about the body.[27] Together these factors preclude an even or widespread distribution of expert knowledge. Is it any wonder, then, that even within the same household understandings of the body can vary so significantly?

Medical knowledge in Pelocok is not orderly. There are aspects of it that can be modeled, such as aspects of cultural knowledge, but we must be careful not to organize all the variations and inconsistencies into a neat package. Rural Sasaks' interest in medicine is stimulated by pragmatic concerns, such as how a specific illness can be avoided and treated. What to the outsider might seem like a babel of medical knowledge is experienced by insiders as options for coping with illnesses, any of which might prove useful (Last 1981, 391–92).

Renato Rosaldo suggests that between the order of systems and utter chaos there is a realm of "nonorder" where people actually go about living (1989, 102):

> When in doubt, people find out about their worlds by living with ambiguity, uncertainty, or simple lack of knowledge until the day, if and when it arrives, that their life experiences clarify matters. In other words, we often improvise, learn by doing, and make things up as we go along. (92)

This realm of muddling through, where action, thought, and feeling are simultaneously personal, contextual, and cultural, is nonorder. *Nonorder* is the word that best describes my understanding of the multiple and often knotted strands of medical knowledge to be found in Pelocok.[28]

---

27. There are domains of knowledge that are more coherent among rural Sasaks. One of these is the arena of Islam. Islam, based on written Arabic texts, has a firm foundation for coherence. There is a *pesantran* in Pelocok that most young children go to for a year or more to learn to recite the Qur'an. Orthodox Islamic practice is also taught in the elementary school. As I have argued elsewhere, this is not to suggest that Islam as it is practiced in Pelocok is identical with Islam practiced elsewhere (Hay 1997). But Islam, unlike the domain of medical knowledge, does have specific texts and institutions that ground and distribute understandings more coherently and consistently.

28. There are other domains that are more completely modeled by Sasaks and less open to nonorderly actions, including the life-cycle rituals, kinship, and agriculture. Medicine is surprisingly unorganized in Pelocok, but to a lesser extent the domains of politics and religion also invite a considerable amount of "muddling through."

A PLURALISTIC MEDICAL SETTING

Medical anthropologists confronted with the problem of describing multiple medical traditions within a single setting have productively used the phrase *pluralistic medical systems,* or sometimes *medical pluralism.*[29] Kleinman (1980) provides a descriptive model of medical pluralism in which medical systems are categorized into three overlapping and hierarchical spheres: the popular sphere in which laypersons treat themselves, the folk sphere in which nonprofessional or nonbureaucratic healers are consulted, and the professional sphere in which members of organized healing professions are consulted (50–68). This sits uncomfortably with the Sasak materials. In a place where every adult has medical knowledge and some secretly learned *ilmu,* everyone is a specialist who could be called to treat particular ills (see also chap. 6). Indeed, in Pelocok the boundaries between popular and folk spheres are completely blurred, so that only the professional sphere, when a person resorts to a biomedical specialist, stands out as distinct. Yet, to set off biomedical knowledge as distinct from all other forms of knowledge about the body would inappropriately assume a homogeneity among the latter. Ohnuki-Tierney's (1984) model of medical pluralism, which lacks Kleinman's hierarchy based on specialization in medical knowledge, sits better. She suggests that there are different medical systems that interact closely with one another, shaping each system's "form and color" to fit with the "sociocultural milieu of that society" so that ultimately the different systems are complementary rather than competitive (6, 22off.). Certainly, in Pelocok, experts and laypersons are continually interacting, distributing, legitimating, and rejecting ideas of others.

Yet I hesitate to call Pelocok's medical traditions *systems.* Among the two ethnomedical traditions and within the biomedical tradition, of course there are basic systematic relationships in how the body is understood, as well as in illness etiology, diagnosis, and treatment. But a medical system is sometimes conceived as a coherent and integrated whole, as is shown by two classic definitions:

> We can view medicine as a cultural system, a system of symbolic meanings anchored in particular arrangements of social institutions and patterns of interpersonal interactions. In every culture,

---

29. See, e.g., Lieban 1967; Leslie 1977, 1980; Heggenhougan 1980; Cosminsky and Scrimshaw 1980; Brodwin 1996; Finkler 1994b.

illness, the responses to it, individuals experiencing it and treating it, and the social institutions relating to it are all *systematically interconnected.* The *totality of these interrelationships is the health care system.* (Kleinman 1980, 24, emphasis added)

The medical system is *an ordered, coherent body* of ideas, values, and practices embedded in a given cultural context from which it derives its signification. (Kleinman 1973, 208, emphasis added)

For much work in medical anthropology, this emphasis on systematicity and coherence is not a problem given that topics commonly focus on specialist knowledge and practices, which tend to be fairly consistent.[30] It is also easier methodologically to conceive of, research, and describe things that fit together. But, as we have seen, as soon as we turn the medical gaze away from specialists—who in Pelocok do not even have much of a coherent system—coherence disappears into a "hodgepodge" approach to issues of health (Dentan 1988).

A system implies a closed set of orderly elements working together. For the Sasak materials, it makes more sense to use the phrase "pluralistic medical setting" referring to the multiple sources of medical knowledge found in a single geographic area. In Pelocok there are understandings of anatomy and its workings that are held and promoted by distinct individuals, as well as widely distributed concepts, understandings, and habits. Yet, while building semblances of order, I have also made a point of indicating the edges of order by showing that *in going about everyday living each individual person has particular interpretations of what a particular body is, how it becomes ill,* and, as we shall see in later chapters, *in what contexts it is vulnerable, what preventive practices can alleviate those vulnerabilities, and what particular saliencies inform perceptions of particular persons.* It is these particularities in play with personal constellations of knowledge that motivate and make salient people's experiences, understandings, and treatments of illness. We must be careful not to inexcusably systematize actual processes of muddling-through,[31] yet we must explore what patterns do emerge out of the bits of cultural

---

30. For exceptions see Price 1987; Olesen et al. 1990; Romanucci-Ross 1986; van der Geest 1991; Last 1981; Pool 1994.

31. In his ethnography examining interpretations of illness through dialogue in Cameroon, Pool (1994) makes a similar argument with respect to the phrase *medical system.* In addition to criticizing it for the discreteness the word *system* implies (256, 261ff.), Pool criticizes it for being a concept based on our models of biomedicine, thus shaping how people deal with illness elsewhere to our assumptions of what illness and medicine are (260–65).

knowledge, structures, and social processes we find. In short, to understand the lived reality of negotiating a pluralistic medical setting in a place like Pelocok, we must constantly tack back and forth between order and nonorder.

PLURALISM IN A PEASANT SETTING

There are predictable characteristics of the relationships rural Sasaks have with the various medical experts; in particular, relationships with *dukun*s and *belian*s have a similar ease about them, whereas relationships with biomedical personnel like the *bidan* are distinctly different. The difference lies in the ways peasants interact with nonpeasants as opposed to with other peasants.

How can the relations within a pluralistic medical setting such as Pelocok be modeled? Wolf's (1966) notion of peasant coalitions is a promising place to begin. Wolf argues that coalitions are alliances, often temporary, among persons or groups of persons formed for the purpose of coping with pressures and concerns (80). These coalitions can be characterized by many interests drawing people into alliance such as medical concerns, kinship, friendship, and economic ties (a many-stranded coalition) or by a single interest such as just medical concerns (a single-stranded coalition). Furthermore, these coalitions can be made of horizontal relationships, that is, among peasants, or vertical relationships, between peasants and nonpeasants. Many-stranded, horizontal relationships tend to be the strongest, most stable, and enduring relations whereas single-stranded, vertical relationships tend to be the most brittle (81–88). With these concepts in mind, we can return to the Sasak materials, looking at the ways knowledge about bodies is distributed.

In Pelocok, knowledge tends to be distributed among those persons with whom one has many-stranded, horizontal relationships. Laypersons tended to distribute knowledge among kin or within friendship relationships. Amaq Deri would have only communicated his medical knowledge to a son, with whom he would have had filial and economic ties as well as an interest in healing. Papuq Isa distributed her secret healing knowledge only to those with whom she had strong kinship and economic ties, but she would explain how the body works to anyone and in so doing would distribute knowledge through single-stranded relationships. In sum, many-stranded relationships were the norm, and medical knowledge was distributed only to other peasants, never—with the exception of the anomalous anthropologist—to outsiders. Even persons born peasants and raised in Pelocok, like the hamlet mayor, who had rejected all but formal social ties with the community in favor of climbing the governmental ladder, who exclusively used biomedical care, and who, in dress and attitude, became like an outsider, were now outside the loops of ethnomedical knowledge distribution.

In contrast, any distribution of the *bidan*'s biomedical knowledge would have been in exclusively single-stranded, vertical relationships. The relationships would have been single-stranded because she lived separate from the community, avoiding villagers' invitations for social interactions outside the realm of medical care. Because Rini was relatively wealthy, from the larger society, and her medical knowledge was the only one legitimated by the government, any distribution of it to peasants would have been vertical and downward.

Understood in this way, the difference often noted between local medical knowledge and biomedical knowledge can be modeled without resorting to the rhetoric of power. The stability and strength of the relations along which local medical knowledge is distributed give that knowledge over time a wider field of distribution as well as a greater resonance or truth-value precisely because it is secured by other vital social relationships or strands. In contrast, the brittleness of the relations along which biomedical knowledge is distributed, limits the range of its distribution and gives that knowledge less security or truth-value.

As noted in the last chapter, peasants exist only as a subordinate part of a larger, nonpeasant society. Because of this, unlike in Ohnuki-Tierney's (1984) urban setting, medical pluralism among peasantlike peoples that incorporates biomedicine cannot be modeled as a choir of mutually interacting, complementary voices. The different traditions of ethnomedical knowledge do interact and are complementary, whereas biomedical knowledge, because of its vertical direction and the lack of social ties validating it, competes with and (in the case of Indonesia's development goals driving biomedical distribution on Lombok) seeks to supplant local medical knowledge.

— • —

I had come into Pelocok shielded by an array of vaccines, a small first-aid kit, a modest biomedical understanding of anatomy and illness mechanisms, and a definition of health as the absence of biomedically detectable diseases. I had assumed if I washed daily, drank boiled water, and avoided mosquitoes and people who coughed up blood, I would stay healthy. But for people in Pelocok, health was an entirely different matter.

As we have seen, their definition of health is to have the idealized bodies of people with high social status and economic wealth. Because this definition is tied to unreachable ideals, Sasak peasants are always less than healthy. Moreover, their understandings of anatomy, of what the body is and how it operates physically, show some family resemblances, particularly in terms of metaphor use, but overall the ethnomedical traditions available in Pelocok do not follow a single theory of the body. Indeed, the ethnomedical traditions give evidence both of strong personalistic and strong naturalistic understandings of health. The medical pluralism of Pelocok is further complicated by a biomedical tradition. Rural Sasaks have complex relationships with various health experts from whom they gain some of their understandings of bodies. But in a society where everyone is a potential healer, everyone has idiosyncratic medical knowledge. In the end, most people were not concerned with understanding bodies in the abstract. What mattered was preventing and healing illness.

Interlude

Learning to Be Vulnerable

After about a month in Pelocok, I was beginning to find my feet. I had a basic grasp of the language. I knew my way around and was beginning to get a sense of people's lives. I had even collected a couple of illness case studies. Indeed I was beginning to think that living there, inconveniences aside, was quite easy, and the people were not too surprising. One conversation was all it took for me to realize that my feet were not on solid ground at all. Inaq Mol (my "mother") and I sat alone one day on the *barugah*. A *barugah* is an open, raised bamboo platform covered by a roof; it is the centerpiece of every courtyard, the primary site for socializing and visiting. Not every family owns a *barugah,* but the Mol family did; it and the cement floor of their small house were relics of past comparative prosperity. There we sat, silently unsheathing newly harvested rice paddy. It was midmorning and the courtyard was quiet.

Interrupting the silence, Inaq Mol suddenly asked me, "You already [*wah*] want to spend a day and a night with Nyonya Zahrah?" Nyonya Zahrah is the first wife of a respected nobleman who has strong relationships with many of the people in Pelocok, including the Mol family. I was confused by the question. One of the more frustrating elements of the Sasak language is that, like Indonesian, it lacks tenses; time is marked only generally by adding words such as "already" (*wah*), "not yet" (*ndeqman*), "earlier" (*onet*), and "long ago" (*juluq*). Confused and thinking that Inaq Mol was asking if I had already planned to spend the night during an upcoming ritual at the noblemen's house, I answered, "Yes." *Aoq.*

Inaq Mol, sliding between the paddy to sit close beside me and whispering now, asked, "What did she tell you? What small words [*kata kodeq*], words inside the heart, did she give you?"

Realizing that I had misinterpreted her first question, and now more confused, I answered, "There aren't any."

She tried again, "You already [*wah*] want to stay a day and a night with Nyonya Zahrah while at her house long ago [*juluq*]?"

Now completely confused, I answered incorrectly saying, "No, not yet" (*Ndeqman*), when actually I had spent two weeks living at Nyonya Zahrah's before beginning fieldwork in Pelocok, as Inaq Mol knew.

Inaq Mol, not at all dissuaded by what must have been my baffling answers, continued, "What small words do you know? Tell them to me. What do you say in small words, words inside? Words that you use when you go someplace new so that you are not afraid?"

I finally had a glimmer of understanding, saying, "I don't use words like Sasak words. I do use words, but every time they are different. The words are not the same as words in the Sasak way." Fieldwork is much like playing a connect-the-dot game with half of the dots missing. I remembered the whispered words La Nan, the daughter of this family, had made me write down during the first week of my fieldwork. She had told me to memorize them to protect myself. I remembered how La Nan told me that before her father would give her those words, she had had to be alone with him, not sleeping for a day and a night. It seemed Inaq Mol thought that Nyonya Zahrah had imparted the same kind of secret words to me in the same way. Perhaps she got the idea because the day before, while the nobleman and his wife were in Pelocok to invite me to their planned ritual, both of them started telling me about Sasak methods of healing toothaches, headaches, and stomachaches, knowing my interest in Sasak health care and no doubt trying to be helpful. Occasionally in their descriptions they had referred to *jampi* (healing spells) that must be said as part of the treatments.

Inaq Mol continued urging, "You must have words, small words inside your heart. Everyone is afraid of you [*Seleputne dengan takut kence ide*]."

Completely taken aback, I asked, "Who? Who is afraid of me?"

Inaq Mol answered, "Everyone. Everyone says they are afraid to try/test you [*cobade*].[1] Your knowledge is great [*ilmude luet*]. You have complete [knowledge of the] Christian religion, Islam religion, Hindu religion. People are afraid to try [*coba*] you. What are the words inside your heart? You say the words and that is enough. You do not need to worry wherever you go. What are your small words? Make them big." Obviously, conversations I had had, mostly with large groups of people come to check out the *buleq* (white person, foreigner), had made an impression. I had told them I had *belajar* (studied) each of those religions, not realizing at the time that my understanding of what knowl-

1. When speaking of trying or testing (*coba*) a person, what is meant is testing them with magic: sending them a curse and seeing if they are strong enough to repel it.

edge is differed from theirs, thus the significance of my words took on meanings I had not intended.

I answered, "I have knowledge (*ilmo*), but I use no small words like Sasaks."

Inaq Mol insisted, "You must. Say the words, not small but big."

I realized that if I continued to deny that I had small words, she would be convinced that I was lying, particularly because I had said that I had knowledge, which she would interpret logically to mean that I had small words. I did not want her to think I was ungenerous with my knowledge. While I puzzled briefly over the best way to answer her, Amaq Mol and another man came and joined us. Inaq Mol immediately dropped her look of intensity and moved away from me, saying loudly that the price of hulled, uncooked rice was very low now, and she wanted to store the rice rather than try to sell any of it. Obviously the topic of our conversation was supposed to be a secret.

This was a "dialogical breakthrough," a term defined by Attinasi and Friedrich to mean a moment during fieldwork when a conversation results in a split-second and fundamental realignment in the thinking of the field-worker (1995, 39). It was with this exchange that I realized that there was something fundamentally different between me and these Sasaks. I was not afraid, and they were. I went anywhere, blatantly not heeding warnings of dangers, ghosts, and witches, thinking that they were told simply to try to keep me at home as the Mol family pet. I did not imagine that other adults were actually afraid as they walked in their own village. The small words the daughter had whispered to me that would protect me while I bathed, walked, or traveled I had dutifully written down and kept secret. But La Nan struck me as such a silly girl, alternately scolding me, stealing my things, and humbly serving me, I had not taken her seriously. She had been trying to teach me, I saw now, that I was vulnerable. In this exchange with Inaq Mol, it became clear that I *should* have been vulnerable.

I did not see myself as vulnerable because I had continued to assume that I was only vulnerable when my body was exposed to viruses, bacteria, and the like. As long as I avoided unboiled water and mosquitoes, washed myself and my clothes daily, and stayed away from people who coughed up blood, I assumed I would stay relatively healthy, in the biomedical sense of the word. In contrast, these rural Sasaks were somehow vulnerable to other things beyond my ken, and they used knowledge in the form of small words to protect themselves. To begin to understand Sasak health care, I had to unlearn my assumptions about how persons are vulnerable to illness and about how knowledge acts in the world.

— 3 —

A World Full of Dangers

It was dusk in the compound, the time of gathering at the end of the day. Some were out bathing. Others were sitting and chewing betel or smoking cigarettes. Cooking fires were being lit. "*Ape kelakde*"—which vegetable are you boiling for dinner?—could be heard as women ducked into kitchen huts to ask for coals to start their own fires. Voices drifted across the compound in the stillness. "*Lekan embe?*"—where are you coming from?—could be heard shouted from inside houses addressed to the shadows walking by the open thresholds. "*Lekan no daya*" or "*leq gawa*" or "*lekan kontak*" would be shouted back by the people coming home from their fields or the forest. "*Tume wah!*" would be shouted back from inside the woven walls, insisting the person come on in and visit. "*Bareh wah!*" came the usual response, although everyone knew the person would in fact not be coming back later.

I heard Papuq Alus's voice responding "*lekan no lauq*"—from the south—as she passed the kitchen hut where Inaq Mol was cooking and had shouted the usual question through the matted walls. I went outside and followed Papuq Alus to her house. Setting down the basket she carried on her head, she unrolled a soiled and badly frayed mat out on her dirt stoop, and there we sat shelling the beans that would be her vegetable for the evening meal. She had asked me a few days previously to take a photograph of her youngest son, because he was planning to leave to find work in Malaysia; I had come to set the day. I told her of my plan to go into town on Saturday to buy the film, so that on Sunday I could take his picture. She looked up at me, this slip of a woman, and said worriedly that the travel expenses were so high to go round-trip to Mataram and that she couldn't help me pay for them. I agreed that they were high (3,300 Rp = $1.50), but I empathized with Papuq Alus and, trying to change the subject away from the awkward subject of money, I added that I could imagine how lonely I would be if I did not even have a photograph to remind me of a departed child.

Then she said, "Inaq Rodah ordered me to come pound paddy tonight. Pure rice (Indon., *padi suci*). Only women who have stopped menstruating and young girls who haven't started yet can pound and prepare pure rice. Inaq Rodah told me and I agreed to come tonight to sift and pound paddy. This pure rice will be the top rice used in the circumcision in the month of Maulid.[1] But one's thoughts have to be quiet. And one isn't allowed to talk while preparing the paddy, so that it is *suci*. But my heart, my thoughts are not quiet, so I am not going. My son is going away, and my thoughts are so." And she made quick up-and-down movements with her fist in front of her heart.

Many young men from Pelocok and other rural areas of Lombok go to Malaysia to seek work and adventure. Attractive rumors tell of men who marry rich Malay women or who make 20,000 Rp ($10) a day working on rubber plantations. Youths sell cows and borrow money to make the trip, which costs over a million rupiah ($500) if they do it legally. It is an expensive and risk-filled venture. The youths do not concern themselves with the other rumors, ones that occupy those left behind. These tell of men who fall sick with no one to care for them, who are imprisoned for years, and of those who never come home again. Papuq Alus's son had begged to be allowed to go to Malaysia for four months before she relented. A serene and kindly woman, she had taken a liking to me from the beginning, seeking me out for talks and calling me to keep her company while she prepared ritual foods. But the more her son had begged to go, the quieter and more reclusive she had become. As his departure approached, she seemed to waste away before my eyes. She didn't smile any more. She hardly talked to anyone except to speak of her worries about her son's departure, his safety, and the money he would need.

I returned from Mataram on Sunday to find that her son had left ahead of schedule. I could not take his photograph after all. Wanting to see how she was bearing up, I sought her out. But Papuq Alus, I was told, was busy with her petty trade business and had not been home since he had left. She had been sleeping with a niece in Masbagik, coming north to Pelocok to sell pepper seedlings during the day. Three

---

1. The top rice (Indon., *padi atas*) is the cooked rice used to serve the religious leaders (*kiayis*) during any ritual. Although the top rice should be pure for every ritual, no one bothers to insist on such rice except for circumcision and *bekuris* ceremonies: these are the most holy of the life-cycle rituals.

days later, she stopped by our *barugah* (covered platform) to drink a glass of coffee. She looked weary. Alone with her, I asked why she was sleeping in Masbagik.

"My throat is dry," she answered quietly, " My stomach feels empty. It's like that when a child goes to Malaysia. My thoughts are busy [*sibuk*]. If I just stayed home, I would just sit and stare/contemplate [*momot*]. The result would be illness. Better that I am busy and sleep in Masbagik."

THE DANGERS OF UNEASY THOUGHTS

In Papuq Alus's words, we see glimpses of how she *experiences* her body. As a postmenopausal woman, she is *suci* (pure, clean). Her purity makes her a member of a select group of females that can be called upon to prepare the special, sacred rice for rituals. Yet this purity of body is corrupted by the unease in her thoughts. One's thoughts should be peaceful in parallel with the purity of one's body. The restlessness of her thoughts, that she portrays with the jerky movement of her fist in front of her heart, would be communicated to the rice thus nullifying the purification process.[2] Papuq Alus speaks not of the content of her thoughts as affecting the rice, but of their tone. A serene state of mind works with the purity of her body to make pure rice. An uneasy state of mind works against the purity of her body, corrupting the rice. She chose to stay at home alone that night, thereby also alerting the community that something was not right with her, by not going to prepare the rice as she had promised.

After her son leaves, Papuq Alus again describes her thoughts as busy, uneasy. Again uneasy thoughts are seen as corrupting, this time threatening her health. She would become ill if she gave in to the uneasiness of her thoughts. Yet now, rather than isolating herself as she did by not joining in the rice preparations, she seeks society. She sleeps at another's house rather than alone at her own. She was very consciously forcing herself to stay active to prevent herself from becoming ill. She feared her busy thoughts would so incapacitate her that she would simply stop functioning, that she would just sit and stare, lost in the maze of her thoughts. She recognized herself as vulnerable to illness because of this and even describes somatic symptoms: the dry

2. Similarly, when a man is weaving a hanging basket to rock an infant in, his thoughts must be serene, and he cannot speak while he is making it. For if he speaks, or if his thoughts are disturbed, I was told, the child will cry and not be able to sleep.

throat, the empty stomach. The departure of her son so worried her, so filled her thoughts, that she was in danger of becoming ill.

Unni Wikan describes a similar case of devastating loss for a young Balinese woman, Suriati (1990). The woman's fiancé dies, and she is brokenhearted. Inside her own house, she cries and moves "as if she were dragging her body behind her" (9). Yet, whenever she went out, Suriati would put on a glittering smile, joking and laughing with those around her. Wikan argues that for the Balinese, sadness "undermines the strength and steadfastness of one's vital force (*bayu,* Bal.)" (8), thereby making one vulnerable to all kinds of illness, both ordinary and supernatural. The goal was to forget one's sadness by seeking to engage normally in society, thereby simultaneously working to prevent illness and overcome the sadness one thinks/feels (Bal., *keneh*).

Like Suriati, Papuq Alus does not cry publicly at the departure of her son. Papuq Alus makes extra efforts to be busily engaged in the activities of society. And like Suriati, the disturbance of her thoughts that would make her "gaze emptily into space" (10) is connected to a physical vulnerability. The movement of Papuq Alus's fist rapidly jerked up and down in front of her heart is a visual image of uneasy thoughts commonly used in Pelocok, an image I think would be recognizable to Suriati. I never heard a Sasak word analogous to Balinese *keneh,* meaning "thinking/feeling." But uneasy thoughts portrayed with a movement indicating a pounding heart corroborate my intuition that Sasaks, like Balinese, are not bothered with a Cartesian duality. Unlike Suriati, however, Papuq Alus made no effort to put on a "clear, bright face" (17). She did not pretend her thoughts were calm enough to pound rice, nor did she hide the fact that she was sleeping in Masbagik because she was so disturbed by her son's departure. Nor does Papuq Alus seek to forget her sadness. It is important for Sasaks to never forget anything because forgetting is a lapse in memory and knowledge, and therefore a degeneration that, in its extreme, leads to death. Finally, for Papuq Alus, by her own description, it is her uneasy thoughts that make her vulnerable to illness, not the waning of vital spirit that accompanies sadness.

Sasaks are not Balinese. This needs stating for two reasons. First, because the Balinese are among the darlings of anthropologists, and seeing a case like Papuq Alus, so similar to the better-known case of Suriati, one could overlook the differences and assume incorrectly that the cultural knowledge they both worked with was the same. Second, we are interested in what develops out of praxis, out of what people do, how they manage their own concerns and the welter of events they come up against. Praxis in no way precludes cultural models and structures (Bourdieu 1977b). Indeed, praxis is culture's lifeblood. But if we begin with overarching assumptions of the culture as basically Indonesian based on classic ethnographies from Java and Bali we set ourselves up to see a picture that doesn't fit with Sasak expressions of what their own experience of living is actually like (Paul 1989, 4, cited in Wikan 1990, 14).[3]

Papuq Alus was filled with anxieties before her son's planned departure, yet she chose to stay home and, after I left, was alone for the rest of the evening, because her son didn't come home until very late that night. Papuq Alus could have easily gone visiting, as she was wont to do, rather than staying alone that evening. She did not speak of herself as vulnerable to illness then, but only as having too many uneasy thoughts to be quiet (*tenang*) enough to make pure rice. Yet a few days later, after her son's departure, she avoided being alone at home because she was now vulnerable. Why the change? Why was she not vulnerable to illness by staying at home with her busy thoughts before his departure and so vulnerable to illness afterward? One can not argue that either choice was more culturally appropriate than the other. Both were perfectly acceptable by social standards. The only difference is in Papuq Alus's *experience of herself.* Whether her anxieties were greater after his departure or whether the immediate reminder of her empty house was simply too much for her we can not know. What we do know is the significance she placed on the turbulence of her thoughts. They had reached such a peak for her, that she was in danger of becoming ill. It was the dangerous uneasiness of her thoughts, not her son's departure, that directly made her vulnerable to illness.

The last chapter presented the ways in which rural Sasak understand bodies. This one attempts to explore how they *experience* their bodies. Or, to be more precise, it attempts to give a sense of how they are aware of their bodies as they go about everyday living. Everyday living is a difficult task. As we have seen, economic concerns weigh heavily on people's minds. On the other hand, economic concerns are so constant, they do not seem to matter much. Rather it is the other cares that can pervade one's thoughts. For Papuq Alus, her concern about losing her child to Malaysia grew like a cancer, blighted out her smile until finally she had to leave her home to keep from succumbing completely and becoming ill. *Vulnerability is the experience of oneself as open to harm,* as

3. Among these classics are Bateson and Mead 1942; Belo 1960; C. Geertz 1960, 1965, 1973; H. Geertz 1961; and Peacock 1987.

open to the possibility that illness will enter (*tume*) and rise up (*taik*) into the body. It is the personal sense that one has something to be worried about, that illness is just around the corner.

THE PROBLEM OF VULNERABILITY

Vulnerability, the experience of self or the perception of others as open to harm, is a slippery subject. Initially, I had intended to close this chapter with a massive "Vulnerabilities" table with gender and age variables down the side and vulnerabilities across the top: middle-aged women are vulnerable to A, B, and C; middle-aged men are vulnerable to X, Y, and Z. But this table kept unraveling. One middle-aged woman would be vulnerable to A, and one would not. And what to do with the one middle-aged man who was terribly vulnerable to black magic, not because he was middle-aged, but because he was overproud, strong, and handsome, had married too many times, and had no friends? A table with enough caveats to be accurate would be too unwieldy to be useful. No, vulnerability cannot be understood in tabular form. One experiences vulnerability when assessing self relative to the perceived environment. Moreover, like Papuq Alus, one's own strength waxes and wanes over time and space. While this assessment may not be verbalized it often is voiced with the phrase *ndeqku bani*.

NDEQKU BANI

"I am not brave enough" (cf. Wikan 1990, 82). I heard these words everywhere from nearly everyone with a frequency of use inversely proportional to age and standing in the community. "I am not brave enough to bathe there." "I am not brave enough to talk with him." "I am not brave enough to go there alone." Why were they not brave enough to walk around in their own landscape by themselves?

On the other hand, I was *bani* (brave). It never occurred to me not to be. Certainly at times I felt unsure and uneasy, but I took it that that was part of my job as an anthropologist. I was continually asked when going places—to the river to bathe or to a different compound to visit—if I were *bani* to go there alone. My answer of "yes" always seemed to startle people. One night, halfway en route to a death ceremony with a young woman as my only companion, my flashlight died. There was no moon in the glittering sky, and the path we walked was pitch-black.

Saying "*ndeqku bani*" my companion pulled my wrist toward the next house to find someone to deliver us to the ceremony with a flashlight. Past experience told me it would be a half-hour minimum visit, and I was eager to get to the ceremony that had no doubt already started. I told her it didn't matter, that we should walk on, and that the path was not difficult. She walked, clutching my arm the whole way. We arrived and she told all about our misadventure, and everyone was amazed at how brave I had been. A *kiayi* scolded me for venturing out in the dark, saying that it wasn't allowed, it was too dangerous.

Then it dawned on me that being *bani* had connotations different from the positive ones I was used to. No one but me ever went to bathe completely alone. No one slept alone. No one ever went outside at night without some kind of light. No one would go visit and accept food and drink at a non-"relative's" house.[4] No woman but the very old and wrinkled would ever travel alone, or live without a husband or father to protect them. Being alone was perceived as reckless and dangerous.

Indeed, I came to realize that not being brave is usually considered a good thing. Not being brave means, particularly for a female, that she is modest, conservative, obedient, and not a risk-taker. Children—male and female—are also encouraged not to be brave. Not to go down certain paths because of *selaq* (cannibalistic witches) there. Not to go out at night. Not to go anywhere alone. People—men and women alike—are encouraged not to travel. One should not visit different areas of Lombok or Indonesia. One should be afraid of being among strangers because "we don't know their hearts." Fear is not a negative quality.[5] People without fear are considered either enormously powerful with potent knowledge themselves or stupid persons who do not know that the world is full of dangers.

Such fear, particularly the fear of other people, has serious implications inhibiting the development of coherent and integrated cultural systems. Suspicion and distrust of others do not create an atmosphere conducive to close interaction and the sharing of some kinds of knowledge. Ethnomedicine in Pelocok is pluralistic and largely nonorderly partially because fear inhibits the open communication necessary for a society to develop consistent ideas among its individuals. So rural Sasaks tread lightly in a world teeming with dangers seen and unseen.

---

4. Any person can be designated as a relative, and fictive kin ties are invented if pressed.

5. Cf. "Children *should* feel afraid in the dark" (Keeler 1987, 66, emphasis in original).

COMMON ARENAS OF VULNERABILITY

If my being *bani* surprised people, it was simply because I was *bani* when many (although not all) people, particularly young women, in Pelocok would not have been. The experience of self as open to harm is a personal experience, a personal interpretation of one's own experience of self. Nonetheless, there are spaces, times, and circumstances when expressions of vulnerability are not surprising. It is *not* that a person is automatically vulnerable given these spaces, times, and circumstances. Rather, certain situations are generally understood to be dangerous (Indon., *bahaya*), and in them, if a person says *ndeq ku bani*, no one is taken aback. In discussing these situations, if pushed, people will say the danger is of becoming ill (Indon., *sakit*), and it is these situations of potential danger for illness that I outline below. *Cultural knowledge* is the term I use to identify information that is held in mutually recognizable forms by a majority of people within a community or society (cf. Shore 1996, 11). That is, most people in Pelocok have understandings, intuitions, information, that, when expressed verbally or nonverbally in any particular context, most people would recognize or at least respect even if they did not hold identical understandings and intuitions. Sasaks refer to such cultural knowledge as "*Ngeno wah sere iteh*" (This is the way of Pelocok), "*Ngeno ongkat baluqku*" (That is what my great-grandparent said), or "*Ngeno kata dengan laiq*" (Those are the words of the ancestors). Thus, if a confused anthropologist asks "Why this?" and these or similar phrases are offered as answers, the enlightened anthropologist can think, with some justification, "Aha! This is an area of cultural knowledge."

Dangerous Times

As in many places of the world not yoked to the ticking of clocks, there is a slippery, imprecise quality about time among Sasaks. The vague movement of time is only punctuated by annual rituals, the Friday Islamic prayer (which most men in Pelocok attend), and the five daily calls to prayer issuing from the mosque (which only about half a dozen people heed).[6] In everyday experience, the vague movement of time is

---

6. Unlike ordinary people, *kiayis* and ritual specialists do keep some track of the passage of time in order to reckon auspicious days for elective rituals and to identify the current month and year important in name-giving and in annual rituals. But the counting is never precise, and days can be added or dropped to accommodate the wishes of authority figures or to reach a consensus for when to celebrate a ritual.

unremarkable with two exceptions: the potentially dangerous times of dusk and of rituals. Dusk is the time for gathering at home after a long day's work. It is the time to wash off the grit of the day, thus cleansing and purifying the body. It is a quiet time, but also a dangerous time. It is considered dangerous to continue to work at dusk, and parents are careful that their infants are not outside at dusk, otherwise they would become *sakit* and cry until dawn. A *kiayi* reading from his book of secret knowledge verified that dusk —the time between *asar* (the late afternoon Islamic prayer, about four o'clock) and *magrib* (the evening prayer, about seven o'clock)—is a highly dangerous time, when there are many *malik* (taboos, dangerous powers).[7] Another man, Papuq Junin, once explained to me his secret calendar for calculating auspicious days and times. He too noted that one of the five periods of most days is dangerous. But unlike the *kiayi,* he argued that the period changed according to what day of the week it was: for example, on Mondays and Fridays the dangerous time is at midday, and on Thursdays, there is no dangerous period at all. But Papuq Junin added that most people do not know the calendar and think that dusk is always dangerous because it is the death of a day.[8] Perceived dangers of dusk do not prevent parents from entertaining guests, children from gathering fodder for cows, or adults from finishing a harvest. But, without a compelling reason to do otherwise, people prefer to be quietly bathing or playing with children in the compound come dusk.

Far more dangerous than dusk are certain months of the year. There are twelve months of the Sasak year, corresponding to the orthodox Islamic calendar: Rajap, Rowah, Puasa (Ar., *Ramadan*), Lebaran Belo,

---

Women's menstrual cycles do *not* measure time, because they are so irregular. It was not unusual for a nonpregnant, nonlactating, premenopausal woman to experience amenorrhea for up to five months. The lack of regularity was perhaps due to the anemia and low body fat common among women, or perhaps due to inappropriate estrogen levels in birth control pills and implants as one woman in Pelocok suggested. According to official records, 30 percent of households had women that used one or another kind of hormonal birth control.

7. The *kiayi* also noted the meanings of other times of the day: "Early in the morning is *ramai* (friendly, crowded). *Panas lapar* (hot hungry, midmorning) is *turun resiki* (the coming down of blessings or good fortune). At *butung tenari* (midday) it is a good time to plant crops. At *asar* (late afternoon) there are *kuleh* or *malik* (taboos, things that are forbidden). And *magrib* (after sunset) is *suwung* (there is nothing)." There is an obvious correlation with the five daily prayer times of Islam, but I do not know whether Islamic teachings in the Qur'an or the hadith (a collection of commentaries on the life and words of Muhammad) remark on the metaphysical circumstances that surround each prayer time in this way.

8. In the Islamic world, it is typical for days to be reckoned from dusk to dusk rather than by the Western system of reckoning them from midnight to midnight.

Lalang, Lebaran Kontak, Bubur Puteh, Bubur Abang, Mulut (Indon., *Maulid*), Suwung Tembeq, Suwung Tenggah, and Suwung Tuntut. All but four of these months are marked by annual community rituals known in Pelocok to be essential in the Islamic religion (*rukun Islam*). Only the two Buburs—Bubur Puteh and Bubur Abang—are considered times of particular vulnerability.

Throughout Lombok, these two months between the journey to Mecca for those on the hajj and the celebration of the prophet Mohammed's birthday, are named Bubur Puteh (White Rice-Porridge) and Bubur Abang (Red Rice-Porridge). In all urban areas and a number of rural areas as well, these months are empty of rituals or concerns; it is life as usual. But in Pelocok and some other rural villages, these months are filled with *malik* (taboos) that everyone knows and everyone follows. No one marries. No one builds houses, kitchen huts, or other kinds of shelter. No one travels any further than the market town, and certainly not to the sacred ground of the volcano. No one celebrates any life-cycle or other rituals that can be postponed; even birth and death rituals are quieter and smaller than at other times. In Pelocok and a few other rural places, on the 15th of Bubur Puteh and on the 5th of Bubur Abang, each *kiayi* has a *rowah* (ritual feast with prayers)[9] for each Bubur respectively.[10]

When I asked why these months were particularly dangerous, I received vague responses that they were dangerous already (*bahaya wah*), that the ancestors had said so (*ngeno ongkat dengan laiq*), that this was when the jinn and other spirits were active with their own rituals (*kane jim dit baket begawai luwet*), or that this was when humans were originally created (*kane waktu mamaq dit ninaq temiaq*). According to *kiayis* and ritual specialists (*tukang adat*), the Buburs are months of creation: the white is the semen and the month of male creation, the red is menstrual blood and the month of female creation. Therefore these

---

9. In Pelocok, people used the Arabic *rowah* for ritual feasts, called *selamatan* in much of the Indonesian literature (i.e., Geertz 1960) and called *kenduri* in the Malaysian literature (Colson 1971).

10. Victor Turner suggests that calendrical rituals are rituals that affect the entire community and often focus on status reversals: rituals to end droughts, famines, and plagues (1969, 169ff.). Among the Sasak, all of the calendrical rituals, including the rituals of Bubur Putih and Bubur Abang, are associated with the Islamic religious calendar. These rituals are requirements (*rukun*) of Islam, and failure to conduct them would lead to misfortune for the community. Thus they are rituals of maintenance, not reversal. It is also significant that, unlike the environs of the Ndembu, where Turner worked, Lombok, particularly in its northern half, is fairly constant climatically. Droughts, famines, and plagues do not occur cyclically. Thus, annual rituals of reversal in Turner's sense would not be necessary.

are the months when people must be the most respectful and show gratitude by not busying their lives with projects, travels, and unessential rituals. Allah, jinn, the dead ancestors, spirits, and *dewas* become angry, and sickness or death happens to those people who have forgotten the warnings of their ancestors—and here people in Pelocok point fingers at people in Masbagik and other areas of Lombok who do not remember (Indon., *ingat*) the taboos of the Buburs. In addition to avoiding taboos, using water (to pat on one's head) and betel chew (to dot on one's forehead) are sanctified during the ritual celebration of Bubur Abang in order to provide additional protection against illness and to atone for any insults that one may have inadvertently committed during the two months.

Even newborns are vulnerable during the months of Bubur: should an infant have the misfortune of being born during the 20 days between the ritual celebrations of Bubur Puteh and Bubur Abang, it is said that that person will go crazy unless each year he eats the ritually sanctified white and red porridge made at the respective Bubur celebrations. These porridges are served in little boats made out of banana leaves and fastened with needles "to prick the thoughts of the child so that it will not go crazy." Why are newborns vulnerable to madness if born during this time? An old man hinted an answer to me, saying that after the Bubur Puteh ritual the world was unbalanced and everything was incomplete until the celebration of the creation of females with Bubur Abang. These months are times of pronounced vulnerability to illness, when everyone avoids dangerous practices and seeks the medicines (*owat*) of the Bubur rituals if they perceive themselves or their children to be vulnerable to illness.

The cycles of days and the cycles of months, year after year, bring with them periods of relative vulnerability. To suggest that Sasaks continually worry about being vulnerable during these periods would grossly exaggerate reality. During the months of Bubur, people do not violate the most overt taboos, and they are careful to gain the protections of the Bubur rituals, but all without undue concern, just as people in urban America avoid the downtown streets at night that they might navigate during daylight.

Dangerous Times of the Life Cycle

In comparison to vulnerabilities of dusk and the Bubur rituals, the vulnerable periods in a person's life trajectory are treated with more overt concern. There are four such periods that are recognized as periods of relatively higher vulnerability to illness: pregnancy and birth; the first seven or nine days after birth for both mother and child; the years prior to circumcision; and the period after the death of someone else.

Sasaks enumerate life-cycle rituals beginning with marriage rather than birth because, as they say, how can you have a child if there isn't already a marriage?[11] The pregnancy that is supposed to follow is considered a dangerous time when the woman and the unborn infant are susceptible to illness and death.[12] A woman's first pregnancy is considered particularly dangerous, and it is to ensure the safe delivery of the child that a *besumbut* ritual is conducted. In the *besumbut,* the prospective parents are ritually cleansed, the health of the child is ensured, and the pain and danger of birth are prevented. Yet, the nervousness of the expecting couple determines how seriously they take the ritual. More often than not, husbands do not show up at all, and their part is played by a female friend. Husbands' lack of concern about their wives during pregnancies is not unusual, and they would often say that it is nothing to be pregnant, that women are used to it.[13] In contrast, pregnant women and their parents are typically very careful to make all of the correct preparations for the *besumbut* ritual. Still, there are women who do not, presumably because they do not experience their pregnant selves as particularly in need of protection. For example, the ritual bathing of one young couple was ill-prepared: the amount of money in the *penginang* (a kind of offering basket) for the spirits was incorrect, grated coconut for the cleansing had to be borrowed, and at the cul-

---

11. The moral implications of this question suggest that sexual intercourse never occurs without the social legitimation of marriage. Premarital or extramarital intercourse is not supposed to occur, but of course it does. If such sexual relations result in pregnancy, in most circumstances the family of the woman will force the father to marry her immediately. Neither the couple nor the child of such a union is stigmatized. Only once while I was in Pelocok did a woman become pregnant while unmarried and remain unwed. This woman was a divorcée who had had a relationship with a married man from outside Pelocok. Her family was unable to force a marriage, and the woman had her son out of wedlock. Gossip did follow her, but neither she nor the child was socially ostracized or condemned. With rare exceptions then, Sasaks follow the ideal, and marriage precedes or coincides with pregnancy.

12. Pregnancy is perhaps the most commonly noted occasion for experiences of vulnerability for many peoples (e.g., Peletz 1996, 216; Davis-Floyd and Sargent 1997).

13. Although this view is inaccurate according to maternal mortality rates, it is also understandable given reproductive histories in which women routinely give birth to as many as 14 or 15 children. On the other hand, men may respond thus as a defense against their own helplessness in protecting their wives and children during pregnancy and childbirth.

mination of the whole ritual, when the pregnant woman is supposed to fall back in a stream and break a raw egg over her head to ensure an easy delivery, it was discovered that she had forgotten to bring an egg! That portion of the ritual completely skipped, the children tore into the ritual foods while I sat with the *belian* who whispered to me that too many requirements had been incorrect so that the *besumbut "ndeqne jari"* (hadn't taken hold, hadn't happened). When I asked if it would be repeated, she said, no, that she did not think it mattered to them. I suggest that it did not matter because that pregnant woman did not sense herself in any danger.

Other pregnant women and women in their childbearing years, however, do consider themselves particularly vulnerable to illness and death. As one woman ill and pregnant with her third child said:

> The first, third, fifth, seventh, ninth, and eleventh childbirths are the hardest. Those are the ones when you can die. And I am afraid to die. I was so tired with the first child; I almost died. I am tired with this one. Even if I walk just a short distance, I am tired. I am afraid that I may die.

During my sojourn in Pelocok, over two dozen women spoke quietly to me of their fears of illness during pregnancy and dying in childbirth. Women who had had difficult past births told of how they avoided pregnancies altogether because they were afraid of dying during childbirth. Others spoke of how their children always die inside, and therefore they didn't want to have any more. These fears clash with the high cultural value Sasaks place on children: all adults are supposed to want children, moreover social adulthood, economic strength, social status, and security in old age all depend upon having children—the more the better. Some women expressed no concern about the vulnerabilities of pregnancy and birth, others expressed mild or strong concerns yet continued to have children almost annually, and other women's fears made them avoid pregnancy or, if pregnant, become preoccupied with a terror of dying. Concerns magnified whenever another woman died during childbirth, because then all pregnant women were considered highly likely to follow the dead woman and die also.

The vulnerabilities and fears do not end with successful childbirth. From the time of birth until the *molang-malik* life-cycle ceremony, both mother and child are officially in a period of high vulnerability that is concluded with *molang-malik* (to put an end to *malik*, taboos, dangers).

The ritual also ends the period in which the child has a symbiotic connection to its mother: whatever the mother does during this time can directly affect the well-being of the infant. Indeed, the ritual must await the falling-off of the umbilical stump—symbolizing connectedness to the mother—as well as the gender-appropriate number of days after birth.[14] During this period, the mother and child are considered very susceptible to illness in general, but also to the particular illnesses of *taget* (shock, surprise), *panas dalem* (internal fevers), and *sakit daraq* (blood sickness, resulting if all the woman's "dirty" blood does not come out). Although midwives, husbands, and family members usually encourage new mothers to follow at least some of the taboos for this period, women tend to decide for themselves which taboos need to be followed and which can be ignored. For example, after giving birth a woman must not lie down until the *molang-malik* ritual; otherwise both mother and child will become extremely ill.[15] In one instance a *belian*, Inaq Hapim, who had had government training, told the new mother, Inaq Sederi, just to lie down, that it didn't matter. Inaq Sederi was quiet, yet after the *belian* left, she told all the neighboring women what the *belian* had said, concluding by saying, "I am not brave. I will sit just like I did with all my other children so that we will be healthy" (*"Ndeqku bani. Tokol wah aku, sepertin kenca seleput kanakku akit ite sehat doang"*). Even though she was told by an expert that she and her child would not be vulnerable if she lay down, Inaq Sederi experienced herself as vulnerable and rebelled against the *belian*'s government-taught instructions. In another case, five days after Inaq Teli gave birth, I overheard this conversation between Inaq Teli and her young sister-in-law:

> *Sister-in-law:* When I had my baby, when people left the room, I would cheat. I would lie down. It wasn't a problem [she laughed].
>
> *Inaq Teli:* I am not *bani* to lie down. I cheated once when this one was born [indicating her three-year-old second child] and she was very sick for a month. I'm not *bani* to lie down this time.

---

14. The appropriate numbers of days are seven after the birth of a girl and nine after the birth of a boy. Seven and nine are numbers that occur frequently in ritual contexts.

15. Instead of lying down, postpartum women sit up with their legs extended straight out in front. They are supported by cotton pillows, both underneath them and against their backs.

Here we see two women. One did not experience herself or her child as vulnerable after giving birth and therefore "cheated" and lay prone. The other woman, learning from her past experience when cheating corresponded to her child's illness, regarded her new child as vulnerable if she lapsed again. The mother's and child's health during the period between birth and the *molang-malik* ritual are largely the mother's responsibility: she will follow the taboos only if she experiences a vulnerability.

Only in one particular is the child's vulnerability not left to the mother's guardianship. A person's name must fit (Indon., *cocok;* Sas., *kenak*). An ill-fitting name leads to illness. Some say that the name must fit with the *dewa* (god, spirit, shadowy twin) living within the person. Others say that the name must fit with the self (*dirine*). Thus names are things that matter, not for aesthetic or social reasons, but for reasons of health. The *belian* must come up with a name that will fit the child, and the *kiayi*, who does the actual naming, is finally responsible to be certain the name fits. At the moment of naming, the culmination of the *molang-malik* ritual, it is not at all uncommon for discussion to arise about what name would best fit the child. Names are chosen based on the date and circumstances of the child's birth. Thus, most often people are named for the day of the week they were born on—Ahap (for Ahad, Sunday), Senin (for Monday). But for infants born under unusual circumstances, names are given to fit with these circumstances—a child whose father died during the pregnancy was named "Left-Behind," or a child who was born outside of Pelocok was named "Find home." If the child's name fits, the child's vulnerabilities significantly decrease; if it does not fit, the child will become ill. For example, a child now known as Lo Mah was originally Lo Jan. His name was changed because "Nothing could go through his skin" and "He did not want to get big. His name did not fit." The impenetrability of his skin and his inability to become fat were given various ethnomedical treatments, but, when these repeatedly failed, his name was changed, and "after that he has been only healthy." Fit is determined post hoc, according to the absence or presence of later illness.

After the *molang-malik* ritual, everyone assumes that the name fits, and that the child's vulnerability is decreased dramatically. Nonetheless a child is not out of the woods until it is *bekuris*ed, and, if it is male, also circumcised (*besunat*). These rituals of purification, conducted together, result in full membership in the community of Islam (Ar., *ulama*). For girls, the *bekuris* alone is necessary, but boys must be cir-

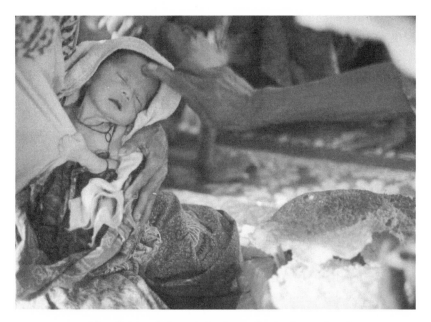

FIG. 5.   Naming an infant (who later died of unrelated causes) during the *molang-malik* ritual (1994)

cumcised prior to the final cleansing of the *bekuris*.[16] Until this final cleansing, children are considered particularly vulnerable to illness. When a child became ill, I frequently heard a parent exclaim that it was ill because it was not yet pure, meaning it had not yet undergone the *bekuris* and *besunat* rituals. Most parents were not brave enough to cut the hair above the fontanel until after these purifying rituals, because cutting it was not allowed according to the words of the ancestors (*Ndeqne kanggo wah, ngeno ongkat dengan laiq*). On the other hand, parents were also not eager to get these rituals over with; if conducted too soon, the child would also become very ill. A girl may be *bekuris*ed at any time after she is named, although parents prefer to wait two or three

16. I heard rumors of female circumcision among other groups of Sasaks, both rural and urban. Indeed, I visited some of these communities, and they described the procedure to me, but I never witnessed it. It was described as a minor shaving in the clitoral region. An eyewitness told me that in one hamlet a Chinese coin—which has a small square cutout in the center—was placed on the child's clitoris and prepuce. Whatever flesh came through that tiny hole was shaved off with a knife. From these descriptions, the circumcision would be classified as a minor clitoridectomy with probably at most a tiny portion of the prepuce removed.

years until the child is said to be "ready" (*nyiap*). Parents are even more concerned about their boys who must be not only "ready," but also "big enough" (*cukup beleq*) to be circumcised and *bekuris*ed. Many said that a boy may not be circumcised until he can walk, usually after 14 months, but others preferred to wait until boys were "big," that is, between three and six years old.[17] Thus parents walk a fine line. On the one hand they are concerned about their young child's vulnerability until the child is ritually purified, and on the other, they are concerned that conducting these rituals too early also jeopardizes the child's health. Neither of these rituals is elective, nor did I see any "cheating" or inadequate preparations for them. Sasaks consider it absolutely essential for one's entrance into Islam as well as for one's health that these rituals be performed correctly.

The five life-cycle rituals—beginning, with marriage—are understood to carry a person safely through his major life transitions and periods of greatest vulnerability. Yet there is one other period connected with a life trajectory that is dangerous: the first nine days after another person's death or the period until that dead person is given his or her main funeral ritual. It is widely believed that after death the *dewa* or the *nyiwa* (soul, self) is separate from the buried corpse, but it stays in the neighborhood to hear the farewells of family and friends, to gather all the blessings and belongings it will need to live in the afterworld (Ar., *aharat*), and to participate in the funeral ceremonies.[18] If the funerary preparations are incomplete, or the belongings whose essence is given to the dead are inadequate, the dead person is said to be forced to live as a child of a prostitute in the afterlife (*Indon.*, *anak pelacur*): someone uncared for, shunned, desperately poor, and ridiculed. Thus, the recently dead person often bumps into living people, either unintentionally or, if some funeral preparation is incomplete, deliberately. Every time a ghost bumps into or speaks to a living person, that person becomes ill with *ketemuq*—meeting a ghost. Usually *ketemuq* is simply a sudden stomach pain, but it can have almost any sudden physical symptom (see chap. 5). If all of the funeral ceremonies and preparations are correct and on time, then on the ninth day after

17. In the 1950s and 1960s, circumcision was conducted at puberty for men, just before marriage at the ages of 12 to 15. Today, in the urban areas of Lombok, circumcisions tend to be held when a boy is between the ages of 6 and 10.

18. The word *dewa*, like most words beginning with *d*, often was softened into *nyewa* in everyday use. *Nyewa* is extremely close to the word *nyiwa*, and in everyday usage, there was great slippage between them. In use, both words, more often than not, referred to the same thing, whether they were defined as god, spirit, or soul in Indonesian.

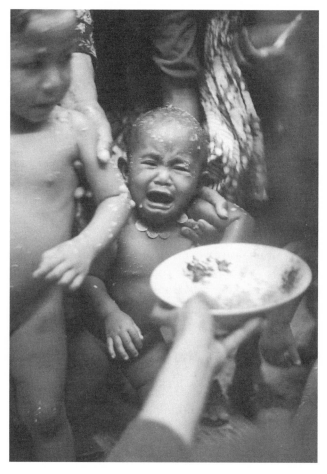

FIG. 6. A girl undergoing the *bekuris* ritual (1995)

death the ghost is given all of the belongings he or she will need in the afterlife and leaves. But until that time, all the living are vulnerable to becoming ill with *ketemuq*. Some people realize that meeting a ghost is highly probable at funerals, and do not worry about trying to prevent the unpreventable—how can one avoid bumping into something one can't see? Others do worry and avoid walking down secluded paths in the area or being alone in the compound, for ghosts are rumored not to linger in large crowds. Thus, both the living and the dead are at risk—the living risk illness and the recent dead risk an incomplete afterlife if the rituals are inadequately performed.

Of Seclusion and Society

Thus far we have explored the temporal contexts of the calendar and life cycle, within which expressions of vulnerability are frequent. But there are other arenas of vulnerability that are not limited by time. Two such arenas that complement each other in their contrariness are those of seclusion and society. Contexts of isolation and highly social contexts frequently triggered statements of *ndeq ku bani* (I am not brave enough) among people in Pelocok.

As mentioned above, ghosts are thought to frequent isolated paths and sit in solitary corners. But ghosts are not the only malevolent things to haunt isolated places. Ask anyone in Pelocok, the most timid child or the bravest man, and he will enumerate the beings that haunt their landscape. The landscape is teeming with ghosts, jinn, *badak* (spirits), Satan, *selaq* (cannibalistic witches), and *dewas* of various trees, mountains, and springs[19]—and each of these is potentially very dangerous to one's health. Ghosts, jinn, *badak,* and *dewas,* may cause illness accidentally, particularly the jinn who are reputedly great pranksters but whose pranks often result in injuries to the living. These spirits are also very sensitive to insult by the unwitting human who bumps into them, walks past without dipping her head in politeness, does not answer requests, or in some other way slights them. Such insults are avenged in illness—anything from a mild case of *ketemuq* to a hard illness (*sakit kras*) that may lead to death. Satan is another spirit who causes illness, but as a temptation (*coba*) or test of one's faith rather than as an act of revenge for an insult. All of these unseen spirits ignite anxiety in most people; therefore, believing in the strength of numbers against unseen foes, rarely does anyone in Pelocok go to any isolated place alone.

The malevolent being that is most feared, however, is *selaq. Selaq* are cannibalistic witches, rumored by some to be humans turned bad or, by others, spirits in human disguise. Initially, I had thought warnings of *selaq* frequenting this path or that stream were just stories to scare children. I was mistaken. Adults among themselves would say things like: "*Selaq* are all over here. Oh I'm not brave to go out at night" or "Between here and home there are lots of *selaq*. We can't go alone" or "It's not allowed to sleep in the field huts. Dangerous. There are a lot of *selaq* in the fields. Mostly at night." Once I asked Inaq Mol how she

---

19. Once I challenged a *kiayi* about these beings, asking how they all fit with the Islamic faith. He smiled at my simplicity and replied that of course they were all jinn. There are different names for them, just as there are different names for different kinds of people, but they were all people.

knew there were *selaq* on one particular isolated and heavily shaded path, and she answered, "I know already. When we walk on a path, if our hair rises, eee, there are *selaq* there. Dangerous" (*"Ku tauq wah. Lamun ite leq langan dit taik bulune, eee, ara selaq ito. Baheye"*). A solitary place combined with a somatic sensation led to her conclusion that she was in danger, she was vulnerable. As I learned the paths and spaces said to hide *selaq,* I noted that men, women, and children alike would walk far out of their way to avoid being alone on those stretches. Even the bravest and proudest men in the village cowered at the thought of going to a streambed alone at night. Early on, still ignorant of my vulnerability to *selaq,* I suffered one night from an acute case of diarrhea. Rather than wake the household, I hurried out of the house too noisily and stumbled down the steep path leading down to the creek. Not more than ten minutes later, I returned home to find a house of concerned faces. After hearing my embarrassed tale, the father scolded me saying: "You can't do that. Don't do it again. Go as two people, not by yourself. There are *selaq* down there at night. Lots of *selaq.* It is dangerous." The next morning, my escapade was all over the compound, and I spent the day listening to warnings of *selaq*s' murderous tendencies, scoldings against going anywhere alone, and exclamations of *"ndeq ku bani."* The spaces in the landscape that the introvert in me found to be refreshing escapes from the continual togetherness of village life were for them spaces of vulnerability.

Not only solitude in the landscape, but also solitude within oneself threatens health. The word *quiet* in both Indonesian and Sasak is *sepi.* The noun form, *kesepian,* means "lonely" or "loneliness." Companionship, being with another person, is never *sepi,* even if the people do not exchange a word but sit silently at opposite corners of a covered platform staring in different directions. *Sepi* is having no one around. When a compound is *sepi,* silent and empty of people, a lone person is thus *kesepian* (Indon.), lonely.[20] And loneliness is said to make one ill, to make one thin, to make one's thoughts too busy.[21] "I am not brave

---

20. I am not arguing that these arenas of potential vulnerability are unique to the rural Sasak. The equation I make above between being alone in the landscape and vulnerability to illness caused by malevolent, unseen beings is common in many places (e.g., Wikan 1990). Similarly the equation of being alone with being lonely is not particularly unusual (see, e.g., Shore 1982).

21. After I had returned from a brief trip to Bali to lecture, Inaq Mol said she had dreamed about me while I was gone, had seen me washing my clothes in a stream by myself. I told her, indeed, I had washed my clothes while I was there. Then Inaq Mol asked: "What did you do in Bali?" I answered following a convention of politeness implying that I missed my Sasak home, "During the day I taught about Sasak customs. But at night I was alone. There was no one with me. I ate alone. And I was lonely."

alone" (*Ndeqku bani mesaqku*) was a phrase I heard frequently from children, women, and younger men in astonished response to my sleeping, bathing, visiting, walking, and traveling alone. I suggest that they experience not simply a desire for continual companionship but also a fear of being alone with themselves. For without a companion, they say, people have a tendency to stare into space and *momot* (contemplate) until they become sick because of their longing for others or their uneasy thoughts. When a newly weaned toddler began to lose weight, his recently divorced mother came to me, asking for medicine. When I asked what was wrong, she answered, "He is ill. He doesn't want to get big. Very thin since his father left. It is lonely at home. He misses his father" ("*Sakit iye. Ndeqne meleh beleq. Kurus gati sejak berangkat amaqne. Sepian leq baleh. Kangenne*"). Similarly, my "family" worried incessantly about my weight loss and scolded me for being alone too much, thinking too hard, and missing my American family too much (cf. Ferzacca 1996, 497).[22] In a place where people equate health with fatness, and weight loss with illness, my increasing thinness was an illness resulting from being alone too much.[23]

Likewise, loneliness is seen as the context that promotes uneasy thoughts. Uneasy thoughts, as we saw with Papuq Alus, lead a person to experience himself or herself as vulnerable to illness. One woman, after a thief had broken into her house stealing items while she slept alone, went to a clinic to get an injection because "I was sick, my thoughts were too busy" ("*Aku sakit, pikiranku sibuk gati*"). She interpreted her experience of being so uneasy in her thoughts as an illness

---

Then Inaq Mol said, "I thought you were sick. But that must have been it. You were lonely."

22. One particularly memorable scolding came from a young teenager. I had closed my eyes to retreat from a conversation, trying to remember the meaning of a particular Sasak word. After a moment, the boy drew me back to the social world by saying: "Don't think so hard! It will make you sick." Indeed, it took me months to convince people that I really was all right when I sat alone writing up field notes. Thinking hard or perusing one's own thoughts was almost never condoned in Pelocok. The one exception I experienced was in discussions about cosmology when Inaq Mol, trying to convince me of her point of view, would say: "Think about it. And think again. And think one more time. And you will understand it is this way." This necessarily solitary activity was antisocial, opening a person up to the harms of being alone and also the danger of insulting others who wanted to be social.

23. My own explanation, which I never shared with them, was that the food cooked in Pelocok was less than appetizing (ranging from bland to barely tolerable), and I had difficulty eating around malnourished children. Sasak adults and the youngest child in a household always receive the best foods, with leftovers doled out to the other children, because children are said not to need vegetables and proteins as long as they are full with rice.

that needed a biomedical remedy. There are of course people in Pelocok who seem content to be alone, who live alone or work alone some of the time. Yet most people I knew were uneasy about being alone. "When there is someone with us, we are happy. There has to be a companion. People of Lombok like to be with our friends. It doesn't feel good otherwise. If we are alone, we are lonely" (*Munne are kencene, demun ite. Harus are kencene. Dengan Lombok isa lamun kenca batur ite. Ndeqne maiq munne deq are. Lamun mesaq, ite sepian*). There are varying degrees of solitude, but in general Sasaks are more comfortable with others than alone, partially because companionship acts as a buffer against the vulnerabilities of solitude.

On the other hand, socializing also creates vulnerability because "we do not know the hearts [Indon., *hati*] of others."[24] In their talk about ghosts, spirits, and witches, Sasaks show a concern about that which is hidden from view. That which is hidden, which one can not see, is potentially dangerous. Similarly, Sasaks are concerned with the hidden hearts of people. I frequently heard phrases like: "They appear nice, but only Allah knows their hearts" (*Gitaqne sola laguq Allah doang tauq hatine*), "It is not allowed to be alone among so many people whose hearts we do not know" (*Ndeq de kanggo mesaq-mesaq kenca dengan luwet ngeno si hatine ndeqne tauq*), "She is beautiful, but the heart, I don't yet know" (*Jeneng iye, laguq hatine, deqku man tauq*). Hearts hide intent: unseen and unknown hearts are the unknown and unpredictable intentions of others.[25] Sometimes, the concern has to do with potential physical violence. Word of mouth, the occasional transistor radio, and later television fueled fears that murder is a commonplace and daily occurrence in distant places like Mataram, Bali, the Netherlands, and America.[26] Strangers are feared for the potential violence they might

---

24. This concern with not knowing others' hearts as a euphemism for not knowing someone's intentions is also common among the Balinese (Wikan 1990). Literally, *hati* (Indon.) means liver, but people refer to it as English speakers refer to the heart, and translations from Indonesian often translate it as heart.

25. Here hearts are again linked with what a Cartesian would categorize with mind, namely, intent, which supports my claim that a mind–body duality is not supported by Sasak life-worlds. It is also worth noting that Sasak concern with the possible negative intent of others being hidden by beautiful faces calls to mind the negative connotations of hypocrisy in the United States. Hypocrisy is not a widely noted concern in the Indonesian literature (exc. see Wikan 1990), where the concern tends to be about what is displayed—the outer expressions—rather than the inner feelings (e.g., Geertz 1973).

26. Transistor radios were fairly common possessions in Pelocok, with one in approximately every three households. But because the radios were powered by batteries deemed too expensive to buy regularly, they were silent more often than not. In 1995, a handful of people in Pelocok paid to have electricity brought to their houses

intend: "They come to visit us. They seem happy to be with us, but they want to kill us. We do not know their hearts." Crowds of people from distant places who gather for large rituals in Pelocok are always treated with generous hospitality but also caution: "We do not know them. They look nice, but how are their hearts? We do not know. Dangerous." Similarly, some people in Pelocok are wary of those in neighboring hamlets, even though they are long-term acquaintances. In one conversation, Inaq Mol and her daughter warned me of people in hamlets not a half-mile from Pelocok:

> *Inaq Mol:* It is good you are here, Eron [Cameron]. If you had gone to stay in X or Y or Z, there you have to pray five times a day and night. If you don't, they will kill you [she made a motion, drawing her hand across her neck].
> *La Nan:* If you don't fast. If you don't pray one day, they will get together and say you are dirty. And they will decide to get rid of you. They will kill [Indon., *dibunuh*] you. People there are very bad. They act nice, but their hearts are not Islam. I am not brave to go there.
> *Inaq Mol:* Don't stay there. You can visit but not alone and do not spend the night. Here you are safe. Nothing will happen to you. They are not brave to come here.

To my knowledge, no one from Pelocok has ever been murdered.[27] Murder in Lombok, even in urban areas, is extremely rare. Yet, not infrequently in crowds of strangers or in spaces outside the confines of Pelocok, women and men expressed concern about being killed by strangers or acquaintances whose hearts are not visible.

This sense of vulnerability to the intentions of others is an everyday experience because it is also difficult to know the hearts of neighbors and friends. *Ilmu* is the knowledge any particular person has, but the word is used most often by Sasaks to refer to secret and powerful knowledge, including the knowledge of black magic.

(mostly by the illegal pirating of power). Of these, the hamlet head and one other family were wealthy enough to buy old televisions. These televisions were turned on constantly and situated on the front stoops, so that anyone could sit in the dirt of the compound and watch. The broadcasts were in Indonesian, which many people could not understand, but they would watch anyway, commenting on the visual images.
27. One young man was killed in a distant village, but he provoked it by attempting to steal a cow. Unlike murder, cattle theft is a common problem in Lombok. If a thief is caught in the act, he or she is typically mobbed by villagers and killed without any resulting rebuke from the law.

According to the Balinese, the people of Lombok—particularly East Lombok—have very strong black magic (Wikan 1990; Gerdin 1982). Black magic causes illnesses through poisoning food or drink. I heard only four illness etiologies point to intentional poisoning, but maybe two dozen warnings were given to me not to eat the food prepared by so-and-so. I was warned that some women had things against various members of my family (jealous of the married daughter, angry at the mother, resentful that I lived with them, insulted by the son-in-law), and some women's cooking was feared simply because *hatine lenge* (their hearts are bad). I was seen as needing these warnings because it was noticed that I would go blithely visiting (*bekedeq*), stopping at any person's house I came across and partaking of anything my hosts insisted on offering me. I suspect that normal people in Pelocok were not as vulnerable to food poisoning as I was considered to be, because most people only visited their close friends and family—people whose hearts they already knew to be good.

The other kind of illness-causing black magic is curses.[28] Curses are sent directly from one person to another, and, in order to direct a curse, one need only whisper that person's name.[29] The Balinese, who also have a great fear of curses, spend a considerable amount of energy picking up strands of hair and fingernail clippings so that these will not be used as mediums for curses (Wikan 1990). In comparison, all Sasaks I knew were much more relaxed about the danger of curses and certainly never concerned themselves with collecting strands of hair and the like. Any insult—being a stingy host, being boastful, flaunting possessions, marrying someone else—can provoke another person to send a curse. Curses result in unusual illnesses (*ndeq biese*) that are extremely difficult, if not impossible, to treat. As battles between the *ilmu* of two people, curses can be warded off or returned to wreak havoc on the original sender, if the intended victim's *ilmu* is stronger than the sender's. Thus, the more *ilmu* a person has, the more vulnerable that person is to curses sent by those he interacts with daily, but also the more likely that those curses will be thwarted. Nonetheless, because *ilmu* is usually something secret, one can never be sure who has the

---

28. Love magic, in the forms of pills and potions sprinkled on the loved one's food, was considered a precipitating element in most marriages. The reluctant "victim," whose own *ilmu* was not enough to ward off the love magic, would suddenly fall in love (*jatoq cinta*), and the couple would marry (see also Ecklund 1977; Cederroth 1981; Krulfeld 1974). Love magic, depending on one's point of view, could be either black magic (*ilmu bedang*, black knowledge) or just *ilmu* (powerful knowledge).

29. Curses are directed with names, because a name is intimately and inherently fitted to a person.

strongest knowledge. "It's not possible for us to see the inside of people" (*ite ndeqne bauq gitaq leq dalem dengan*): the humblest, most self-deprecating person might have the strongest *ilmu* of all.[30] The *ilmu* of neighbors and friends poses a potential threat to one's health.

Sasaks are caught between a rock and a hard place. On the one hand, they are vulnerable when alone in the landscape or just alone within themselves. On the other hand, they are vulnerable to the violence of strangers and the secret knowledge of friends. All things being equal, however, people prefer to be with friends and family rather than alone or in crowds. They simply live with the dangers of black magic.

The Auras of Things and People

Then there is the threat of *kemalikan*. *Kemalikan* is the illness a person gets if they are disrespectful of *malik*. *Malik* I defined earlier as "taboo." But in Pelocok, people also use *malik* in sentences like: "Rinjani is full of *malik*" (*Sobol malik leq Rinjani sino*), "If a person walks past you [meaning me] without excusing themselves, they are intentionally disrespectful and will become ill with *kemalikan* because you are full of knowledge" (*Munne are si lewat laguq ndeqne tabeyan ide, tular manuh ngeno ampokne mesti kemalikan, kan ilmu ide sobolan*), or "His belt has not been washed for a long time. It needs to be washed. That is why you are *kemalikan*" (*Sabukne suwe-suwe ndeq tebesoq iye. Perlune gati. Ngeno kan ide kemalikan*). One can understand how a volcano might have many taboos. It is more difficult to understand how an unintentional slight on another person's knowledge would result in illness. How is illness caused automatically by my slighted knowledge, if I do not send a curse and am perhaps unaware of the disrespectful action? How can an inanimate thing—a belt—cause the same illness?

I suggest that *malik* can also be understood as a kind of aura that

---

30. In a conversation with La Nan, the daughter of my "family," she pointed to the fading poster of the Nine Wali Songgo (Islamic apostles) wedged into the matted wall and told me about the millennium when every person will have to choose among the Wali Songgo. The wisest one, the one who will save the people of Lombok if chosen, is the one who looks the worst, she warned: old, bent, ugly, humble, unwashed, and wearing tired black clothing. Although appearance is prized, appreciated, and bespeaks potent *ilmu* in Pelocok, there are also strands of cultural knowledge that argue that the opposite is also true—the most humble appearances and attitudes bespeak potent *ilmu*.

As a further aside, Geertz discusses the Nine Wali Sanga as Javanese apostles credited with bringing Islam to Java (1968, 25ff.). Posters of the same drawn figures abound in both Javanese and Sasak homes suggesting that the Wali Songgo that Sasaks claim as their own apostles are given the faces of Wali Sanga printed in Java.

emanates from potent, powerful, wise, or sacred sources.[31] This aura has an agency of its own so that if one is disrespectful of it, it retaliates automatically by producing the illness called *kemalikan*. Thus, if while climbing the volcano someone fails to use its special language (*Bese Rinjani*, which consists of a different vocabulary for a number of nouns and verbs), that person will be struck down automatically with a potentially fatal case of *kemalikan*. If someone is intentionally disrespectful of me, even though I couldn't care less whether or not the person said "Excuse me" (*tabey*) as he passed, he would automatically become ill with *kemalikan*. Or if a sacred/powerful object (Indon., *pusaka*) has not been washed or purified recently, it will automatically lash out with *kemalikan* at any and all who come within a certain radius of it.[32]

The awareness of *malik* translates into an experience of self as vulnerable to *kemalikan* in sacred spaces, around people with strong *ilmu*, and near objects of potency. With the exception of sacred spaces like the volcano Rinjani that is obviously full of *malik*, the *malik* (read potent aura) of people or objects is hidden. The wealthy, socially respected, and obviously knowledgeable people (like experts—*kiayis, dukuns, belians*, gurus) are well-known, and one can be careful not to be disrespectful of them. But the *ilmu* of a humble, quiet, self-effacing person is more difficult to gauge, and if someone is intentionally disrespectful assuming that person has no potent *ilmu*, the offender may come down with *kemalikan*. More perplexing yet is avoiding being within the radius of the potent aura of sacred objects, because such *pusaka* are almost always kept secret, hidden away within a wall or in the rafters of a house. Older people are suspected of having many *pusaka*, but young people have them too. And certainly, one can not avoid going to visit the houses of friends and family, *pusaka* or no. To further complicate matters, the *malik* of people and objects ebbs and flows. A newly purified *pusaka* will cause no one harm, indeed it protects people from harms, including illness. Likewise, people are not consistently *malik*, for their potent *ilmu* can become more or less powerful, as they receive and give away *ilmu*, or as their *ilmu* is occupied battling with curses.

Given these contingencies, people seem to experience vulnerability to *kemalikan* variably. Everyone I ever talked to about the volcano spoke

---

31. Similar understandings can be found elsewhere in Indonesia, particularly with regard to kings and presidents (e.g., Anderson 1990), and volcanoes and *pusaka* (e.g., Pemberton 1994; Hefner 1985).

32. *Pusaka* can be any object that has been handed down from one's ancestors. The most common *pusaka* among Sasaks were knives, palm-leaf books, and belts or strips of cloth.

of it with great reverence, giving lists of what one may not do on the volcano, including having sex, speaking loudly or making much commotion, asking questions about what is this or that, using nonvolcano vocabulary, or complaining. Climbing it with a group of 20 people from Pelocok, I readily noticed that everyone, from the *kiayi* to a young girl, all carefully followed all of these *malik*. Ignoring them on Rinjani, the most sacred space on Lombok and equal—according to some—to the sacredness of Mecca, automatically would cause death. I was told numerous gruesome stories of people who had died while climbing the volcano because they were intentionally disrespectful (*tular manuh*).

Concern over the auras of other people was more variable. Persons who were older and/or more confident in their own *ilmu* were less likely to excuse themselves or even duck their heads when walking past anyone, except strangers who might take it as an insult and retaliate with curses. In contrast, La Nan, my married "sister," was inordinately humble, bowing her body so that her hands almost touched the floor anytime she walked past anyone of her size or older. It is of course impossible here to distinguish between showing respect out of good manners, out of concern for potential poisons or curses, and out of concern about the potent aura potentially causing *kemalikan* of others. Never did I hear a person say that they feared getting *kemalikan* from others; but an individual might say simply that he was not brave enough to approach so-and-so, or she was not brave enough not to act politely. Only after a diagnosis of *kemalikan* would an ill person lament that it was because he had been with so-and-so earlier or because she had not made enough coffee to give so-and-so a glass earlier. But *kemalikan* from people was never very serious: a few days of terrible itching, or red and swollen eyes. Similarly, the *kemalikan* one suffered from being within the radius of a potent object when it needed purifying was mild: itchy patches, puffy eyes, or tripping and falling. In one case, a woman's prolonged labor was said to be due to a potent knife hidden in the mat wall above her head. In the handful of times I witnessed the handling or washing of a *pusaka*, only the object's owner was brave enough to touch it, with echoes of *ndeq ku bani* resounding from assembled family or close friends. The object itself was always treated with extreme gentleness and care, nor was it allowed to turn one's back on the object while it was out of its hiding spot. Yet under usual circumstances the object was hidden and ignored. After all, one could not stop visiting a favorite friend or cousin simply because one suspected she had many potent objects stashed away. Only when people who frequented a certain compound started becoming ill with *kemalikan* did I ever hear people talk about avoiding that place until the owners had taken care of the *malik* of their *pusaka.*

Places, people, and things have auras that can cause illness. However, concern about being disrespectful of these auras is generally back-grounded in most people's thoughts unless they are making pilgrim-ages to sacred places like the volcano or are already suffering from *kemalikan.*

The Second World

Alam kedua (the second world) is the space where the dead live and that the living visit when they dream. Whereas in the everyday world (*alam ita,* our world) auras and spirits are invisible, in the dream world they can be seen. If they are seen, the dreamer may become ill. When one dreams, one interacts with the spirits, ancestors, and auras with all their secret knowledge and potencies. In other words, while asleep, people are vulnerable to becoming ill just as they are vulnerable to *ketemuq* and *kemalikan* while awake. Inaq Mol explained it to me once thus:

> *Cameron:* So there are two worlds. One we can see and one we can not see, where the dead live?
>
> *Inaq Mol:* Yes. Think about it. And think again. And think again. And one more time. And slowly you will understand.
>
> *Cameron:* So if I suddenly become ill with *ketemuq,* because I met a dead person, it is while walking I meet the second world?
>
> *Inaq Mol:* No. It is in your dreams. In dreams one meets a dead person and gets ill. When you dream, your body remains asleep, but you go to the *alam kedua.* There you can meet peo-ple who have died. If you dream you meet an ancestor, you will get ill. Also there you can meet people from far away. For example, it's impossible that you have not dreamed of Rob [my husband]. You meet him in your dreams although he is far away. How it that possible? It is possible because he too is in the *alam kedua.* You meet there. You can talk with him there.
>
> *Cameron:* So when we dream we enter *alam kedua,* we meet dead people and also others who have entered *alam kedua* because they are dreaming?
>
> *Inaq Mol:* Yes. Think about it and think again. And add some more.

Edward B. Tylor would appreciate this conversation, for Inaq Mol's words support his theory of how "primitive" people develop religion (1958). He argues that dreaming about people who have died meant to "primitive peoples" that death was not final, that there is an essence or spirit of the person that lives on after death. It is the belief in an afterlife that is the fundamental motivation for "primitive" religions, according to him. While Sasak religion is certainly not primitive nor is it based on dreaming, dreaming is an important aspect of Sasak cosmology and religion. Dreaming introduces the living to the second world, the normally unseen world.

In her statements, Inaq Mol contradicts my earlier argument that living people can bump into unseen dead spirits in everyday life as they walk around their landscape. Once, returning home later than Inaq Mol after a funeral ritual, I found her treating herself as one would for an illness. When I asked what was wrong, she replied that she had just met a dead person while at the ritual. She had not been asleep and therefore could not have met him in her dreams. I have documented seven other cases of *ketemuq* with etiologies not referencing dreaming. I suspect that direct questions like the one I asked Inaq Mol in the above conversation flustered her; I was asking for a logical explanation for something one knows from experiences, often contradictory. She could not explain how we can meet ghosts who live in the second world walking around in our world; she relied on a dream explanation saying the other was wrong, even though she and others experienced *ketemuq* while in the everyday world.

A major difference between becoming ill with *ketemuq* or *kemalikan* while one is awake as opposed to while asleep is that in dreams one sees who or what caused the illness. If a person comes down with *ketemuq* while at a funeral rite, she will assume the ghost was the person being given the ritual. If a person wakes up with a stomachache, she will review her dreams to identify the dead person she saw in them. In the case of *ketemuq*, identity makes no difference in treatment. But in the case of *kemalikan*, it makes a great deal of difference. A person may either wake up with *kemalikan* or have it already, then identify its source while dreaming. If someone dreams of getting *kemalikan* from a person, he sees which person's aura he has offended and can avoid doing so in the future. The auras of *pusaka* always take the form of a snake in dreams. Not knowing this common interpretation, one day I was telling Inaq Sur about a dream in which a cobra was striking when I awoke in a sweat. Immediately she asked me where the snake was. I told her it was on the path to her compound.

Inaq Sur: Ah, it is my husband's belt. It needs to be washed. If you had gotten bitten, you would be *kemalikan.* It is dangerous for us all here until his belt is washed.

Ah, sabuk sumamaqku. Perlune gati tebesoq. Lamun tegigit, ide mesti kenaq kemalikan, ngenit gati. Bahaya gati gen ite ndeqne man tebeso-qin sabuqne.

Cameron: But I do itch terribly.

Laguq ngenit aku gati.

[Another woman walked into the cooking hut.]

Inaq Sur [to her]: Cameron is *kemalikan.* She dreamt of a snake.

Emeron kemalikan. Iye mimpin ular.

Here, even though I had not been bitten in my dream, my itching meant to Inaq Sur that I had *kemalikan.* When I told the dream and Inaq Sur's diagnosis to a different person, he asked if I had been bitten by the snake. No. Then I was ill with something else, not *kemalikan,* he replied, adding that I should not go back to Inaq Sur's because I was in danger of *kemalikan* there. According to one person, my dream in conjunction with my itchy skin meant that I already had *kemalikan;* according to another, that I was in danger of getting *kemalikan.* The dream was central to both interpretations.

To say that some Sasaks consider themselves vulnerable to illness while dreaming does not mean that they are concerned about this vulnerability. On the other hand, perhaps they are. I am reminded of a woman's astonished reply to my insistence that I sleep alone: "People of Lombok are not brave to sleep alone. We would not sleep well." *Dengan Lombok ndeq bani mesaq-mesaq bedum. Ndeqne bauq maiq bedum mesaqne.*

The Dangers of Forgetting

The final arena commonly known to be full of dangers is one's own mind. The mind is dangerous because it can forget. Forgetting is dangerous because the lapse in memory and knowledge, in its extreme, leads to death, as we will see. For now, we limit ourselves to those lapses in memory that trigger illness.

Victor Turner mentions that for Ndembu in Africa, if ancestors are "forgotten" they will return and plague the living (1967, 10). He implies that forgetting means negligence of duties toward ancestors, which they then retaliate. Half a world away, the same applies for rural Sasaks. One must remember to put out food to welcome dead visitors at every ritual. One must remember all of the *rukun* (Sas., customary guidelines or requirements) of burial and the eight different mortuary rituals, so that the dead will not be a child of a prostitute (Indon., *anak pelacur*), meaning a person forgotten by the world. To be forgotten makes the dead angry, and they will "come and give an illness, a very bad illness. One that lasts and does not go away." It is not the errors in rituals that anger the ancestors, but the forgetting.

Errors happen frequently. After I had been to enough rituals to know what to expect, at almost every ritual I would ask a *kiayi* or *tukang adat* (ritual specialist) about something that appeared odd. More often than not, the reply was, "Yes, well it is not quite right, but it doesn't matter." There is a certain degree of laxness in performing the rituals, even mortuary rituals. For instance, if a family did not purchase enough bananas or other foodstuffs, the *tukang adat* would tell the *kiayi*, "I know it is not right, but this is all there is," and the *kiayi* would invariably answer, "It doesn't matter. It will be good enough." Almost anything can be fudged over, but it may not be "forgotten." If the food tower for the dead is taken out without calling attention to its shortcomings, the *kiayi*s would scold people saying *ndeqne kanggo lupaq* (it's not allowed to forget) and send them scurrying to correct the fault. Or if a family with the financial means lets an inordinate amount of time slip by (usually four months or more) before hosting a life-cycle or mortuary ritual, a *kiayi* would scold them for "forgetting." It is the act of forgetting that is the problem. And it is the act of forgetting that ancestors are said to punish with illness. If a family without means "gives" the dead person only an old mat to sleep on, an old set of clothes to wear, and a cracked pot to cook in, the ancestor will not be angry. But if a family with means does these things, fellow villagers will gossip behind their backs of how they have forgotten their dead and will surely become ill.

In addition to remembering the ancestors, one must also remember one's religion. As Muslims, all Sasaks believe in Allah. Allah is the Supreme Being, the maker of fate (Indon., *nasib*).[33] He has the ultimate power over illness and health. Pelocok is a place where many of the actions typically associated with being Muslim are largely absent:[34]

---

33. The Sasak concept of fate is complex. While Allah had preordained all that will happen, this does not diminish either agency to act in the world or motivation to attempt to change situations (see Hay 1998b, 1999; see also Krulfeld 1966).

34. This absence is the source of much criticism by the majority of Sasaks on the island, who tend to call the people of Pelocok and similar areas in Lombok "pagans." The latter retaliate by saying that the majority are not real Muslims for they have forgotten many of the *rukun*s passed down by the ancestors. In actuality, there is an enormous continuum of Islam as it is practiced on Lombok. But the more orthodox Muslims are intolerant of what they imagine to be (and what often is) the laxness of

no more than a handful of people pray daily, no more than a couple of dozen people fast for the entire month of Ramadan, people pilgrimage to the sacred volcano Rinjani, saying that "Rinjani is better than Mecca" (*Rinjani sola'an dit Mekkah*), and men and occasionally women drink alcoholic palm and rice wines. In other ways people in Pelocok are devout, committed to their beliefs of what makes a good Muslim and following what they understand to be Islamic *rukun* (religious law). The most important among these are to have a good, clean/pure heart and never to forget one's faith in Allah. Indeed, the essence of a good heart is remembering Allah. But if one forgets, even momentarily, Allah will give that person illness. As one woman said about the illness of her stepson: "He forgot [*ndeq ie ingat*] Allah. For one moment while he was drinking palm wine, he forgot. If he had constantly remembered, it is not possible that he would have become sick. Even if the food was poison. Even if the drink was poison. But he forgot. He believed more in shamans [*dukuns*] than in *Tuhan* [Indon., lit., father, another name for Allah]. He did not remember, and so he was given [*te'embeng*] illness." Remembering Allah at all times, believing in His power above all others, can ward off even the most potent of illness. But if one forgets one's faith for even a moment, Allah is understood to issue a reminder in the form of illness.

Nor may one forget oneself. In acute attacks of disorientation or drunkenness, people flock to the side of the ill person, worried because that person has forgotten everything. Anxious bystanders whisper among themselves: "He doesn't remember anything" (*Ndeqne ingat ape-ape iye*) or "She has forgotten herself" (*Lupaq dirine wah*).

One memorable night Amaq Sunin became drunk (Indon., *mabuk*) on palm wine. When I arrived, he had already vomited a great deal and looked listless, leaning back into the supporting arms of a male neighbor. He was just drunk—the word *mabuk* circling the growing crowd—and I could not see what all the fuss was about. Why didn't they just let the man sleep it off? Instead he was surrounded by worried faces.

They called in two different people to treat him. His wife held his hand, a constant stream of tears flooding her cheeks. His mother sat watching a few feet away, her face contorted, occasionally sobbing, with tears in the crevices of her cheeks. Sunin himself was crying. For a moment he would be quiet, then his face would contort drastically, his whole body tighten up and shake. As suddenly as it started, it would

---

practice by some who call themselves Muslims. The social and political tensions along the moveable boundaries of who is and who is not a Muslim are often palpable on Lombok.

stop again. One neighbor treated him by mouthing silent words over a glass of water and then, taking the water in her mouth, sprayed it in a fine mist over Amaq Sunin's body. A few moments thereafter another neighbor mouthed silent words over a bowl of water with sirih leaves and, taking the leaves, slapped them on Amaq Sunin's head saying "Remember! Remember your name! Remember your self!" (*Ingat! Ingat arande! Ingat diride!*). Amaq Sunin started to chant to himself, eyes closed and swaying, *la illaha illa allah*—the Arabic chant associated with death in Pelocok, when he wasn't shaking. Sunin's wife began sobbing, dropping his hand. Tears were now in Inaq Mol's eyes as well, as the younger children cowered in the corner of the room.

Over Sunin's chanting, Amaq Mol, Sunin's father-in-law, knelt and took the hand of the intoxicated man, saying in a stern, strong voice: "Remember your name. Remember! Remember your wife. It is not allowed that you forget. Remember yourself!" (*Ingat arande! Ingat seni-naqde! Ndeqde kanggo telupaq! Ingat diride!*). These order-pleas to remember went on for a full five minutes. I heard tense voices in the room say: "He does not remember," "He does not know how to remember." Finally, Sunin opened his eyes, sat up, and taking a sirih leaf, smeared it with lime.[35] He held it in front of his face, mouthing words and blowing onto it, occasionally interrupted by a contortion of his body and a horrid sound as if he was cracking his back just by the violent tensing of his muscles. Gradually he calmed down and announced in a loud voice, "Satan is gone" (*Satan lampaq wah*). Amaq Mol then grasped his daughter's hand, giving it to Amaq Sunin saying: "This is Nan. She is your wife. Do you remember?" Sunin smelled (Indon., *cium*) his wife's hand.[36] Tears were dried and faces relaxed as Sunin drifted to sleep.

Many Sasak men, and occasionally women and children, drink alcohol, usually *tuaq* (palm wine tapped directly from the *now* tree). While it is perfectly acceptable to drink heavily, one should not become drunk, one should not drink to the point of forgetting. Amaq Sunin's announcement that "Satan is gone" is interesting because it was totally ignored by everyone gathered, even in discussions of the event the following day. The statement implies two things: first that Amaq Sunin was

---

35. Sirih leaves, lime chalk, and betel (areca) nuts are always handy in a rural Sasak home, usually stored in a box on the floor near where people are sitting.

36. Kissing with lips to show affection is a relatively recent adoption of European ways in Indonesia. *Cium*, which Indonesian dictionaries translate as "to kiss," is more closely translated as "to sniff or smell a person's skin" and is considered a sign of affection and intimacy. While kissing can be seen among younger, urban generations in Indonesia, *cium* in the classic sense is the only overt physical expression of intimacy I ever witnessed in rural Lombok.

possessed by Satan through no fault of his own, and second, that Sunin was strong enough to win the battle with Satan and make Satan leave his body. For pride's sake—and Amaq Sunin is a very proud man—he tried to promote an interpretation of his acute episode that made him faultless and strong. His statement was ignored. Immediately after Sunin fell asleep, the adults present had a discussion, counting the number of glasses he had drunk and repeatedly observing that one should not drink to the point of drunkenness. They knew he had been intoxicated, but the drink alone had not made him ill—after all, those drinking with him had drunk as much or more. No, Sunin's acute illness had been due to his forgetting.

Why should forgetting cause such concern? People genuinely were afraid Amaq Sunin was going to die, not because he had drunk too much but because he had forgotten himself. He had forgotten who he was and what his social relationships and responsibilities were. He even had to be reintroduced to his own wife! It was this forgetting that brought on his episode, and it was by remembering—by people sitting with him ordering him to remember who he was—that he was healed.

The concern with remembering is a constant one for rural Sasaks young and old, male and female.[37] People rarely say they have "forgotten" this or that—at most, if directly challenged about something inconsequential promised but not produced, a person will respond "I forgot a little" (*Lupaq sekecet aku*). But people strive never to forget anything, inconsequential or not. Ritual specialists are the people the community relies on to remember all the important *rukuns* of rituals, thereby protecting the health of all from the vengeance of "forgotten" dead. But people are ultimately responsible for themselves, to always remember who they are as social and religious persons, because forgetting brings acute illness or death.

NOTABLE ABSENCES

There are two items that are notably absent from this list of sources of vulnerabilities: epidemics and poverty.

Epidemics do occur in Pelocok, and people recognize them as times

---

37. This is in contradistinction to much of the rest of the Southeast Asian realm in which the ethnographic literature overflows with an emphasis on forgetting. From kinship-name amnesia to forgetting the dead, the goal is to achieve harmony by forgetting. This makes the Sasak emphasis on remembering all the more interesting. It is explored theoretically in chapter 8.

when everyone becomes ill with the same thing. Although I do not know of any recent epidemic that left a large number of deaths in its wake, older persons tell of an epidemic in the early 1940s that filled a cemetery with half of Pelocok's population. Yet nowhere in my materials do I see evidence that even some Sasaks feared epidemics or were anxious about being near others who were ill. Why should this be so? I can suggest three partial answers. First, as we have seen, rural Sasaks do not seem to have a well-delineated concept of contagion. Second, vulnerability to illness has much to do with personal potency and knowledge (*ilmu*), thus making proximity to another ill person irrelevant. Third, Sasaks have a strong notion of fate (*nasib*) reflecting the will of Allah, which is used post hoc to explain how potent persons sometimes become ill. As Amaq Mol replied to my questions about contagion, persons get ill in epidemics because it is the will of Allah. A sense of vulnerability to fate would be fruitless, for how could one oppose the will of Allah?

Likewise, no evidence has emerged from my materials that would suggest that rural Sasaks experience themselves as vulnerable because of poverty and hunger. In one sense, this contradicts my earlier argument that Sasaks perceive themselves as less-than-healthy in part because they are not fat and wealthy. Yet being thin, poor, and usually hungry is the normal state of things in Pelocok. Outsiders recognize this instantly as poverty. Rural Sasaks recognize this way of living as poverty, too, but only in moments when they compare themselves to wealthier and fatter outsiders. Must not the experience of vulnerability have another imaginable experience of invulnerability? Experiencing oneself as vulnerable implies that there are times and spaces lacking the negativity of vulnerability, or at least that one perceives other persons who for some reason are in a normal state lacking the negativity of vulnerability. How can one be vulnerable because of poverty when that is all one knows? How can one imagine its absence long enough to *experience* one's self as vulnerable because of it?

Equally, perhaps rural Sasaks do not perceive themselves as vulnerable to the dangers of poverty because they have developed a kind of immunity to its dangers. Being an outsider, I was constantly warned of the dangers of living with them—of working too hard in the fields, eating too much chili paste and not enough meat and eggs, and sleeping on the ground with anything less than four mats. I was vulnerable to the ills that inevitably came from living like they did. They, however, were used to them (*ita biese wah*). Being used to (*biese*) something was understood to impart immunity. As a comparatively wealthy outsider, I was assumed to not be used to manual labor, spicy foods, and sleeping on the ground. Without that prior experience, I was vulnerable to what they considered the dangers of poverty. Interestingly, toward the end of my fieldwork when my father came from America to visit me in Pelocok, especially bland foods were prepared for him, and I was expected to sleep on the floor so that he could have my sleeping platform; while I was now used to spicy food and cold temperatures, my father was assumed not to be. I had acquired the immunity of experience. Experience with poverty has made Sasaks feel themselves immune to any dangers it might have.

I suggest that epidemics and poverty are sources of illness that outside observers—those well-versed in biomedical notions of contagion, and well-used to the luxury of a full stomach—would ascribe to rural Sasaks. But as I have tried to show, it does not follow that rural Sasaks experience or even perceive these things as something to which they could or should be vulnerable.

Personal Factors
Informing Vulnerabilities

To summarize, there are seven arenas in which rural Sasaks commonly experience themselves as vulnerable to illness. Hidden dangers abound during times of the day and months of the year, during periods in everyone's life, while alone or with others, while awake or asleep, and even within one's own mind. In short, there is not a place or time that is absolutely safe. Yet not everyone experiences himself as vulnerable in all these arenas. Each person's experience of vulnerability to illness varies according to his own sense of his *ilmu* in relation to that of others, his awareness of potential dangers, and his personal past experiences.[38] For example, I twice watched Papuq Isa argue loudly with the *kepala dusun* (government-paid mayor with high status, wealth, and government-backed power), blatantly scolding him for trying to circumcise two of her grandchildren in his upcoming circumcision ceremony.

---

38. As with the Sasak, our sense of our own vulnerabilities varies according to our sense of self relative to others and our environment, the knowledge we receive, and our personal experiences. AIDS in this country provides a perfect example. Early in the 1980s, when newspapers said it was a disease of gay men, straight people gave it little thought. When it became known that the HIV virus could be transmitted with any bodily fluids and anyone could carry the virus dormant for years, panic struck nationally, funds were poured into AIDS research, condom campaigns exploded in the media, dentists began using gloves and masks, blood used in transfusions began

Other people typically argued only circumspectly with the *kepala dusun,* remained silent, or made innumerable excuses to avoid doing whatever was requested. Outright arguing with him was simply not done. Discussions with others who had succumbed to agreeing with the *kepala dusun* after he had disregarded all their excuses always included the sentence *ndeqku bani*—they were not brave enough to argue with so powerful a man. Yet this ancient slip of a woman was *bani;* as she told me later: "I am not afraid of him. He might have the knowledge of the government, but I have the knowledge of the ancestors" (*Iye ndeqne takutanku. Ilmu iye ilmu pemerintah, laguq, ku are ilmu dengan laiq*). She perceived herself *at that time* as invulnerable to any harm he could retaliate with. Yet, at another time when he had come to sign up a grandchild to receive a polio vaccine, she remained silent. Papuq Isa did not approve of vaccines or injections of any kind because she thought they blocked blood flow and made a body vulnerable to brittle bones, yet in this context, only a month later, she did not argue. Her sense of her own strength relative to the *kepala dusun*'s had changed for some unknown reason. Now she was not *bani*. This suggests that vulnerability is dynamic as a person's experience of self changes; remember, Papuq Alus did not perceive her uneasy thoughts about the departure of her son to Malaysia as dangerous one week but did the next.

Similarly, as a person's awareness of potential dangers changes, so does one's sense of vulnerability. For example, after Inaq Marni gave birth to a deformed fetus, rumors flew among women that the *Pil* (birth control pills) had caused the deformities. For weeks, the safety and possible ill effects of various birth control methods were discussed among women, and packets of pills, half used, could be seen in rubbish heaps. Their interpretation of the cause of the deformities triggered a fear formerly unknown. As another example, in a discussion about cosmology, a young male friend told of his uncertainties of vulnerability to *ketemuq:*

> Until the ninth day ritual, the soul stays near. Some people say that souls live on Rinjani, but I am not sure. But I know that dead people always come home. And that is why people can get ill from *ketemuq. Ketemuq* is not a matter of dreams. Some people say so,

---

to be carefully screened, and marches and quilts alerted the nation to its vulnerability. Now, with decreasing numbers of annual AIDS cases in the United States (although the numbers are growing exponentially elsewhere), with more scientific knowledge of the disease, and with almost no family or circle of friends untouched by it, fear has ebbed in this country. For a fuller account of Americans' changing perceptions of immunity see Martin 1994.

but it is not. It is if the soul talks to us, says our name, but we don't hear it, we get sick suddenly. It's very frequent just after someone dies. Or for instance, if you come to visit and I do not offer you something to drink and my father who is dead, comes in and sees this and says "Why haven't you given her something to drink?" I don't hear it, but I will get sick. *Ketemuq.*

From these words, it is unlikely this man experienced dreaming as making him vulnerable, but apparently he perceived himself as vulnerable to *ketemuq* during the period after a person dies and also at any time when he fails to act according to proper social etiquette. If at a later time his understanding of cosmology changes, his experiences of vulnerability might also change.

Third, experiences of vulnerability are strongly informed by personal past experiences. Indeed, if a person's past experience gives reason for current fears and vulnerabilities, that person is never questioned. No one will sit down and try to "reason" with the person, saying, as one might in the United States, "Don't worry, it will not happen again." So when Inaq Budin was eight months pregnant with her second child and made the arduous climb up the sacred volcano "so that my child will be healthy" (*Adit bayakku sehat*), no one tried to talk her out of it, no one tried to convince her that the painful death of her first child would not be passed on automatically to her second. She feared she was vulnerable to bearing children that died.[39] Such personal vulnerabilities might stem from one's own sense of self—no one would ever say to Inaq Budin that she might have somehow been responsible for her first child's death. Inaq Budin alone sensed the vulnerability within herself. Such vulnerabilities also can be the result of conversations—participated in or just overheard—that created etiologies for illnesses experienced. When Amaq Mill returned ill from visiting the neighboring island of Sumbawa, everyone gathered together, worrying over his fevered body, and in discussions they diagnosed his illness as *penyakit Sumbawa* (the sickness of Sumbawa). "Some people, they go to Sumbawa, and nothing happens to them. Others, they go, and they get sick unto death," an old *dukun* said. Long after Amaq Mill had recuperated, I asked him if he planned to return to Sumbawa. He responded that he was not brave enough to do so because he would get ill again. His illness, diagnosed in a dialogue, became an experience of

---

39. The child was born healthy with no signs of developing the illness that killed Inaq Budin's firstborn.

illness that informed his later sense of his own vulnerabilities. In essence, in spite of general arenas of vulnerability, the experience of self as vulnerable to illness is personal.

On the one hand, there are arenas of cultural knowledge about vulnerabilities that inform to greater or lesser extents many peoples' experiences of vulnerability, thus implicitly arguing that these experiences are significantly socially constructed. On the other hand, there is dramatic intracultural variation in both knowledge about and experiences of these vulnerabilities, strongly emphasizing that vulnerabilities are personal, contingent, emergent, and informed by social dialogue. In improvising and muddling through daily concerns, cultural knowledge and personal knowledge about vulnerability lose their scholastic distinctiveness because knowledge and experience are always interpreted by someone in a particular context with particular experiences, motivations, fears, hopes, and worries.

VULNERABILITY AS A SUBJECT OF STUDY

Most medical anthropological literature inscribes the knowledge of experts, the biology of disease, illness narratives and ideologies, ecologies, etiologies, diagnoses, treatments, or the politics of health care. What is strangely missing is a *foregrounded* concern with vulnerability—how potential illness is experienced and understood prior to its reality. In the Sasak case, how people interpret and cope with illness only makes sense in light of their attention to vulnerability. I am reminded of a colleague from Emory University, who, a month after returning to the States from fieldwork in a tropical area, had an acute episode of abdominal pains, chills, and fevers that landed her in a major hospital. For two days, doctors tested her for all kinds of diseases except malaria, even when she herself suggested it. Malaria was not among the possibilities, according to the attending doctors; it was not something to which someone in Atlanta was at risk, even though she experienced herself as vulnerable to it, and indeed, that is what she had. My argument is that notions and experiences of vulnerability affect critical aspects of health care. Recognizing vulnerability and any corresponding preventive measures are essential to understanding how people manage health.

In contrast to vulnerability, risk is a frequent subject of medical anthropological inquiries examining the probability statistics for acquiring a disease. A clear distinction between vulnerability and risk is long overdue, as a cursory look through the collection of articles in the otherwise exemplary *Culture and Depression* shows (Kleinman and Good 1985). Four of the articles used the term *vulnerability* in one-sentence references to experience: persons' experience of themselves (Schieffeln 1985; Shweder 1985) and what others thought their experiences of vulnerability should be (Marsella et al. 1985; Good et al. 1985). Two articles used the term in references to externally determined factors of probability for disease (Kleinman and Kleinman 1985; Carr and Vitaliano 1985). The term *risk* is also used in three articles to indicate externally determined factors of probability for disease (Kleinman and Kleinman 1985; Marsella et al. 1985; Good et al. 1985). Notice that some usage implies an interchangeability between the two terms, so that when we come across "vulnerable individuals" or "personal vulnerability" (Marsella et al. 1985, 313; Kleinman and Kleinman 1985, 468), we are unsure exactly what is meant. The muddled usage suggests that vulnerability and risk are not matters of consequence. But for people experiencing it, vulnerability is a weighty matter deserving precision in our discussions. Let the term *risk* be defined, in keeping with the articles cited above, as the external assessment of the objective probability of acquiring a disease. Risk is something that can be statistically quantified, a process that, for example, can result in lists of "risk factors" that aid in diagnosis. In contrast, vulnerability is the subjective experience of personal susceptibility to dangers.

In addition to the citations above, ethnographic accounts that refer to vulnerability rarely include more than a passing sentence here and there. For example, in her ethnography on Wana shamanism, Jane Atkinson mentions Wana vulnerability during dreams, from bumping into spirits, and to sorcery attacks, noting that women and children are more vulnerable than men (1989, 60, 61, 106, 112). As another example, in an article about an outbreak of Kyasanur Forest disease, a tick-borne virus, Mark Nichter says that vulnerability was linked to cosmological irreverence or immorality, spirit malevolence, "unknowable karmic debt," overexposure to heat, entering the forest, prior acute illness, bad stars and planets, or the presence of the illness in a family member or a royal family member (1992, 230, 232, 234, 235, 236, 237, 243, 245, 247). Such references to vulnerability swirling ungrounded in anthropological writings seem to bespeak concerns with vulnerability entered faithfully into field notes but not completely analyzed.

With the recent interest in personhood and conceptions of self, there has been an increase in more detailed discussions of vulnerabilities usually explained through a disruption, depletion, or loss of life force.[40] Yet these insights into the vulnerabilities of personhood are seldom explored in terms of salient health concerns that shape and inform actions and interpretations. Exceptions can be found in Massard 1988, Inhorn 1994, Wikan 1990, Tsing 1993, and Laderman 1991. These works emphasize the importance of noting variability within and between groups, detailing how and why persons are vulnerable in certain contexts, emphasizing experience, and tracing how vulnerability shapes treatment. They highlight the value of emphasizing vulnerability in order to understand how persons manage their health.

Our understanding of vulnerability among the Sasaks would have been ontologically incorrect had I begun with a discussion of personhood, using it to rationally explain vulnerabilities. Vulnerabilities overlap some of the understandings of body discussed in chapter 2, and they overlap some understandings of personhood discussed in chapter 4. But mostly vulnerabilities are socially informed personal experiences. Looked at in this way, the problem of vulnerability raises important questions for understanding how health concerns are managed. How is vulnerability personal? What does it mean to experience one's self as fragile? To what extent is it shaped by previous experiences of illness, and to what extent does it shape later illness experiences? In short, how do people experience vulnerability in their lives, and how do those experiences affect how they manage their health concerns?

These are salient questions for understanding Sasak health care. Indeed, the scattered references to vulnerability for other peoples suggest that these are salient questions in many areas of the world. Atkinson (1996) tells of a letter she received from her former field site, and in the friend's plea for her to return we can hear the implicit awareness of the fragility of life. He wrote: "Don't take a long time before coming to see us. If it's long before you come, not many of us will remain, because we will have all died out" (190).

LIVING VULNERABLE LIVES

This chapter has emphasized the personal experience of vulnerability, but vulnerability is also strongly social. A person will be scolded for building a house during the months of Bubur Putih and Abang, not doing all the *rukun* correctly for rituals, or walking through certain

---

40. See, e.g., Desjarlais 1996, 144–45; Pollock 1996.

spaces alone at night.[41] In casual conversations, people will warn each other that it is dangerous to travel outside of the immediate area or that Papuq Y has so many potent objects hidden away that it is wise not to go to his house too frequently. Daily one hears other people express vulnerabilities beginning with the words *ndeq ku bani,* or telling illness stories of how they met a dead parent or ate the poisoned food of a spiteful neighbor. Also in memorizing secret words or watching others' preventive practices, one learns of potential vulnerabilities. Yet, even such explicit warnings, observations, and teachings of others do not simply accumulate. Each person interprets, judges, ignores, and, in short, goes about what Obeyesekere has called the work of culture, to see what of this knowledge fits his experience or is worthy of consideration at a particular time (Obeyesekere 1990). It is this process, with all its complexities and contingencies, that shapes whether or not a person experiences himself as vulnerable in a given, current context.

Vulnerability to illness is not always a foregrounded concern; rather, at certain periods, moments, or contexts, a person experiences herself as vulnerable. It is a personal, emergent, and dynamic experience. One night, a woman is not brave to walk alone to go watch a favorite television program on the lone set three minutes away, and the next night, she comes in late from the fields and goes bathing alone in complete darkness without a thought. A boy who had walked a certain path home from school every day for months suddenly changes his route after hearing that *selaq* are said to inhabit the path. A man who drinks to the point of forgetting refuses alcohol altogether for a month, and then gradually starts again, but now with careful moderation. Life's cares change. Self-perception and the perception of others and the world changes. Experiences of vulnerability can become habitual, or they can become backgrounded, changed, or regarded as irrelevant.

EXPERIENCES OF VULNERABILITY AND MANAGING HEALTH CONCERNS

Experiences of vulnerability are personal and variable, but experiencing oneself as vulnerable in at least some arenas is a universal for rural Sasaks. For them, because the world is experienced as fraught with dan-

---

41. Just as in the United States when a person will be scolded for walking in the rain without a hat or umbrella with the warning that he/she will catch a cold.

ger, vulnerabilities perpetuate illness etiologies that point to everything
from birth control pills to ghosts. The world is full of dangers. Because
one of those dangers is fear of other people's knowledge, Sasaks are
unlikely to share *ilmu,* including ethnomedical understandings, spells,
and small words (*puji*). Moreover, whatever is shared is shadowed by
the suspicion that the most potent *ilmu* is kept secret. It is kept secret
because people's health depends on whether they have more and
stronger spells and small words relative to others, including neighbors
and friends. Suspicion and fear perpetuate perceptions of danger and
inhibit a forum for the public accumulation of knowledge about healing. Instead, in whispered conversations people try to convince others
to give them small words so that they might better cope with their own
vulnerabilities.

— • —

It was a little over a month after Papuq Alus's son departed for Malaysia.
I was in a field helping with a rice harvest, when a young child came
running up and told me that Papuq Alus had a letter from Malaysia and
wanted me to come home. Let it not be bad news, I remember praying
to whatever gods could hear as I hurried home.

Papuq Alus's smile was dazzling as she urged me to read the letter
written in Sasak to her. Her friends in the market town had read it for
her already, but she wanted to hear it again. He wrote that it had been
an exhausting two-week trip to the border of Sumatra, and then there
had been some minor difficulties getting a work visa for Malaysia. But
he now had a job working on a rubber plantation. He had a place to
stay, enough to eat, and he was healthy (*sehat*).[42] He asked after his
mother, her health, and the health of others in the compound. Papuq
Alus was radiant. She asked me to write him a response. At her dicta-
tion I wrote: "I received your letter. Thank God you arrived safely. I am
healthy. Everyone is healthy." She could think of nothing else to say to
him. She had told him all that was important. "You are healthy and safe.
I am healthy. Everyone is healthy." That night, for the first time, she
slept in her house. She was completely alone, but no longer vulnerable.
Her thoughts were finally easy.

---

42. As we have seen, while in Pelocok, people tend to describe themselves as less than
healthy. But the emphasis on being well in this letter and Papuq Alus's response were
about easing one another's worries and communicating that no one was at death's
door. In a place where death is never far away, the primary concern is that a traveler
return home alive to find those he loves also alive.

～ 4 ～

Agents of Coping

How does one cope in a world full of dangers? In a world where everyone is less than healthy, in a world where there is no certainty that one will be alive a few weeks hence, in a world where people are rarely brave and experiences of vulnerability are common, anxiety is part and parcel of everyday life. How then do people manage to get through the daily tasks of living?

The word *anxiety* does not have a Sasak equivalent. But *anxiety* most succinctly captures what Sasaks mean when they express—through actions or words—that they feel vulnerable. Anxiety is "a reaction to the danger of a loss of an object" (Freud 1959, 95). For our interests here, it is a reaction of "uneasy suspense" to a perceived threat to the health or safety of oneself or a loved one (Rachman 1998, 2). Most of the substantial psychological literature on anxiety focuses on psychological disorders. Recent attention to examining normal levels of anxiety has suggested that anxiety motivates the highest focus of neural functions, including memory, toward integrating information for anticipatory behavior against the perceived threat (e.g., Luu et al. 1998). In other words, anxiety compels people to seek a way of coping and does so by focusing memories on the problem at hand.

In this chapter we examine how people cope with experiences of vulnerability. Illness in both its presence *and* its absence stimulates anxiety in people and motivates action. In the presence of illness, anxiety motivates people to seek treatment. In its absence, experiences of vulnerability prompt preventive actions and treatments; the trick is to find an agent that knows how to do so. To know in the Sasak sense of the word *tauq* is to have agency, to be able to act on the world, including to be able to act meaningfully on concerns about health.

Agency has come into the limelight of anthropological writings in the last two decades because it allows people to be active in constructing their societies and realities. Coinciding with this is a flourishing of studies into personhood and self. So far, I have avoided confronting these topics directly, yet they emerge at every turn. Bodies are uniquely marked by persons' lives. Understandings of bodies are personal constellations of various traditions of knowledge. Experiences of vulnerability are unique to each self. Out of these discussions emerges the sense that there is something about Sasak persons that is vital to how they cope with health concerns.

EXPLORING THE RELATIONSHIP BETWEEN PERSONHOOD AND HEALTH

Recent anthropological literature on issues of personhood abounds,[1] yet it remains a murky topic partly because of a lack of consensus about definitions. I understand a person to be a socially constituted being, whereas a self is an awareness of an "I."[2] A person encompasses a sense of self, but not vice versa. In other words, an awareness of an "I" can exist outside of a social world with which one interacts in a meaningful way.[3] The distinction is important for the Sasak materials, but in reviewing the relevant literature, which often does not draw so fine a line, I use personhood as a gloss for both concepts.

The relationship between personhood and health has been partly explored by medical anthropologists. Some have detailed how concepts of personhood can be derived from experiences of illness or vulnerability (Laderman 1991; Wikan 1990), and conversely how illness can be illuminated in the light of personhood (Roseman 1991, 1996; Pollack 1996). The relationship between personhood and health can be further explored through three questions. First, to what extent do concepts of personhood make a person anxious about his health? Sec-

1. The idea of the person was first brought to the fore in anthropology by Marcel Mauss (1985), and recent cognitive anthropology has loosely defined the person as a social and embodied being. This definition gave rise to three questions: How do beings become persons (e.g., Conklin and Morgan 1996)? Are persons bounded individuals or unbounded, permeable social entities (e.g., Geertz 1973)? And how are we to understand persons as multiple, context-dependent, embodied, and ever-changing (e.g., Ewing 1990; Kondo 1990; Mageo 1995; Wikan 1996)?

2. See Desjarlais 2000 for much fuller and more detailed definitions based on the distinctions of philosopher Amelie Rorty. See also Kondo 1990, for a highly influential and careful study of the self.

3. Social outcasts who are utterly ignored, such as the homeless or alien anthropologists, are denied or stripped of their personhood even though they may still have a sense of self (Desjarlais 2000; Geertz 1973, 1983).

ond, do concepts of personhood change in response to experiences of vulnerability and illness? Third, to what extent do those concepts enable a person to cope with those experiences?

The importance of personhood in other Indonesian ethnographies implies that Indonesia is a good place to seek answers to these questions.[4] Overall, the discussions center around a concept of *semangat* or *sumange'* (Indon., life force, energy, vital spirit; Bal., *bayu*) that is considered fundamental to life and health.[5] For example, Errington (1989), writing about the Luwu of Sulawesi, argues persuasively that vulnerability is based on the measurable strength of one's *semangat*. If one's *semangat* is low, not only is illness a possibility, but so is social and political degradation. *Semangat* is a quality that is partly inherent and partly a matter of individual pursuit and negotiation. People constantly attend to their *semangat*, trying to protect and strengthen it, thus maximizing one's potency as a person and minimizing susceptibility to physical, social, and political harms. In Sulawesi and elsewhere, Indonesian personhood is characterized by a constant concern with maintaining control over one's body and one's expression in social situations by nurturing *semangat*.[6] Illness is a sign that one's life force is weak.

It is difficult to describe the sheer panic I felt upon rereading these Indonesian ethnographies and realizing that I didn't know the Sasak word for *semangat* or if they use the concept at all. I had read about *semangat* before fieldwork, but I forgot about it once among Sasaks. Before leaving the field, I reviewed my materials for major holes; but my sense of Sasak personhood felt relatively complete—certainly not like it was missing its most crucial element. Yet, *semangat* is so important to other peoples in Indonesia and Malaysia, how could the same not be

---

4. For early studies in culture and personality see, e.g., DuBois 1944; Bateson and Mead 1942. More recent studies have emphasized how elements of personhood are manifested in politics and symbolic systems such as ritual performance, etiquette, time, and language use (e.g., Peacock 1987; Keeler 1987; Kipp 1993; Kuipers 1990; Traube 1986; Geertz 1973, 1983; Hoskins 1996).

5. See, e.g., Keeler 1987; George 1996; Laderman 1991; Barth 1993. Fabrega's (1980) description of the ladino concept of *consistencia* appears similar to the notion of vital life force described here.

6. Tsing's (1993) account of the Banjar offers a minor exception in that they do not seem concerned with a life force or *semangat* as much as with reason and rationality as forces through which the boundaries of the body are maintained and protected. The Meratus Dayaks offer another exception to my description of "Indonesian personhood," because for them, persons become vulnerable when there are closed boundaries around themselves, and it is by maintaining social and cosmological connections that vulnerabilities can be kept at bay. The Sasaks, in comparison, have vulnerabilities both when the boundaries of their bodies are penetrated and when those boundaries are closed to social relationships.

true for Sasaks? How could I spend almost two years there and not know the answer? Panic flourished.

Then I realized that if *semangat* were as important to the Sasak as it was to the Balinese, Javanese, Luwu, and the rest, I would have to know it. As Polanyi argues, tacit knowledge is available to those who do not have it through clues, through tangible and palpable events and reasons that point to the tacit (1958; Polanyi and Prosch 1975). The tacit casts shadows on cave walls that all can see, even the densest anthropologist. If in two years of fieldwork there was no evidence, overt or tacit, of *semangat* or a similar life force among people in Pelocok, chances are good that such a concept is not salient for them.[7] Thus, we must start from scratch to understand Sasak personhood and their agency in responding to threats of illness. In so doing, we must bear in mind that the person need not be the only locus of agency (Ortner 1984; Keane 1997).

MULTIPLE LOCI OF AGENCY

Indeed, the Sasak materials show that in coping with health concerns, the relevant locus of agency may be an individual person but it can also shift to the community at large or to a potency that transcends both individual and community, namely, *ilmu*. The community consists of persons, but in significant ways a person can not act alone to cope with vulnerability and must rely on the agency of others in the community. *Ilmu*, secret knowledge, is of course known by a person, but as it is knowledge learned from others (people or spirits) it is social, and because it has a constant truth-value, it transcends both and becomes an agent in itself. Here I endeavor to balance an understanding of Sasak persons, with an understanding of society and with transcendent truth, showing how the locus of agency to cope with a world of dangers shifts among these three.

SASAK SELVES

It is selves who experience vulnerabilities—"*I* am not brave enough"— therefore we must begin with how Sasaks construct them. The use of

---

7. I was doubly reassured when rereading other ethnographies on Sasaks that also have a total absence of the concept and the word. Some individual Sasaks may have a concept of a life force, but it is certainly possible to examine Sasak personhood and agency without one.

teknonymy, which involves changing one's own name with the birth of each new generation, might suggest that Sasaks have little sense of unique selves (Geertz and Geertz 1964). Moreover, all rural Sasaks are poor Muslim peasants, which is a defining aspect of self, but not one that suggests uniqueness. With serial monogamy a normal practice, even marital status matters little. There are, however, three things that do matter and that define unique selves. One is the strength of one's social relationships and the number of one's offspring. Indeed, I suggest that Sasaks use teknonymy not to reduce importance of the individual, but to esteem it, by noting the honor of having offspring (see also Barth 1993). The second thing that matters is one's own experiences, histories, and memories. The third thing is the completeness and potency of one's *ilmu*. These three ingredients—key social relations, personal pasts, and *ilmu*—are what determine a unique sense of "I," and they are the three things that can substantially change in one's life. Economic status and religious affiliation do not change, and changes in marital status are given little social weight. But families can grow and die. Past experiences can strengthen and weaken one in the present. Knowledge can be gained and forgotten. These are the changes that can threaten one's definition of self, and anxious anticipation of negative changes in these is what produces experiences of vulnerability. Family members can become ill. One's past illnesses or memories of a child now gone from home can make one weak and ill. Forgetting knowledge leaves one naked against the unseen dangers of the world. These three defining concepts of Sasak selves make them prone to vulnerability.

Individual Agency

As long as a person can remember, his self can take action to cope with experiences of vulnerability. There are everyday acts of prevention that circulate among rural Sasaks that one can use without calling upon the help of others to ease one's sense of vulnerability. Indeed, prevention of perceived dangers permeates nearly every aspect of daily activities.[8] From how one bathes in the morning to how one walks home at night, illness prevention is part and parcel of everyday actions. Some actions seek to make a person pure and clean to prevent illness. Others involve the humoral concepts of hot and cold in which an even temperature is

---

8. For a detailed discussion of Sasak everyday and ritual prevention practices see Hay 1998b, 222–68.

maintained through specific food intake or avoidance, and the warmth of water one bathes in. Others follow the logic of homeopathic medicine, such as drinking a red tea to replenish red blood. Still others seek or run from biomedical medicines. Some are drawn from Islamic teachings, others fly in the face of orthodox Islam. And then there are some, like using a pinch of worms on one's forehead to prevent illness from meeting a ghost, that confound any category or logical connection. Some of the preventive practices, like drinking crushed brick, are consciously done when the sense of vulnerability is sudden, novel, or particularly keen. But most practices do not entail a break in daily activity; they are habits. While many approach habitus status—actions that are familiar throughout a community and commonly interpretable with similar, widely distributed meanings (Bourdieu 1977b, 78–80)—others are personal habits not widely distributed. As such, they are difficult for an outsider to learn, and I would frequently ask myself, "Does that action done in that way mean something, or is that just the way he does things?" At other times, I stumbled unexpectedly across habits of prevention when I got scolded for putting wood in the fire the wrong way or for planning trips during Bubur Abang. Indeed, knowledge about preventive actions is usually not secretive; it is openly distributed through scoldings and warnings of illness. For example, children learn that the only correct way of putting wood in a cooking fire is "feet" (large end) first; otherwise, they are warned, they will get ill. Only a handful of older people specified that the children themselves would not get ill, but that this manner of putting wood in a fire prevented breech births. This, like many everyday preventive practices, is learned so as to become a lifelong habit.

To what extent do people engage in such preventive actions? Most Sasaks use some of them daily. But while some practices are used with great frequency throughout the community, others are rarely used. Let us not forget how everyday life is lived in Pelocok. It is jumbled, with people crossing paths and sharing gossip at every turn. Preventive practices are passed person to person in the contexts of seeing them done or hearing of the vulnerabilities of others. For example, after climbing the volcano, I laughingly told Papuq Junin of my exhaustion during the climb. Papuq Junin replied, "Didn't they rub garlic on your knees? No? Amaq Mol, he still does not know everything. He is so strong, he does not need the garlic, but other people need it. It makes you strong, so that your legs do not hurt. Inaq [Mol], why didn't you rub garlic on her knees?" And Inaq Mol replied that she hadn't known about the garlic, but in the future, yes, she would be sure to use it on herself and anyone climbing with her.

Moreover, the preventive practices were frequently contradictory. In 1994, before the childbirth clinic arrived in Pelocok, seeking biomedical injections was only used as a last resort to treat an illness, never as a form of prevention. Injections were generally considered dangerous to one's health because they were thought to block the flow of bodily fluids and make bones brittle. But those who had relatives in the market town did sometimes seek preventive injections and would come back to Pelocok telling how injections had kept them fat or strong or virile. By 1995, after the clinic opened, more people, though certainly not all, sought preventive injections. One woman, after telling me at length that one must avoid injections in general while pregnant in order to prevent illness and a difficult labor, went on to tell me—with no apparent sense of contradiction—of how she had had four injections during her pregnancy that she credited with making her childbirth easy and her infant healthy.

Prevention is an everyday part of Sasaks' lives. Trying one form of prevention in no way discourages a person from trying any others that might promote immunity as well. When a person experiences himself as vulnerable—whether it be a persistent vulnerability or a new vulnerability—he has recourse to a wide variety of everyday preventive practices, some he already knows about, some he learns from the words or actions of others, and some, perhaps, he comes up with on his own.[9]

THE SOCIAL PERSON

At the same time, selves are not islands entire of themselves; Sasaks are necessarily social entities. Persons belong to a category called *manusia* (Indon., humans) whereas beings who are giants without apparent social skills (like the contemporary European tourist) or who wear no clothing (like Sasak images of people from Kalimantan and Irian Jaya) are only debatably human.[10]

---

9. I do not know of any specific examples of persons creating practices or medicines of illness prevention. But people often claim to create new practices or medicines for treating illness—often through knowledge gained in dreams—and I would not be surprised if preventive practices are sometimes formed in the same way.

10. The ambiguous status of tourists became clear one evening in a crowd of neighbors gossiping about a group of tourists they had seen. A young woman told in all seriousness how she had seen a tourist squatting in the forest a few days ago, and after he had left, she went over and found, to her utter surprise, a pile of excrement there. She concluded with the awed statement, "Only then did I know that tourists are humans too!"

Not only must one know what are assumed to be basic social proprieties, one must be someone's family or friend. People (*dengan*) do not matter in one's world. They have no ties; they are not of concern. I was frequently told not to visit certain hamlets because the people there "are just people" (*dengan doang itoh*) not friends, not family of Pelocok. Persons matter; they are part of one's world. People (*dengan*) from elsewhere do not. Nonetheless, strangers can easily be made persons through imagined kinship links. I was family because, as La Nan once explained, her father's ancestors had gone to America and I was their descendent even though I did not know it. She asserted, "Kakak Ameron [Older Sister Cameron] has to be family, if not, it is impossible she would be able to come here and live with us." All marriage spouses, regardless of their origins, typically are made "cousins" through a distant ancestor. As long as one is perceived as kin, one is family (*keluarge*), not just people (*dengan doang*). Within the idiom of kinship, Sasaks identify persons and construct social relations. It is by way of kinship— real or fictive—that *ilmu* is distributed, healers are chosen, and decisions are made in times of crisis.[11]

Moreover, it is one's status as a person, as a member of the community of families enmeshed in one another's concerns, that legitimates both one's experiences of vulnerability and one's agency for coping with problems. Those outside one's social networks, those who are just people (*dengan doang*), not only do not matter, they are untrustworthy, unpredictable, and not people with whom one can interact openly and comfortably. Because peasants are at the bottom of the socioeconomic totem pole, most of those who are *just people* are wealthier, better educated, and of higher social status. When interacting with them, rural Sasaks do not expect to be invited to sit in chairs or to eat with their hosts. They do not expect to be talked with as an equal. They acknowledge and enact their status at the bottom rung of the socioeconomy. For their part, most outsiders assume rural Sasaks to be backward, stu-

---

11. Kinship and its importance in anthropological thought are too complex to discuss here. Rather, I refer to David Schneider's critique, which argues that kinship is based on a questionable Western assumption that blood is thicker than water (1984). Kinship in terms of actual blood relatedness has some importance to the Sasak in terms of inheritance, the strength of emotional bonds, reciprocity expectations, and the distribution of secret knowledge (see also Ecklund 1977). Kinship as terms of address (which may or may not reflect blood relatedness) marked everyday social relations with emotional bonds, responsibilities, and the distribution of knowledge, including secret knowledge. Being able to address someone as mother, father, sibling, child, or grandchild creates a social relationship, a pattern of interaction and mutual concern; it changes someone from being just *dengan* (people) into a person who matters.

pid, and unable to change. Peasants are assumed to lack agency—otherwise why would they still be peasants?—and therefore must be taken care of by the state. When rural Sasaks seek biomedical aid, they do not express feelings of vulnerability or claim any knowledge of what could treat an illness. They are deferential, passive, and silent. Outside the world of peasantry, rural Sasaks lose something of their personhood.

Outside their world, they are no longer agents who can act on their vulnerabilities and ills. In encounters with *just people,* rural Sasaks themselves become—if only temporarily—who they are assumed to be. The defacement of personhood happens less in biomedical encounters within the rural world, for while one's personhood might be questioned within clinic walls, outside of them, one's personhood is immediately restored. Because the medicine of local clinics can be avoided or sought easily, even if once sought the patient does not interact equally with the clinician, this structural advantage affords biomedicine as a viable option for acting on one's anxieties about health. But in contexts where rural Sasaks have to travel to towns beyond their social world to seek care, their personhood, their sense of mattering socially, suffers to such an extent that they assume that they have no agency in managing their own health and rely solely on the advice and acts of others.

Yet, in their own world, rural Sasaks work together to address the anxieties of one of their own. An experience of vulnerability or illness is not just a problem of self but a social concern.

Social Agency

As soon as a person expresses a feeling of vulnerability or illness, the locus of agency shifts at least in part to the community at large. Hughes (1963) argues that all health concerns are public concerns (see also Landy 1977). Hughes's interest was in public health, but his argument fits the Sasak data. Once a vulnerability or illness is expressed, it becomes a social matter—a concern to anyone among one's kin that learns of it. Acting on the vulnerabilities or illnesses of others is more than an obligation; family and friends want to ease the anxieties of those they care about.

When the vulnerability or illness is commonplace, others' actions are relaxed. For example, when a young man worried about becoming ill while traveling, an uncle recommended he have a ritual bathing. When a woman complained of a headache, one neighbor boiled her a cup of coffee while two others interspersed their gossip with suggestions of different treatments. Social interest parallels the level of anxiety the vulnerability or illness stimulates, but, even if people just make simple suggestions or offer a drink as a remedy, those who hear the complaint do something.

When a vulnerability or illness is more serious, word spreads throughout the community quickly. When someone is vulnerable, people act to pad the social environment and make suggestions of preventions. In the case of illness, family and friends will gather, keeping the ill person company for days or weeks at a time, suggesting possible illness names, and offering treatments. The community gathers, and in gathering it collects all of its resources in one place with the purpose of acting on the illness. Even the dead are involved, for they too can seek the name of an illness or suggest treatments and pass these on to the living through dreams. As we shall see, social interaction is crucial to naming and treating illness.

Rituals of Prevention

Rituals are another form of social agency to prevent illness. For our purposes, I understand a ritual to be the performance of meaningful actions by a ritual specialist.[12] Thus a person can not prevent some ills without the aid of other persons. Rituals are essentially social. Anthropologists have spoken of life-cycle or life-crisis rituals as processes organized to change a person's state or status within the community, revealing along the way a culture's most salient symbols, values, structures, and paradoxes (e.g., Van Gennep 1960; Turner 1967, 1969; Barth 1975). But life-cycle rituals are equally organized to conduct a person *safely* through the major, culturally recognized crises of life.[13]

---

12. Differentiating rituals from everyday or mundane stylized gestures is a complex undertaking, one largely beyond the scope of this inquiry. For our purposes, a rather simplistic dichotomy—separating actions based on whether or not they were conducted by a ritual specialist—is sufficient. In Pelocok, where everyone has prevention and healing knowledge, anyone may perform stylized gestures or actions meant to prevent illness. But Sasaks themselves do not dignify such actions with the verb *begawai* (to perform a ritual, to work the ritual object/purpose), for a *begawai,* a ritual specialist—either a *kiayi* as religious leader or a *belian* as healer-midwife—must be in charge of the event.

13. Even when this aspect of life-cycle rituals is acknowledged, it is usually considered inconsequential. For example, Firth details two pregnancy rituals that the Tikopia, a Pacific island people, explicitly say are conducted to prevent problems during childbirth. But Firth argues, "The real point seems to lie in the economic and social accompaniments of the rite" (1967, 56). While his functional argument fits rationally with the data presented, why was the stated reason for the rites—prevention of problems during parturition—not considered worthy of scholarly interest? Firth himself

Each of the five Sasak life-cycle rituals incorporates aspects designed to prevent illness and danger during moments of transition. These experiences of vulnerability motivate and make vital the rituals aimed to conduct a person safely through life's transitions.[14] Other Sasak rituals aimed at illness prevention are engaged in only by persons who feel themselves vulnerable. Ritual forms of illness prevention are those practices explicitly said to prevent harm or maintain health that must be carried out by a ritual specialist: either a *kiayi* or a *belian*. A *kiayi*, as a religious leader, is responsible for all of the concerns of death and Allah, and the *belian,* as midwife, is responsible for all of the concerns of the living. These are specialists who communicate through prayers and spells with spirits, ancestors, gods, and Allah to invoke protection for the people who feel themselves vulnerable.[15] The life-cycle rituals must be done regardless, but as with the couple who were unconcerned about their pregnancy, even these may lose their preventive power if a person does not consider herself vulnerable enough to attend to the necessary details.

The common thread running throughout most of the ritual preventive practices is that they entail some sort of spiritual cleansing. Water sanctified by a *kiayi* in prayer is poured or sprinkled on people and sometimes drunk; this process is referred to with the word *mandi*—to bathe. It is the same word used for everyday, mundane baths, however, ritual *mandi*s are not aimed at cleaning the body. The purpose is to make the person pure or holy (*suci*). A pure person would be worthy of the *dewa* that inhabits her, unlikely to insult dead ancestors or other spirits, and generally immune to illness from supernatural causes. The pinnacle of the ritual *mandi* is the moment when the *kiayi* pours out the

hints why elsewhere when he refers to "these ideas, which, irrational to us, appear to the Tikopia to have received empirical verification" (45). It is the concern with portraying the Other as rational, by Western definitions of rational, that stops Firth as well as others from exploring the significance of well-documented instances of preventive ethnomedicine. I suggest that we look for significance where the people we study tell us it is. This is not to argue that more abstract analyses of data have no place, rather to question the ethics of searching for a "real point" while ignoring the salience of the ritual for the people who perform it (e.g., Gorlinski 1997).

14. Experiences of vulnerability are not the only motivators for the life-cycle rituals discussed. Stated religious and cultural requirements, social expectations, and mundane joys and entertainments of rituals are also significant motivations for the rituals. But the preventive aspects of the rituals are very significant.

15. *Dukun*s, like *belian*s, communicate with spirits, ancestors, souls, and gods. Yet *dukun*s are not considered prevention ritual specialists. The reason for this might be the common association between *dukun*s and black magic (and thus, their ambivalent reputation as a source for healing and for harm). Or perhaps *dukun*s' expertise is strictly with treating illnesses and does not extend to preventing potential future ills.

purifying water into the hands of those who feel vulnerable. This moment is most dramatic at the *mandi kubur* (ritual bathing at the grave of an ancestor) when, after a series of prayers, the *kiayi* takes a kettle of water and, whispering words over it, waters the grave three times in a trail from its head to its foot. He then raises the kettle so that the water pours over the heads of screaming infants and playful children and into the cupped hands of the more serious women and men who stand at the foot of the grave. While he pours, the *kiayi* says: "So that you will be healthy, so that you will grow big, so that you will have a long life" (*Adiqne tauq sehat . . . adiqne bau beleq . . . adiqne panjang umurde*). Through the water, the living are connected with their dead ancestors and receive their blessings. Water purifies so that the world's dangers can not touch the living.

The other kind of ritual cleansing is called *belanger,* which involves rubbing the hair with a mixture of grated turmeric and coconut. *Belanger* is a part of every life-cycle ritual as well as the burial ritual and at assorted times when people experience themselves as vulnerable. The differences between ritual *mandis* and *belanger* are that (1) ritual *mandis* are only done by *kiayis* whereas *belanger* are done by *belians* or by laypersons, and (2) ritual *mandis* require preparation and relative expense whereas *belanger* is easily available. Both *belanger* and ritual *mandis* are practices that make a person *suci*, thereby lessening their vulnerabilities.

After these spiritual cleansings, rituals tend to conclude with a spot of betel chew placed on the forehead (*bubus*). The betel is chewed by the ritual specialist and spat onto a clean betel leaf. Then the ritual specialist mouths words (*ilmu*) onto it and marks the person's forehead. The only explanation for the *bubus* marks was: "So that it is known that one has been cleansed and is pure" (*Adiqne tauq wah temandiq, wah suci*). *Bubus* marks only followed rituals aimed at preventing harm and maintaining health. They are stamps of immunity.

In their emphasis on making persons pure, these rituals are practices of illness prevention. We have examined the ways Sasaks use the word *suci* as a metaphoric description of spiritual grace and health. Purity coincides with health, long life, strength, and wealth. Once, watching a family anoint themselves with the water of a ritual *mandi,* I asked the ceremony's purpose. The *kiayi* answered: "It is for the soul [Indon., *jiwa*] and the body [Indon., *badan*]. To make one more healthy. To make sure one stays healthy. But also for the soul in the afterlife. It's to guard against the possibility of being sick or of a problem with the soul.

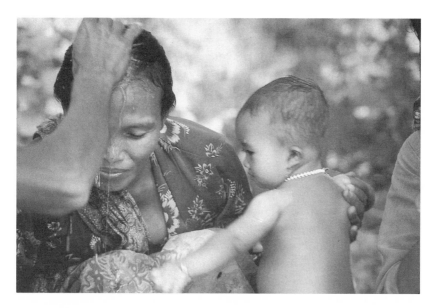

FIG. 7.   A ritual bathing to prevent illness at the grave of an ancestor (1994)

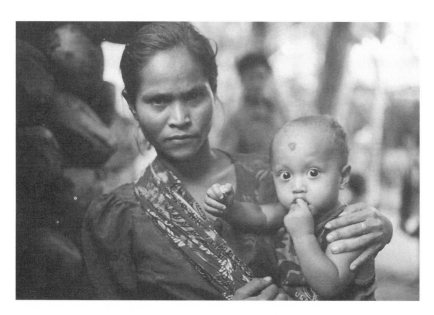

FIG. 8.   The stamp of immunity (1995)

It is also good if one goes on a long trip. As a blessing before going on a long trip, it is good."[16]

To what extent do people actually seek health through these ritual forms? Life-cycle rituals were universally practiced in Pelocok, and so it is difficult to know for whom illness prevention was a foregrounded concern and for whom it was a side benefit. But participation in the other rituals can suggest an answer. Aside from Lebaran [Ar., *id 'al fitri*], the day that marks the end of the Islamic fasting month, on which most households bathe ritually at the grave of an ancestor, *mandi kuburs* were fairly rare. Of the six young men who left to find work in Malaysia, half had a *mandi kubur* before embarking. Of the hundred and some boys who were circumcised, I know of less than ten who had a *mandi kubur* beforehand, and these were the boys of parents concerned about being forced by social politics to join circumcision ceremonies before their sons were ready (*siap*). Otherwise, there was a *mandi kubur* when two men were initiated as *kiayis* and another one when an older man decided he needed one so that he would "always be healthy." The *mandi kuburs* as well as other non–life-cycle forms of ritual prevention were not weekly or even monthly occurrences. Among the people I knew best, the infants and young children received some sort of ritual cleansing between five and ten times annually, teenage and adult women were ritually cleansed two to six times annually, and teenage and adult men were ritually cleansed once or twice annually. The age and sex disparities in participation in ritual preventive practices match the overall expectations of vulnerability we saw in the last chapter.

Biomedical Preventions

Local biomedical clinics, provided by the government (consisting of "just people"), offer rural Sasaks another option for coping with vulnerabilities. Biomedical methods of prevention through everyday practices such as cleanliness, nutrition, and avoidance of risk behaviors (smoking, sexual promiscuity) are, with the exception of cleanliness, generally ignored among rural Sasaks. Nonetheless, some will seek biomedicines to cope with their vulnerabilities.

Aside from seeking pills from traveling medicine men, Sasaks occa-

---

16. The *kiayi* answered this question using Indonesian terms, which might explain the implied Cartesian dichotomy, a distinction that gets muddier in the Sasak lexicon. Certainly at least some people some of the time thought and spoke of bodies and souls as separate entities. At other times, those same people would describe uneasy thoughts as making them ill, suggesting a more unified understanding.

sionally go to clinics asking for pills or injections to alleviate experiences of being less than healthy. For example, once word got out that the *bidan* had pills to increase one's blood (pills for low blood pressure), people who felt weak, not brave enough, and generally vulnerable flocked to her clinic seeking those little red pills. Those who received them took them whenever they felt weak rather than at regular intervals. The pills were understood in terms of homeopathy and humoralism: their red color indicated that they increased one's red fluid (blood), thereby bringing bodily fluids into balance and making one stronger and less vulnerable.

But even when people experienced no anxieties regarding health themselves, political pressure, the tactics of biomedical development, and the words of an anthropologist could influence people to seek biomedical forms of illness prevention. In 1977 the Indonesian Ministry of Health established a national program of immunization that recommended that all children receive vaccinations against polio, diphtheria, pertussis, tetanus, measles, and tuberculosis. In Pelocok in 1994, I was aware of only a handful of children who had ever had a vaccine; newborns never got tetanus inoculations. In 1995, with the arrival of the clinic, the Bu Bidan would march into the home of a newborn, pick him up, and inoculate him against tetanus before anyone could stop her. On the one hand, people were wary of injections because they disrupted humoral balances, weakened bones, and didn't make any difference in any case. On the other hand, with the ease of getting injections now, people wondered whether injections could make their children less vulnerable.

Then in August 1995, a yellow banner was hung across the porch of the clinic announcing the upcoming immunization campaign (Pekan Immunisasi Nasional—PIN) against polio. On September 13 and again in October, all children under the age of five were to be immunized with the oral polio vaccine.[17]

A month before the scheduled day, the hamlet head went around issuing "invitations" that served the twofold purpose of telling parents that they were required to bring their children for immunization and

---

17. It was a political program, and unsurprisingly immunization also became a matter of local politics. Initially, the plan was to have the immunizations at the hamlet head's house, which boasted a large porch and yard, rather than the much smaller health clinic lying directly across the street. Site size was a minor factor in this plan. At this time, a large faction of 93 households was seeking government papers to secede legally from the jurisdiction of the rest of Pelocok and establish their own independent hamlet head. Pelocok's current hamlet head, Amaq Rudi, was doing everything in his power to undercut the secession and reestablish loyalty toward himself. Hosting

of making an immunization record for each child. I happened to be visiting Papuq Isa, the *belian*, when Amaq Rudi, the hamlet head, came to invite her grandson. He began by taking out some very official-looking papers and asking Papuq to confirm information on her grandchild— his approximate age, sex, parents. She answered impatiently, then asked what it was all about. Amaq Rudi replied that it was so the child could be listed as a recipient of medicine (*owat*) against "pinus." She wanted to know what kind of medicine. He answered "vitamin," to which she replied that her grandchild didn't need any vitamins. He told her that it was mandatory and handed her the immunization record card. I asked what "pinus" was, and he answered, "Pinus is a sickness of children." Amaq Rudi had mistaken the PIN name of the project for the name of the sickness. But it didn't matter to Papuq Isa who was no more concerned about pinus than polio.

Not only did the *belian* and the hamlet head not know what polio was, no one I spoke with knew about it (cf. Nichter 1996). Over the next weeks, a steady trickle of women stopped to ask me what the vaccine was for and if it was really necessary. Some people were obviously hesitant about it, the more so the younger their children. I encouraged everyone I spoke with to get the inoculation, describing polio as a horrific illness and the vaccine as certain protection. I had seen polio victims begging too often on the streets of the provincial capital to be impartial. Thus did I undermine some suspicions of biomedicine, becoming an authoritative voice outlining vulnerabilities about which, beforehand, these rural Sasaks had no ken.

On vaccination day, the national immunization program proved a success. By 10 A.M., a total of 225 children had been immunized, and the record was being scanned for any delinquents. Amaq Rudi was angry that some had not come. As soon as he wandered off, his wife came over. I asked her where her four-year-old son was for his immunization. She smiled, "He does not want to take it" (*ndeqne meleqne*). Then she told the record keeper to just write her son's name down as if he had been vaccinated! The following month 203 children were reimmunized, again not including the hamlet head's son. As with any form of prevention, parents judged whether the vaccines "fit" (Indon., *cocok;*

---

a program that would bring everyone to his house would severely undermine the symbolic support of the secession. Papuq Junin, the leader of the secession movement, recognized this ploy and adamantly refused to allow anyone from that area to attend. After much ill will, the vaccination site was moved across the street to the health post.

Sas., *kenak*) their children. About 20 children became feverish and lethargic in the days after the vaccine. Their parents said that the medicine did not "fit" them, and they were not taken back for the second dosage in October. These parents were brave enough to stand against the hamlet head when he rebuked them, because they now knew that that medicine did not *fit* their child.

I estimate that of all eligible children, roughly 86 percent were inoculated in September and roughly 76 percent received the second inoculation. Why the large turnout for immunity to an unknown disease if my argument is correct that people seek preventive practices because they experience themselves as vulnerable? First, the inoculations were free of cost. Second, they promised to protect children from harm. Finally, there was political pressure to have one's children immunized.

Martin suggests that "accepting vaccination means accepting the state's power to impose a particular view about the body and its immune system—the view developed by medical science" (1994, 194). Martin assumes that accepting a particular medicine means accepting the ideology behind it. Not at all. No one—neither the government *bidan* nor the hamlet head—ever attempted to explain that the children were given vaccines and what vaccines were about. The serum was described only as vitamins or medicine. There was no education about or acceptance of a biomedical ideology. Although most people in Pelocok were confused as to why their children should have the "vitamin," they did not question the government's right to insist that they be immunized. Nor were they bothered by the government's endorsement of biomedicine. From a Sasak perspective, what matters is whether something works. In chapter 2, we saw the complex, multiple, sometimes contradictory understandings of the body that Sasaks hold without the slightest sense of cognitive dissonance. If people experience themselves as vulnerable to illness, they are as likely to have a ritual cleansing as they are to go to the clinic for an injection. It matters not that each of these preventive strategies has behind it a different ideology and understanding of the body. What matters is the possibility that they might work. By choosing to go to the local clinic for the inoculation, rural Sasaks did not lose their agency to act on their ills. Rather, they used the government's endorsement of biomedicine to get free vitamins for their children that *might* make them grow big and strong. Thus part of Sasaks' agency to act on their anxieties about illness is their ability to take advantage of the opportunities offered by the larger society of outsiders.

AGENCY AS PERSONAL AND SOCIAL

The locus of agency to cope with vulnerabilities and illnesses can be both individual and social. People are capable of coping with health concerns without resorting to others or even mentioning the concern. But, because selves are formed within the community, through continually participating, interpreting, playing, and caring with others, selves are constantly in-the-making within a social world. A person is essentially both a self and a social being. And thus, what are the words family and friends say to encourage a person at the point of death to live? "Remember your self! Remember your family! Remember your children! Remember!"

Recall Papuq Alus, whose uneasy thoughts threatened her health and who prevented illness by staying busy and sleeping with relatives. Upon the departure of her son, she experienced her *self* as vulnerable. In this new context of loneliness and worry, her self was susceptible to harm. She expressed this vulnerability to others through words, through a more melancholy demeanor, through the movement of her hand in front of her chest, and through her strategy of prevention that kept her from sleeping at home. And people did respond to her differently, now that she was vulnerable. We were gentler with her, more careful to smile or offer her coffee when she passed. We spoke of her when she was not there, noting how thin she was, how she didn't smile anymore, how she so rarely came to the compound to visit. After a while, some neighbors grew critical, saying that she needed to get back to her normal life. Others defended her in her absence, imagining how they would be if their child left. Even after Papuq Alus received the letter from her son and began sleeping in her house again, her loss was not forgotten by any of us, regardless of her decreased experience of vulnerability. For many of us in the compound, our practice of seeking her out so that she would not be too much alone slipped into daily habit and did not change, even as time dulled the sharpness of her experience, and other concerns took precedence. Papuq Alus's experience of vulnerability and her strategies for preventing illness affected who she was as a person; together she and we around her acted on her sense of vulnerability and reformulated Papuq Alus-as-person and our relations with her.

Persons only make sense as beings-in-the-world (Csordas 1994): multiple, ever-changing, and constantly responding to their complex contexts overflowing with people and cares, words and experiences. In a world where health is always tenuous, illness always lurks just out of sight, experiences of vulnerability are universal, and illness prevention is a part of everyday life, being in *this* world informs personhood. Health concerns are integral in defining who rural Sasaks are, and integral to any understanding we might have of them. Papuq Alus's experience of vulnerability informed and motivated who she became as a person after her son's departure. Her personhood—her particular circumstances that left her alone when her son left—informed and motivated her experience of vulnerability. Vulnerability and personhood mutually inform and shape each other; I will argue that both of them shape and are shaped by experiences of illness. But as beings-in-the-world, persons, their vulnerabilities, and their illnesses are not entire of themselves. Health concerns, once expressed, become the concern of society. Society offers life-cycle and other rituals of prevention for coping with vulnerabilities. It offers biomedical clinics that people can try to take advantage of. Finally, it responds to others' vulnerabilities, reshaping interactions to protect vulnerable persons. Person and society both are agents in coping with vulnerabilities and can be shaped by them.

EXPLORING THE AGENCY OF *ILMU*

Agency tends to be thought of as a capacity of individuals or groups, but among Sasaks, knowledge itself has the potency to act. *Ilmu* is considered a crucial element of many societies in Southeast Asia, and it is often connected with illness in the form of spells and treatments (e.g., Peletz 1996, 158ff.; Geertz 1960, 88–89; Atkinson 1989, 52–76ff.).[18] But, in these other places, *ilmu* seems to take a back seat to *semangat* (life force, spirit of life) in discussions of vulnerability, strategies of prevention, and experiences of illness. Among the Sasak, however, more than personal or social agency, it is the agency of *ilmu* that resonates with vulnerabilities and illness.

Defining *Ilmu*

I had initially translated *ilmu* as *knowledge*. But Sasak *ilmu* acts differently than English *knowledge*. In English, we speak of knowledge as some-

---

18. Based on research in urban Java, Ferzacca argues that the word *ilmu* there is increasingly reserved for scientific knowledge and the knowledge of academic disciplines, while *ngelmu* refers more to the mystical practices of knowledge discussed here (1996, 217–18).

thing we *share*, implying that it is unlimited, intangible, that it does not diminish in the telling of it. Indeed, from elementary school into adulthood, persons in America who express knowledge, who say something even if that something is wrong, are generally considered wiser and more engaging than those who are silent. In Lombok the opposite is true. For the Sasak, *ilmu* is a limited, tangible entity that does diminish in the telling of it.

Ilmu is limited. That is to say, for rural Sasaks, perfect and complete human knowledge was once possible. The ancestral *datu* (kings) and *wali* (religious apostles) had complete and perfect *ilmu*. They knew all things, never became ill themselves, never truly died,[19] and could heal all illness with their words. But although they taught others some of their *ilmu*, their teachings were never complete. Some *ilmu* was always hidden from their pupils, thus to this day people lament the incompleteness of their *ilmu*. As Papuq Junin, a man respected for his extensive *ilmu*, once whispered to me, "My great-grandfather had a lot of *ilmu*, but he did not give it all to me" (*"Bageq ilmu baluqku laeq, laguq ie ndeqne sere buet mbengku ilmune"*). Within families, dead parents and grandparents are suspected of not passing down all of their *ilmu*. Some people, like the *dukun* Amaq Deri, have no intention of distributing any of their *ilmu*. The result is that some *ilmu* is always lost with each generation. Because *ilmu* can be gained in dreams from dead people or from one's own *dewa*, *ilmu* is not irretrievably lost to humans in theory, but in practice, it is lost. *Ilmu* now is greatly diminished from its perfection in the past.

Ilmu is tangible. By this I mean that *ilmu* is something a person owns.[20] When speaking of people with *ilmu*, Sasaks are far more

---

19. People loved to tell stories of old of how kings and *wali*s had appeared to die, but never really did. Some vanished in the shrouds before they could be buried. Some vanished from their graves, as people who had sought to prove their deaths found out. Only when a body vanished was it certain that that person was someone sacred, a king or *wali*. Some of these stories took place in centuries past, but others more recently. Inaq Mol claimed that the father of one *kiayi* in Pelocok and the father of a nobleman both vanished from their respective shrouds after they had "died." More commonly, I heard tell of Multiwali, a renowned teacher of Islam (*tuan guru*) who was supposed to have died in the 1920s or 1930s and whose grave site lies in a cemetery a 45-minute walk to the southeast of Pelocok. Yet, the day after his burial, when someone decided to dig up the grave to see if he had really died, his body had vanished, leaving just the shroud.

20. But it is ownership in a different sense than one owns a house, because *ilmu* is integral to one's being, one's potency in the world. There is nothing quite analogous to it in American understandings, although one could consider it rather like a person's kidney. A person's kidney is integral to her. While she can give away one kidney and continue to live, she is herself weakened by the loss.

inclined to say, "He has much knowledge" (*Iye are luet ilmu*). Only in sentences implying *ilmu* but not using the word as an object did I hear people say, "He knows a lot" (*Tauqne iye luet*). Usually, *ilmu* is conceptually *owned* rather than *known* (cf. Siegal 1978, 20). Likewise, *ilmu* is something one gives (*mbeng*) and is given (*te'embeng*), it is not something perceptually that one *shares*. Indeed the Sasak language does not have a word comparable in meaning to the English *share*. Rather, *ilmu* is a commodity, and one described as *mahal*, expensive. When Inaq Sahim gave me some small words (*puji*), she always prefaced her teaching with these or similar words: "This *ilmu* is the expensive thing. Here we are all poor. There is nothing. But with this *ilmu*, it is enough. You do not have enough money to buy it. If others come and offer money, I will not give it to them. It is too expensive. But I care about Eron and therefore give you my *ilmu*." Although *ilmu* is not usually purchasable, if a person is selected to be given *ilmu*, norms of reciprocity apply, and the receiver is obligated to reciprocate in some way with money, gifts, labor, and/or social attachment. For example, one wife boasted of how her husband had been selected to receive *ilmu* so expensive that it had cost them dearly: 144 old coins, a full-sized cow, and various articles of clothing.

Ilmu is a commodity in another sense: it ideally does not change in content as it is given by one person and received by another. *Ilmu* is not interpreted, it is memorized. *Ilmu*, either in the form of small words (*puji*) of harm prevention or spells (*jampi*) of illness treatment, is given by another person or in dreams. The receiver's job is to memorize the lines, word for word.[21] It does not matter if the words are understood. As we shall see, words used in *jampi* are sometimes completely mean-

---

21. The Sasak emphasis on memorization dovetails with the emphasis on memorization in the study of the Qur'an. Unlike the Bible, which is written by men, the Qur'an is the direct word of Allah given through angels, memorized by Muhammad, and then written down word for word by scribes. There are even some words, abbreviated letters actually, such as "Alif, Lam, Mim" (Surah 2:1) in the Qur'an that have no clear meaning (Ali 1989, 122–24). As one Islamic scholar, lamenting the lack of understanding most Muslims have for the words of the Qur'an, wrote: "The ambition of every Muslim is to read [recite] the *sounds* of the Arabic Text" (Ali 1989, xix, emphasis in original). As the words of Allah, merely repeating those sacred words has potency in the world. For example, al Kursi, as Sasaks referred to al Quraysh (Surah 106), was recited by people to themselves when they felt vulnerable, and a written version of it was even hung in two Pelocok households as a sort of amulet protecting the house. This Surah is about the tribe of Quraysh, the people who are the guardians of Mekkah, and who therefore have the particular protection of Allah against hunger, war, and other dangers. The character of Sasak *ilmu*, then, corresponds strongly to the Islamic understanding of the Qur'an, with the one exception that although the Qur'an is open to all, the Sasak *ilmu* is ideally secret, known only to one or a few persons.

ingless. Meaning is not important, but the way the words are strung together is vital, and for that reason *ilmu* is precisely memorized (see also Atkinson 1989, 52–53). *Ilmu* then is an object, an expensive commodity that ideally remains unchanged as it is given and received.

Ilmu diminishes in the telling of it. It is *not* that in telling *ilmu,* the *quantity* or *content* of one's own *ilmu* diminishes. Ideally, the quantity—how much one knows—and content—what one knows—remain the same, regardless of how many people know it. But the *quality* of the *ilmu* diminishes with each telling. Quality does not refer to the rightness or correctness of the content of *ilmu* (although that too is suspect). Rather, quality refers to the potency inherent in it. For Sasaks, as well as for other Indonesians, all *ilmu* has inherent potency, or, to use Anderson's term, power (1990).[22] It has the potential for efficacy in the world.[23] For example, *ilmu* in the form of small words is apotropaic so that the more one has, the less vulnerable one feels, and the more brave one can afford to be. But in order to guard the efficacy of one's *ilmu,* its distribution must also be carefully guarded. Generally speaking, the more secretive the *ilmu,* the fewer the people who know it, the more potent it is. Inversely, the more common the *ilmu,* the more people who know it, the less potent it is. Secrecy is the key to safeguarding the potency of *ilmu.*

Recall my confusion when Inaq Mol wanted me to tell her the small words (*puji, kata kodeq*) that enabled me to be brave wherever I went (see interlude). Small words are the mantras or spells people say to protect themselves. They are small because, like all *ilmu,* they are mouthed rather than spoken aloud when used. The potency of small words and other kinds of *ilmu* depends on their secrecy. For this reason, *ilmu* is transmitted in whispers. It is given to a child isolated with the parent for a day and a night. It is shared between spouses when all the doors are

---

22. The inherent connection between knowledge and power that Sasaks make is *not* the same thing as Foucault's well-known position of knowledge/power. Foucault uses a historical and political perspective drawing heavily on Gramsci's Marxism to argue that certain ideas when adopted by those with political and social authority can dominate and subjugate other ideas to such an extent that they can change whole social systems, such as criminal justice, gender relations, and mental health care (Foucault 1965, 1972, 1977, 1978, 1980). Sasak *ilmu* in the sense I discuss it here is potent, it is able to act on the world, preventing ills, deflecting curses, and treating ills. In later chapters, I discuss the authority and legitimation that *ilmu* can have in society—an argument that dovetails marginally with Foucault—but that should not be confused with the inherent potency of *ilmu* discussed here.

23. This potency for efficacy of *ilmu* fits within the vast anthropological literature on the power of words (e.g., Lévi-Strauss 1963; Malinowski 1948; Mauss 1975; Tambiah 1968).

shut and the compound is silent. It is taught to a fictive granddaughter in the dead of night, barely breathed so that an eavesdropper will not overhear.

Ancient Papuq Isa lived in the poorest excuse for a house of any in Pelocok, and I loved the place. Four enormous pillars supported an old wooden *lumbung* (rice barn). Between the ground and the bottom of the *lumbung* was a small bamboo platform, where she treated her patients, ate her meals, welcomed visitors, and hosted overnight guests. Along the back was a bed, a separate raised bamboo platform, and around the whole were hastily erected walls of woven split bamboo.

Although I had apprenticed myself for a long time to Papuq Isa as a *belian* and healer, it was not until the last two months of my fieldwork that I asked her to give me *ilmu*. The first night I went to spend the night at her house, her son and a friend of his were there. We chatted until it was late, then the two men lay down to go to sleep, and Papuq Isa lowered a pink cloth separating us on the bed from the men. By the light of a wick stuck in a tin-can-turned-lamp, she whispered that I should open my notebook and began telling me a spell (*jampi*).

Before she gave me the second line, she lifted the cloth and found her son's friend, paper and pencil in hand, trying to write down the overheard words. She scolded him, saying that she did not want to tell him *jampi*, and dropped the curtain. Twice more she caught him; the third time she said angrily that she would stop telling me anything because of his eavesdropping. Apparently shamed, the man went outside and Papuq turned to me with a playful grin, whispering, "Listen. He'll go outside and sit there and listen to us." We blew out the light and crept silently outside to find him huddled by the outside of the wall. She told the surprised man to go off to his own house. We watched him trudge out of the black compound, then we curled up next to each other to ward off the cold and went to sleep. After one of her many coughing spells that interrupted our sleep, she lit the light and, barely aspirating at all, gave me 23 *jampi* and *puji*.

This mode of transmitting *ilmu* in secrecy fundamentally affects both its accuracy and its value. Secrecy means that one can not check with others later to see if one memorized it correctly. Pride in one's memory—to forget is to be vulnerable—prohibits returning to one's teacher. The result is variation. For example, La Nan taught me a *puji* to keep me safe from someone intent on killing me that she claimed to have learned from her mother. Inaq Mol and her sister Inaq Sahim separately taught me *puji*s for the same purpose, which they were given by their mother. Their mother, Papuq Isa, taught me a *puji* again for the same purpose. All of these were slightly different. Either my genealogy of the *puji* is wrong, or it had been altered in each transmission. For Sasaks, alterations degrade the value and efficacy of the *puji*. Sasaks recognize that this happens, and for as long as the teacher is alive, it is the teacher whose *ilmu* is most highly regarded, even when the student's *ilmu* is said to be "complete" (*buet*).

Given this, one might ask why the *ilmu* is not just written down. The easy answer is that the majority of people in Pelocok are illiterate. But even as more people can write and try to learn *ilmu* first by writing it down, *ilmu* must enter (*tume*) a person to be potent. Words on a page do not do the trick. So my various teachers each admonished me to memorize the *ilmu* they gave me. Inaq Mol insisted: "Study. Study until you know them [small words] completely. They have to enter the wind inside us. Once they are in the wind [pointing to her stomach] nothing will happen" ("*Belajar! Belajar aditne buet tauq. Harus iye tume angin ite. Wah ito, ndeq mbe-mbe*").[24] La Nan insisted that I eat the paper on which the *ilmu* had been written so that it would always be in my heart. Papuq Isa told me that once the words entered (*tume*) me, I would never have to worry about when to use each one, that it would just come to me. *Ilmu* enters persons. It enters their hearts and stomachs and their wind (*angin*).

Ilmu, this learned knowledge, enters and becomes integrated within one's entire body and being. I am reminded, "In all learning, one is changed, becoming someone slightly—or profoundly—different. . . . What is learned then becomes a part of that system of self-definition that filters all future perceptions and possibilities of learning" (Bateson 1994, 79). For Sasaks the change in person that occurs when one acquires *ilmu* is more profound; it is not just a person's outlook, perceptions, and interpretations that change. In a world without presumed Cartesian duality, knowledge and thinking are intimately bound up with hearts, stomachs, experience, and illness. It is the person's being—their bodies, their definition of self in relation to a dangerous world, their potency to act in that world, and others' perception of them as potent persons—that changes with *ilmu*.

---

24. In chapter 2, we saw how the Sasak idiom for a cold is *masuk angin* (Indon.), which translates as "entering the wind." By both syntax and using the Sasak word *tume* (to enter), Inaq Mol is indicating that *ilmu* must become part of a person's internal wind or breath. It is not wind that enters as with a cold, it is knowledge entering an element already inherent in the person.

The Pride of Ilmu

Ilmu shapes persons and can prevent and treat illness.[25] As we will see, it is so crucial for coping with unusual illness that it adversely colors interactions between rural Sasaks and biomedical personnel. For this reason, it is important to understand something of the confidence and value Sasaks place on it.

One lazy morning, Amaq Mol and I were engaged in a lengthy discussion of Lombok's history, its kings and apostles (*wali*). When Amaq Sunin walked into the house, he tried to change the subject away from these beings with their complete *ilmu*. I brought up the *wali* again, to which Amaq Sunin replied: "In America you have airplanes with bombs. But Lombok is rich in *ilmu*. With *ilmu* alone, Lombok could destroy your planes with bombs."

Ilmu is potent against the most powerful of forces. *Ilmu*, in Sunin's statement, could stop a military air invasion. The *ilmu* of the people in Pelocok can also stop any interference from the Indonesian government, as I heard Inaq Sahin say: "That is why the government doesn't come to bother [*ngganggu*] us here. We have *ilmu* that makes them not pay attention, they pass us by. Pak Kadus [the hamlet mayor] is full of *ilmu*. Because the *ilmu* is so strong here the government doesn't come and bother us here." *Ilmu* can protect an island; it can protect a community.

Recall Inaq Sahim's words: "Here we are all poor. There is nothing. But with this *ilmu*, it is enough." People in Pelocok are enclosed by poverty and peasantry. They bow down to government officials and sit on the ground rather than on chairs when talking with wealthier outsiders. They know they are considered backward, primitive, stupid, and people of the forest by people in larger towns and villages. Yet, in their own estimation, their *ilmu* reigns over all these things. Their *ilmu* is both respected and feared by townspeople, they claim.[26] From their own perspective, Sasak *ilmu* is stronger than the knowledge of any official, doctor, teacher or anthropologist.[27] It is a weapon of the weak

---

25. The role of *ilmu* in preventing illness is discussed above and in chapter 3. The importance of *ilmu* in treating illness is discussed particularly in chapters 5 and 6 and in the Epilogue.

26. Their claims are validated in writings about the Balinese who fear Sasak *ilmu* as black magic (e.g., Wikan 1990).

27. Indeed, my presence was often taken as a compliment to the potency and fame of their *ilmu*.

from an outsider's perspective, but for them, it is their wealth, their protection, and their pride.

The Agency of *Ilmu*

Ilmu has agency in causing as well as preventing and treating illness. In chapter 3, *ilmu* was discussed as something that acted to cause illness of its own accord. If another person slighted someone with particularly potent *ilmu*, the *ilmu* could inflict illness (*kemalikan*) on that other person. The slighted individual need not do or say anything, or even be aware of the slight. In this way *ilmu* has independent agency.

The agency of *ilmu* to act to prevent a threat or treat an illness requires that the *ilmu* be remembered and expressed. Words, in the form of secret spells, must be remembered and mouthed. To this extent, *ilmu*'s agency is dependent on persons. Yet because *ilmu* is always gained orally from others, persons or spirits, its agency is also dependent on accurate social transmission. *Ilmu* ideally is transmitted unaltered from generation to generation and is understood to be timeless. It is not bound by particular context or by the person who knows it at the moment. Its agency derives from a truth-value and potency that transcends the person and the community. The essence of *ilmu*'s agency is in its transcendence of time, its eternal truth-value.

THE COMPLEXITIES OF MULTIPLE AGENCIES

The trick when experiencing anxiety about health is to find the effective agent that knows how to cope (*tauq*) with a particular vulnerability or illness. Sometimes that agent is an individual person habitually doing actions of prevention. Sometimes that agent is the community at large, tossing out prevention suggestions or offering rituals and vaccines. Sometimes that agent is *ilmu*, either one's own or someone else's, which guards against illness and makes illness leave a body. Except in the most mundane, everyday cases in which a person copes without expressing her experiences to others, all three of these agents usually complement each other in acting on a health concern.

If health care could be simply limited to illness and treatments, having a direct effect on a person for only that period in which she is ill, this discussion would be moot. But for Sasaks, health is a constant concern, sometimes foregrounded, sometimes backgrounded, but never out of sight. Death is always too close at hand in Pelocok for the luxury of forgetting that in a week or a month one's self or someone dearly loved could suddenly become ill and die. How people cope with illness in its presence is informed by, and informs, how they cope with it in its absence.

For Sasaks, persons are fundamentally and essentially social, but also fundamentally unique. While this is an oxymoron for the cognitive debates on personhood, it is not an ontological problem. Ultimately, a construct of personhood must look both at embodied persons and beyond them to the concerns that move them and the context within which those concerns must be addressed. In interaction with others, Sasaks construct unique constellations of understandings about the body, vulnerabilities, and preventions. Theirs is a self-in-the-making through continual participation in a community. They cope with life's health cares by remembering both their social integration and their personal constellations of knowledge, by remembering both who they are as social beings and their socially initiated but personally unique collections of *ilmu*. Vulnerability and illness are social concerns. The victim does not suffer alone, but is surrounded by people gently easing social worlds, offering rituals, suggesting treatments, and reminding the victim to live. Yet, paradoxically, participating in society is also dangerous—a danger that can only be prevented by *ilmu*.

Ilmu is vitally important to Sasak ethnomedicine. In so saying, it is worth looking again at the Indonesian ethnographies that, at the beginning of writing this chapter, lined my bookcase and now clutter my desk, lying helter-skelter among my field notebooks. On the book-case, the emphasis on *semangat* looked neat and clean compared to the battered pages about the cares and idiosyncrasies of Sasaks. Yet, cluttered together, the life force so central to personhood among other Indonesians looks not so different from the importance Sasaks place on *ilmu*. Like *semangat, ilmu* is consciously nurtured to protect oneself from harm. *Semangat*, like *ilmu*, is limited and tangible. Also, the signs of *semangat* are similar to the signs of possessing much *ilmu*: virility, tranquillity, prosperity, and glory. However, there are three primary differences between the two: (1) *ilmu* becomes words that act on and change the world; (2) *ilmu* is acquired—it is gained from dreams, spirits, and other persons—and *becomes* integral to a person, unlike *semangat*, which is naturally inherent; (3) whereas both *semangat* and *ilmu* can act automatically, much of *ilmu*'s potency against illness is efficacious only if it is remembered. Having *ilmu* creates immunities, because the potency of *ilmu* can deflect potential illness from entering. But even with the strength of the best *ilmu,* persons are vulnerable because they can forget and become ill. As long as it is remembered, *ilmu* can act.

Ilmu is a defining quality of Sasak personhood and society. In *ilmu* lies their faith in themselves as superior to the larger nonpeasant society, enabling them to cope with their poverty, peasantry, and the condescension of outsiders. In *ilmu* lies their ability to prevent harm and treat illness. Ultimately, it is the characteristics of *ilmu* as limited, tangible, and with diminishing quality that are a cornerstone of Sasak ethnomedicine. The most potent preventive and treatment *ilmu* is distributed selectively only along family lines and in secrecy. While all persons and families have *ilmu,* some have more than others, making *ilmu* dispersed unevenly throughout the community. Moreover, through transmission in secrecy and memorization, *ilmu* is accidentally altered because there is no forum for checking its accuracy. Finally, because of its secrecy, no one knows absolutely what *ilmu* each person has nor how potent it is. This system for distributing *ilmu* fundamentally affects the nature of ethnomedicine.

Pelocok, then, is a place where everyone is a potential healer, and no one's knowledge is discounted. There are multiple loci for agency. Selves, shaped by the experiences of vulnerability and illness, can cope with some health concerns on their own. Society, whose relations are marked by people's vulnerabilities and illnesses, is an essential resource and agent for coping with these concerns. *Ilmu,* itself not altered by vulnerability and illness, is a third potent agent for these concerns.

As we have seen, anxiety focuses neurological processes, including memory, toward easing the perceived threat. Sasaks themselves foreground the ability to remember. Individuals can only prevent harm for themselves if they can remember everyday preventive practices and the small words of prevention. Society acts in response to vulnerabilities by focusing many people's memories on preventative practices, on producing rituals according to the words of the ancestors, and by reminding dying people to live. Finally, the agency of *ilmu,* the ultimate agent rural Sasaks depend upon to cope with their vulnerabilities and illnesses, must be remembered to be efficacious. Remembering is the basic process in the agency of selves, society, and *ilmu* that enables rural Sasaks to cope with their anxieties about illness in both its absence and its presence.

—•—

PART II

Coping with Illness

We have seen that people are busy coping with illness before anyone is actually sick. In their anxieties about and agencies for coping with vulnerability, Sasaks set the groundwork for staying alive in the presence of illness.

We step into the presence of illness by tracing a young boy's illness day by day, which emphasizes the uncertainty of life lived forward and the daily anxiety of not knowing whether the ill child would survive the day. Such uncertainty attends the interpretations, interactions, and actions surrounding this illness, or any illness, as chapters 5 and 6 show. When biomedical treatment is sought, as it was for this boy, interactions tend to result in miscommunication, as shown in chapter 7.

When illness ends in relative health, anxiety dissipates, and people refocus on other concerns. But when illness escalates to the point of death, anxiety also escalates. At the final moment before death, only remembering can keep a person alive. Chapter 8 asks why Sasaks focus on remembering at the moment of death and why, more generally, they must remember to live. In so doing, it looks at the process of remembering itself for theoretical as well as ethnographic insights. Chapter 9 steps back from the anguish of ethnographic detail to summarize and integrate the theoretical arguments that have emerged out of it. Finally, the book adjourns with a discussion of the tragic irony of Sasak medicine.

Case Study: An Ill Child

I first met Lo Budin when he was about four months old. His father, Papuq Junin, introduced the child thus: "This is Small Uncle [*Paman Kodeq*].[1] He will be the one that will grow big in knowledge. He will be the one who will know all the knowledge of the ancestors." Papuq Junin was a senior person in Pelocok, yet he had an ageless quality about him. He laughed often, the smile twinkling in his eyes, as he regaled us with stories or played audiocassettes of his beloved Sasak gamelan music.[2] He was heir to the *ilmu* and *pusaka* of his father and grandfather. Through his paternal grandfather, Papuq Junin claimed relations among the Sasak aristocracy and pronounced himself the keeper of the traditions of the ancestors. He was among the wealthiest men in Pelocok and redistributed the surplus of his wealth (although not the principal of lands and cattle) by hosting large rituals, in much the same fashion as the potlatch ceremonies of the Northwest Native Americans equalize community wealth yet build the status of the potlatch host (Walens 1981). Papuq Junin had been married to three different wives and had proved his virility by siring 11 living children. When I first moved to Pelocok, Papuq Junin's compound on the top of a hill was surrounded by gardens. Within a few months the landscape changed entirely, as he convinced people from hamlets in the south to move and populate his hill with promises of a kind of small communal

---

1. The persistent reference by all the family members to the child as Small Uncle, *paman kodeq*, referred to his social status as projected by his father rather than to actual kin relationships.
2. Sasak gamelan music is slightly different in sound, particularly in its greater use of wind instruments, and much more informal in performance style from the gamelon music of Bali or Java. It was popular in Pelocok but because most people did not have tape recorders, *dangdut*—Indonesian pop music—was more commonly heard blasting from radios.

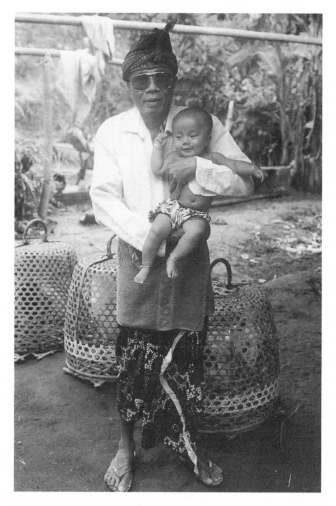

FIG. 9.   Papuq Junin and Lo Budin, before his illness
(1994)

society.[3] With his credentials as a community leader, a senior, virile,
wealthy man, and a man supposedly owning among the most secret

3. What made this community unique—it came to be known gradually as Montong
(little hill)—was the institutionalization of what Papuq Junin said were the ways of the
ancestors in the world of his father. These ways included strict adherence to the
details of Sasak life-cycle, rice, cattle, house, and religious rituals as defined by Papuq
Junin (sometimes hotly contested by local *kiayis*), as well as the institutionalization of
the customary practices of contributing money and labor to the ritual activities of anyone else in the compound.

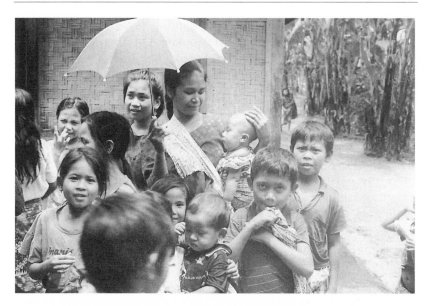

FIG. 10.   Inaq Budin holding Lo Budin under the shade of
an umbrella three months before the onset of his illness
(1994)

and potent knowledge and objects in the region, Papuq Junin was the
most potent person in Pelocok.

Papuq Junin and his young wife, Inaq Budin, absolutely adored the
child. Lo Budin seemed a healthy baby, well-fed and happy. He wore
amulets around his neck and ankles to keep him safe from harm. Once
when he had become mildly ill, his name had been changed from Lo
Sahrun to Lo Budin because his original name had not "fit" him. This
illness was long forgotten, and his parents did not consider him any
more vulnerable to illness than other uncircumcised boys. From the
first, I noted the largeness of his head, but at the time, it was only a
physical characteristic useful for distinguishing Lo Budin from the
hordes of other children swarming around daily.

THE ILLNESS ENTERS

Like all small children in Pelocok, Lo Budin suffered mild colds and
diarrhea from time to time, and on August 20, 1994, when he was
about a year old, he developed a fever and cried more than usual.

On that same day, in another compound, Papuq Junin's sister,[4] the old and highly respected Papuq Sari, took ill. On August 25 she died. Papuq Sari reputedly had powerful *ilmu*. Because of her potency, because she had mothered some of the most progenitive and influential households in Pelocok, and because everyone liked this humble, wise woman, her death struck a deep chord within the community. This chord became dissonance in discussions of who was to have the privilege of hosting her mortuary rituals. By every tradition in Pelocok, the rituals should be hosted by the immediate family and held at the house where the person lived. The evening after her burial, Papuq Junin announced that he was going to be responsible for the ceremonies. He would work with Papuq Sari's daughters, but all the rituals would take place at his house. When someone questioned his right to host the rituals, Papuq Junin responded angrily, "It is decided. I do not want to talk about it anymore."

In the end, because the daughters insisted on their right to host the ceremonies, two sets of rituals were performed: one at Papuq Junin's house and one at Papuq Sari's house. In all conversations I heard, while none dared dispute Papuq Junin to his face, subtle comments made it clear that the religiously significant rituals were those hosted by the daughters, and Papuq Junin's rituals were considered political grabs at the popularity of Papuq Sari.

On August 25, after Papuq Sari's burial, I went with Papuq Junin to see Lo Budin, who had been mildly ill since the first day of Papuq Sari's illness. That day, he had worsened, and Papuq Junin wanted my opinion. The child had a fever of about 100 F and was having trouble keeping milk down. The day before, his mother had taken Lo Budin to get a *suntik* (Indon., injection) from a distant clinic, but he had not improved. I was told that, since becoming ill, he had been treated with various everyday sorts of treatments, including being dotted on the forehead with betel juice (*bebubusan*) and being the recipient of secret healing words (*jampis*) from Papuq Isa (the *belian*) that afternoon. Papuq Junin asked if the clinic might have good medicine for Lo Budin, suggesting that, perhaps because his wife did not know what to ask for, the child had been given the wrong thing. I said that it was possible, and when he asked me to take the child to the clinic the next day, I agreed.

---

4. Or perhaps half-sister by his father's first wife. Tracing the specifics of genealogies is a difficult task for the Sasak, who, like the Balinese (Geertz and Geertz 1964), do not put much store in such things, particularly in such niceties as distinguishing siblings on the basis of the mother, decades after the mothers' deaths.

August 26

Armed with the book *Where There Is No Doctor* (Werner 1992) and a thermometer, I arrived the next morning to find that all Lo Budin's symptoms were gone. Relieved, I looked up the symptoms he had had—fever, vomiting, crying, diarrhea—for curiosity's sake, but found no clear diagnosis. There was certainly no reason to make the trek to the distant clinic. Papuq Junin told me that one of his older sons, Lo Den, had dreamed that the child's name should be changed from Budin to Cili. They had changed it on the spot, in the middle of the night, and surmised that the ill-fitting name must have been the problem. (I continue to use the name Budin here for simplicity's sake.)

Almost as an afterthought Papuq Junin added, "Later we will have a *betemoi* at Amaq Hirin's, too, just to be sure." Amaq Hirin, not a healing expert but considered full of *ilmu*, occasionally did a *betemoi* healing ceremony directed at appeasing a person's *epe* (soul, god, shadowy twin). Papuq Junin seemed certain that the problem of the illness was solved with the name change, but wanted this further healing ceremony as a precaution. As I was about to leave, Papuq Junin confided, "Once Small Uncle is circumcised, I will not worry. But he isn't yet, so when he is sick, I feel sick too." By his own account, then, he felt ill, sick with worry about his ill child who had not yet passed the period of vulnerability prior to circumcision.

Later that day, I spoke about Lo Budin to Papuq Isa, who was very surprised to hear they had changed the child's name. "There was no reason to do that," she said. She went on to explain that the problem was not with the name. The problem had to do with Papuq Sari's illness, because they had both become ill on the same day. Moreover, the child's illness resulted from Papuq Junin's inappropriate insistence on hosting Papuq Sari's mortuary rituals.

August 27

The next day, I watched Amaq Mol treat his youngest son for a sick mouth (*sakit dodok*), diagnosed thus by his mother because he cried constantly. Inaq Mol explained to me that the illness was caused by *pedam* (spirits) in the *baq* (cement reservoir for piped-in water). She added that Papuq Junin's baby was also ill because of spirits in the reservoir. I asked, surprised, if Lo Budin was still ill. Inaq Mol responded, "Very ill. It is a different illness from this one [indicating her son]. The cause is the same, but the illness is different" (*Sakit gati. Lain penyakitne dit ini. Asalne pede, laguq sakitne lain*).

The reservoir had opened just a few weeks before along the main road leading through Pelocok. It held water piped directly from a spring in the distant mountain rain forests. From the day it opened, the women and children exclusively bathed, washed clothes and utensils, and drew water at the reservoir rather than at the numerous streams that threaded through the rice fields. This new structural addition, which everyone praised and used, was now being blamed by Inaq Mol for causing illness in her son and in Lo Budin.[5]

When I went to see Lo Budin, he was rather listless but otherwise did not seem particularly ill. His father complained that he did not want to eat, but that Papuq Isa had already come by and treated him with a *jampi* that morning. When I asked what the illness was, Papuq Junin replied that it had to do with the *dewa* of the reservoir.

I nodded in agreement and then said quietly that I thought Papuq Isa had determined that the illness was connected with the illness of Papuq Sari. I was unprepared for how angry Papuq Junin became: "How could the illness have to do with Papuq Sari? There was no connection at all!" He went on to lecture at length, saying in essence that it was undeniably his responsibility to do the mortuary rituals and that it was impermissible even to suggest that his son's illness was connected to Papuq Sari's death. I agreed that of course he must be right. As quickly as his anger came, it was gone, and he told me of the problems with the reservoir and said that if only it had been placed in his compound rather than along the main road none of this would have happened.[6]

August 28

The next morning, I went to see Lo Budin. He had no fever, vomiting, or diarrhea, but he looked far worse. His eyes were as vacant as if he were sleeping with them open. He would start to cough and just stop,

---

5. Nonetheless, Inaq Mol did not stop using the reservoir or bathing her son there.
6. This was a blatant political complaint. Since the building of the reservoir, Papuq Junin had had an ongoing argument with government powers (the hamlet mayor, village mayor, and subdistrict head) that the reservoir should be placed on the top of the hill in his new community because of the density of the population on the hill and because the community—his community—needed its own reservoir. He never failed to note that the best spot would be in the center of his own compound. Had a reservoir been built there, it would have been a great political and social coup for Papuq Junin.

apparently from exhaustion. He was in serious trouble. I was told that Papuq Isa was treating him with *mul-mul*—a treatment in which sanctified water was occasionally poured on Lo Budin's forehead. The *mul-mul* treatment simultaneously is spiritual, directed at calming the *epe,* as well as humoral, directed at cooling the body to *mul,* the ideal temperature—neither hot nor cold.

I left to seek Papuq Isa and ask why she had changed her mind about the etiology of the illness. Instead, I found her son. I expressed to him my confusion over Inaq Mol's etiology of the spirit (*pedam*) in the reservoir—how did the spirit cause illness? The young man laughed and said that Inaq Mol was wrong, it was not the spirit of the reservoir, but rather the spirit (he used the word *dewa*) of the origin spring that was causing the illness: "The source of the water in the reservoir was not given a ritual. No permission [of the spirit] was asked before the water pipes to the reservoir were built. It's not allowed not to do this. It's not allowed to forget. Papuq Junin, he is a person with *ilmu.* He knows the way to ask permission. But he forgot, so his child is ill."[7]

August 29

It was barely dawn when, on my way to see Lo Budin, I was surprised to see the reservoir decorated with fringed palm fronds. Papuq Junin had decided in the middle of the night to hold a minor ritual at dawn at the reservoir so that the spirit of the reservoir would stop making his son ill—an action that legitimated the reservoir spirit etiology. Papuq Junin told me confidently that these ceremonies would work, but that they needed to be repeated for three days. He added that, once Lo Budin was no longer ill, I could take him to the clinic for an injection so he would quickly become fat and healthy again. I nodded in agreement, while gazing at the listless baby in its mother's arms.

I was deeply concerned about Lo Budin and was, as an ethnographer, very interested in the complexities of the varying diagnoses and treatments that were developing around this illness. At the same time, I was feeling ill and drained myself. Living as an ethnographer in Pelocok was a 24-hour, seven-days-a-week job. I rarely slept more than five hours, and those hours would inevitably be broken by screaming

---

7. Note the use of the word *forget* (*lupaq*). In this case, and in a handful of others, the forgetfulness of one person makes another, weaker housemate vulnerable. Here, Papuq Junin is considered too potent, too full of *ilmu,* to suffer from his lapse in memory by the retaliations of the water spring's *dewa.* Instead the retaliation ricocheted off Papuq Junin onto his very young, helpless son.

babies, cries of theft, 3:00 A.M. rituals, and mice running across my sleeping platform. A diet of rice and tea, with a few vegetables scattered here and there, did little to improve my stamina. But most physically trying—and most exhilarating—was the constant, full concentration of intellectual and emotional energy that went into every waking moment. This situation seemed at least partly responsible for my declining health; the more months I had behind me in the field, the more frequently I came down with colds, fevers, and other ills. Often I was treated in the field by *belians* and *dukuns*, but I learned quickly that if I went to the island's capital of Mataram to buy medications, sleep, eat, and relax for a day or two, I could get back to work much quicker than if I stayed in Pelocok. So, knowing that I would not be allowed to do anything for Lo Budin until the reservoir rituals were over, I resigned myself to lost data and left.

August 31

I came back in the afternoon, weak and feverish but too worried about Lo Budin to stay away longer. The crowd was large at Papuq Junin's house, but no one would tell me why as they greeted me and hurriedly ushered me into the house. "Eron, come sit here by me," came the familiar voice of Papuq Junin from a dark corner of the house. I made my way, bent at the waist as etiquette demands, through the maze of legs sitting in the room. I swept Papuq Junin's right palm with my own in greeting as I sat down and my eyes adjusted to the dim light. Only then did I see Lo Budin arched unnaturally in the arms of his red-eyed mother. He had lost weight, making his head appear larger than usual. His back was stiff and his head thrown back. His limbs and mouth jerked occasionally, erratically. I was horrified. "Small Uncle does not know how to cry anymore. He does not want to eat [masticated rice]," Papuq Junin told me. I asked if he was nursing at all. Inaq Budin replied, "Yes. A little. But he does not want to sleep."

I listened as they told me, with neighbors piping in, of his stiff back, his inability to make sounds, his cold feet, and the wild movements of his eyes and mouth. They told of all of the ceremonies at the reservoir that had been completed, of the treatments of various *dukuns* and *belians*, of their plans to go to the spring itself the next day to do more ceremonies there. Some people spoke of similar cases they had heard about. Some suggested names of *dukuns* or *belians*. After most of the crowd had dwindled away and after promising to return the next day, I went home. Late into the night, I searched for answers in *Where There Is*

No Doctor; the only disease that matched the symptoms I identified was the disheartening one of meningitis (Werner 1992, 185).

September 1

The next morning Lo Budin looked worse, or perhaps the sun just detailed the horrors of his contortions that the night had concealed. I told his parents that he might have meningitis, a very serious illness that needed to be treated by doctors without delay. Papuq Junin said that I couldn't take the infant to the doctor that day because the doctor's medicine would not work until after the ceremony at the spring, which they would have to postpone until tomorrow, because he was needed to supervise the preparations for the final mortuary ritual for Papuq Sari. He concluded by stating that I should take the infant to get an injection the day after tomorrow "so that he will quickly become well."

After hustling between the two mortuary rituals at the different compounds, it was not until late that I had a chance to sit with Lo Budin. Papuq Isa was there. In a moment when everyone else was busy, I asked her quietly what was wrong with Lo Budin and if it was still a problem with water spirit.

> Nah! [In frustration.] None of the healing words (*jampi*) are working. I have tried everything. The healing words are all finished. The ceremonies at the reservoir did not want to work. I don't know. I'm confused. And he [gesturing to Lo Budin with her eyes] is tired unto death. He's so tired. (*Nah! Jampi-jampiq nde-qne jari. Seleput wah ku coba. Buet jampi. Begawai leq baq ndeq mele jari. Ndeqku tauq. Bingung aku. Dit iye lelah gati. Lelah iye.*)

This last point she whispered in a low voice. Whenever Papuq Isa describes a person as *lelah gati*, tired unto death, she expects the person to die.

The two of us reentered the conversation. The room was comfortably filled with a dozen people all focused on the twisted form of Lo Budin. As the discussion moved between the details of the mortuary ritual and the condition of the baby, various suggestions of treatment were voiced. "Order Inaq Sarinah to come here and dance." "Have you already washed the *lontar*s [potent, sacred texts]?" At each suggestion, Papuq Isa took some hair—a small clump of straggly, grey strands near her crown—mouthed words silently, then asked in a clear voice if the dancing or washing the *lontar* would work. Then she would grasp the hair with both hands, pull twice gently, and give it a hard yank. If there had been a loud popping sound, the sound accompanying the scalp pulling away from the skull, that would have meant that the answer was "Yes." But there was no popping sound that evening.

After Papuq Isa had given up divinations and gone home, Lo Budin went into violent convulsions. His head, mouth, eyes, arms, legs, and torso were all twitching around the backward arch of his back and neck. His father, Papuq Junin, instantly initiated a series of treatments for the boy.

The first treatment involved taking the baby outside, bathing him in warm (boiled) water, and rubbing him with garlic (a hot substance). Bringing the baby back inside, Papuq Junin launched immediately into a second treatment of warming his son with fire. Papuq Junin ordered a metal basin and dried coconut shells be brought to him.[8] He built a fire in the basin, then mouthed words over the small bright flames. I do not know how he withstood the heat, but Papuq Junin held his hands *in* the flame for about 15 seconds at a time, then pressed the heat of his hands onto the baby's head and body. Lo Budin was slightly quieted by this time, and he was handed to his mother who tried to nurse him. Papuq Junin blew the fire toward the baby's feet and right hand, each held sequentially. Then after warming Lo Budin's right hand, Papuq Junin took that hand and pressed it against the baby's own forehead. Without skipping a beat, Papuq Junin initiated a fourth treatment by putting on a white headcloth, as worn by *kiayis,* and asking for a bowl of water, betel leaves, and a certain basket. Mouthing words over the water, he took out the contents of the basket—four bundles wrapped in cloth—and dipped them in the water.[9] Then chewing up the betel leaf and taking a mouthful of the water, Papuq Junin sprayed a mist of potent water and bits of leaf all over the baby's body. As a fifth treatment, he called for a bowl of hot coals. He placed a small pebble of incense on the coals, mouthing words as he did so, then, as he had

---

8. Coconut shells burn more intensely, giving off greater heat than wood, and therefore were usually used in religious ceremonies and healing treatments when a quick, hot fire was needed.

9. These bundles were *pusaka.* Their roundish shape and palm size indicated that they were not typical potent objects like sacred texts (*lontars*) or knives (*kris*). They could have been potent belts, strips of cloth, bundles of Chinese coins, or other such things. In any case, what mattered was not what these bundles contained, but rather that whatever they were, they were potent, powerful objects. By dipping them in water, some of their potency was transferred to that water.

done earlier with the fire, he held his own hands in the smoke and pressed them onto Lo Budin's body.

After all of these treatments, Amaq Mus, a man reputedly rich in secret *ilmu,* scooted forward. He took another bowl of water and mouthed words over it. Then, after chewing a quid of betel and holding its red juices in his mouth, he took a mouthful of the water and sprayed a red mist on Lo Budin.

By this time Lo Budin's movements were calm. Papuq Junin sat back, surveyed us all, and, stopping at me, ordered me to take Lo Budin to a doctor the next day. I agreed, but as Papuq Junin began a conversation with Amaq Mus, Inaq Budin and Papuq Sahurr edged closer to me.

Papuq Sahurr: Don't take him to a doctor. Not yet.

Inaq Budin: It's not allowed. It's not allowed until all the Sasak *belian*s are finished.

Papuq Sahurr: Sasak medicine is better than the medicine of the doctor. The medicine there can only make the baby quickly get fat again. It is good at that, but it does not treat the origin [of the illness].

Inaq Budin: Only Sasak medicine can treat the origin. We first must finish Sasak medicine, only then is it allowed to take him to a doctor. That's the way, Eron [Cameron].

Papuq Sahurr: Do not take him tomorrow to the doctor. It's not allowed.

I struggled within myself. I was convinced the child needed to see a doctor as soon as possible, and his father seemed to want me to take him. Yet, the child's mother and great aunt were obviously opposed to it. Finally I agreed to take him, trusting that the father could persuade the others.

Just before I left for the night, Papuq Junin leaned over the still body of his son and said in a clear voice, "*Dendeq lupaq diri, anangku. Ndeq kanggo lupaq diri*" (Don't forget yourself, my child. It's not allowed to forget yourself). It is hard to express the sadness that overwhelmed me as I heard those words that are always—and only—spoken to those one fears may die.

September 2

The next morning, as soon as both dawn funeral rituals for Papuq Sari were completed, I gathered my things so that I could take Lo Budin to the hospital in the distant town of Selong. The child was sleeping rest-lessly, and Papuq Junin greeted me with, "Are you ready to go to the doctor?"

At this his wife, generally meek and soft-spoken, turned on him: "It's not allowed to go to the doctor before one has finished with Sasak *belian*s. It is not allowed to mix them. You can take him to Selong, but I won't."

Papuq Junin was silent for a moment, then turned quietly to me and said, "It is better if we go to the spring and have a ritual for the *dewa* first. Tomorrow he will be able to go to Selong."

That afternoon, I went back and taped the women discussing Lo Budin's illness and asking Papuq Isa and Inaq Mol to "try" various treat-ment ideas by the hair-pulling divinations. Lo Budin looked very bad. His eyes, tongue, mouth, arms, and legs were constantly in motion and out of control. His back and his neck were hard and stiff. Various treat-ments were suggested by the crowd of women, but none were confirmed by the divinations.

Late in the afternoon Papuq Junin and his older sons arrived with water blessed at the grave from an ancestor reputed to be a king in a hamlet to the north. Papuq Junin whispered secret words onto the crown of Lo Budin's head and poured the water over the boy's head and body.

A while later, Amaq Mus, a *dukun,* arrived with water from the spring that supplied the reservoir. He handed the water over to Amaq Mol and mouthed secret words over a coconut shell of hot coals, adding incense to them. While Amaq Mol (as religious leader) prayed silently over the water, Papuq Junin and his wife holding Lo Budin hunched over the smoking incense, trapping it with a cloth over their heads and bodies. After five minutes, the cloth was taken away, but Papuq Junin continued to warm his hands in the smoke and lay those hands on the head and stomach of his son. During this, Amaq Mol dipped his hands in the spring water and laid his dripping hand three times on the crown of Lo Budin's head. Then the three men—Papuq Junin, Amaq Mus, and Amaq Mol—agreed that now everything had been completed for the god of the spring, so I could take the child to the hospital in the morning.

September 3

It was barely dawn, and I was already angry with frustration. Word had reached me through the swift Pelocok grapevine that Lo Budin was *too sick to be taken to the doctor!* Straining to be patient, I went to Papuq Junin and asked what had happened. Amaq Mus told me that he had dreamed that the spring god wanted to be fed *jagung ambon* (a kind of tuber), and for that reason the boy had not yet improved. Then Amaq Mus asked me if Amaq Mol—my Sasak father—had dreamed anything. No, I answered. "No? He's the one that should dream about it" (*Ndeq? Iye si mesti are mimpi gen iye*); Amaq Mus continued, saying, "It doesn't work to mix the medicine of a *dewa* and the medicine of a doctor. It doesn't work. The *dewa* must be finished first, and then one can go to the doctor for a shot" (*Ndeq bau tecampur owat dewa dit owat doktor. Ndeq bau. Dewa mesti cukupin juluq aditne lalo jok doktor gen suntikan*).

Papuq Junin added that the spring god had entered (*tume*) Lo Budin. If a doctor tried to give him an injection before the spring god is calm (*tenang*), the needle would not be able to enter the skin. He concluded saying that I could take him to the doctor after a few more rituals for the spring god were completed. I smiled to hide my frustration and left hoping the child would hang on.

Papuq Isa, the *belian*, sympathetically shared my concern that the child was very ill indeed. Then she told me that the spring god was especially angry and not willing to easily be appeased because people in Pelocok had ignored it for so long. Indeed, she laid some of the blame on her oldest son. Long ago when this son's own child had been ill, the son had vowed to "get water" from that same spring if his child were healed.[10] But he had not done so. "It has happened many times like that to that particular spirit. For that reason, Lo Budin is so ill this time," she concluded.

That afternoon, Lo Budin actually seemed improved. Obviously my diagnosis of meningitis could not be correct.[11] Most of his uncontrolled, jerky movements were gone, and the stiffness in his back had relaxed so that he could sit cradled in his father's lap. When I returned home and told Inaq Mol that Lo Budin seemed to be improving, she asked if he were still opening and closing his mouth. Yes, I replied, but less than before. She replied:

It is like goats. *Bantaq Bembeq* is the name. When the mouth is like this [and she demonstrated by opening and closing her mouth

10. To get water (*byetan aiq*) in this context means to hold a ceremony for a spirit or ancestor at a particular place and bring some water that was sanctified during the ceremony back to anoint a person, usually as affirmation of being healed and protection against future illness.
11. According to *Where There Is No Doctor*, my only source for biomedical knowledge in 1994, once ill with meningitis, a person's condition becomes progressively worse unless treated (Werner 1992, 185).

and sticking her tongue out] like Lo Budin, it is like a goat. Often young children are like that. They have met [*ketemuq*] the head of a sacrificed goat. Inaq [Papuq Isa] forgets about this. But I reminded her earlier today, and her words were "it fits with Lo Budin." (*Sepertin bembeq. Bantaq Bembeq arane. Lamun ngene mulutne sepertin Lo Budin, ngeno sepertin bembeq. Kerung kanak kodeq ngeno. Ketemuq iye otak bembeq wah tebegawaiq. Inaq lupa gen iye. Onet ku ketoq ingatanne, ongkatne "cocok ngeno kenca Lo Budin."*)

September 4

When I went to see Lo Budin, I found Papuq Isa massaging his back. She rubbed his back with downward strokes to encourage the illness to go down and out of his body. Then she mouthed a *jampi* onto his back and covered it with betel-juice spittle. Inaq Budin told me that Papuq Isa's massage had stopped all the vomiting, but that the child's back was still sick. The warmth of his back was proof that the sickness was in the back, making it stiff.

September 5–8

I went again to visit Lo Budin. Papuq Junin told me that he had dreamed that Lo Budin was not yet ready (*ndeqne man siap*) to go to the hospital. He had dreamed that yet another ceremony for the *dewa* of the water spring had to be held first—"*Ndeqman buet kenca dewane*" (Not yet finished with the water god).

I never witnessed these ceremonies at the water spring, because, like most healing ceremonies in Pelocok, there was little *ceremony* involved. Siegal notes that Indonesia generally is remarkable for its lack of healing ritual, and Lombok is no exception (Siegal 1978). Most of these "ceremonies" were conducted by Papuq Junin and/or Lo Den (his older son); only once to my knowledge did a healing specialist, a *dukun* (Amaq Mus), conduct a ceremony. I surmise from experiences witnessing similar ceremonies directed at gods and spirits, that the ceremonies at the spring consisted of mouthed prayers said at the spring while incense smoked. After one or more prayers, the participants ate some of the offered food, chewed betel, gathered water, and headed home.

September 9

Surprisingly, when I arrived Inaq Budin was dressed and ready to take Lo Budin to the hospital. As we prepared to leave, Inaq Budin told me that Lo Budin's circumcision had been postponed from one month hence to early the next summer because Lo Den had dreamed that he met Lo Budin's head, which said that he was ill because he was not yet ready to be circumcised.

The events and interactions at the hospital are discussed in chapter 7. Lo Budin remained in the hospital for 10 days, returning to Pelocok on September 19 with cleared lungs and no seizures.

— 5 —

Naming an Illness

> The important part is knowing what the illness is. If it is
> known what it is, the medicine will work. But if the name
> does not fit, the medicine will not work.
> —AMAQ MOL, SEPTEMBER 1994

> Every illness occurrence, in other words, has a name; the
> problem is to find the correct name, since this usually
> dictates the responses to the occurrence . . .
> —HORATIO FABREGA

THE IMPORTANCE OF A NAME

Getting the name right for an illness is the essential first step in successfully coping with its presence. The efficacy of treatment depends
upon it. As we saw in chapter 2, Sasaks generally are not interested in
knowing about the body and its workings for its own sake. Their interests are motivated by particular vulnerabilities and illness episodes.
Likewise the interest in names—in diagnoses and etiologies of illness—
is motivated by and only discussed with reference to a particular illness.[1]

This chapter does not include tables with lists of illnesses, symptoms,
and treatments. Tables would imply a definitive one-to-one correspon-
dence among these three when actually the meanings of illness names
seem to have a more fluid and contingent character. Moreover, we are

---

1. This pragmatic approach to health care is very common among nonspecialists who
often use syncretic blends of medical ideas and treatments (e.g., Kleinman 1980,
93ff.).

interested in how people cope with their health concerns, which involves looking not for one-to-one associations but for processes of dealing with illness.

How does one name an illness? That is, how does one give a salient label to particular perceived conditions that identify an origin or category? The process of giving illness names is actually quite curious.[2] The first trick is to identify when a person is sick. As Lieban notes, "Health and illness constitute a continuum, and when one becomes the other is often vague" (1992, 187). This vagueness is pronounced among rural Sasaks who are perpetually less than healthy, forever seeking out medicine to become fatter, stronger, and more virile. The line between being less than healthy and being ill often depends on whether or not the ailments can be given a specific name.

Naming itself is the second trick. Names are important. A name legitimates an illness and can become both a personal symbol of experience and a social symbol motivating actions and meaning-making. Yet, one can not base a name solely on a person's experience of pain and illness, because persons' experiences are individually different.[3] Moreover, as we have seen for Sasaks, each person has unique understandings of his or her body, unique experiences of vulnerability, unique social relationships and motivations, and unique constellations of knowledge. Even from a biomedical perspective, bodies are not homogeneous; each is genetically and biologically different. Yet, somehow, despite this diversity, people are able to assign particular perceived conditions with categories and names of illness. The question is how.

Most Sasaks assume that if an illness can be correctly named, treatment will "meet" the illness and make it leave. Looking at the naming processes, I suggest that naming is always a matter of more or less creatively connecting persons, situations, symptoms, and vulnerabilities. In the end, Sasak ethnomedicine is personalistic: that is, who a person is and the vulnerabilities he senses are more important than the symptoms he exhibits.

---

2. I use the word *name*—a translation of the Sasak term—which does not mean that each illness is identified with a specific, already known diagnostic name such as *ketemuq* (illness from meeting a ghost) or *barak* (a swelling illness). Sometimes what Sasaks call an illness name refers to an explanation or etiology rather than a distinct, one-word identification. Thus I use *illness name* as a shorthand for a discrete interpretation or understanding of an illness.

3. For the symbolic nature of illness names see, e.g., Lieban 1992; Turner 1967. For works on the experience of illness see, e.g., Finkler 1994a; Good et al. 1992.

DEFINITIONS

How are we to study and understand the largely nonorderly actions of people in pluralistic medical settings? Here and in the next two chapters we address this question by examining the processes through which people come up with, decide on, and follow through on knowledge that they use to cope with illness. To do this, we must begin with a definition of illness.

The standard definition in medical anthropology defines *illness* in contradistinction to *disease*. *Disease* designates a biomedically categorized physical or physiological disorder. Identifying something as a disease is only significant within the understandings of anatomy, physiology, etiology, and biochemistry promoted by biomedicine. In the biomedical system, there is only one disease for each array of symptoms. Moreover, as an objective event, disease is without inherent meaning. On the other hand, *illness* is the term used to designate all identifications of disorder usually related to physical bodies. Illness may, but does not necessarily, map onto a disease. Illnesses are disorders recognized as meaningful within any particular medical setting. The difficulty with these definitions, useful as they are, is that they tend to privilege biomedical disease as "real" in opposition to the cultural constructedness of illness. In other words, embedded within the terminology are cultural presumptions that place higher value on the objective and scientific over the subjective and cultural.[4] The political weight of the terminology is thus problematic. Actually, because all medical systems including biomedicine are ethnomedical, one could call everything *illnesses*, giving local and biomedical judgments the same value. Here, I do so, reserving the word *disease* to refer to the result of the diagnostic (or name-giving) process used by biomedicine.

In this chapter, I refer to the processes of identifying an illness as *naming* (as opposed to *diagnosing*) for two reasons. First, the word *diagnosis* is defined as "the act or process of identifying or determining the nature and cause of a disease or injury through evaluation of patient history, examination, and review of laboratory data" (*American Heritage Dictionary*, 3d ed., 1996). To the extent that diagnosis is an interpretive process, it is a synonym of *naming;* however as the dictionary makes clear, *diagnosis* implies a biomedical scientific method that does not fit the interpretive processes used by most rural Sasaks to evaluate

---

4. See, e.g., Hahn 1995; Lindenbaum and Lock 1993.

illness.[5] Second, the verb *to name*, a direct translation of the Sasak word *aran*, foregrounds the similarities between naming a child so that its name fits its spiritual being and naming an illness so that its name fits the illness's essence. The interpretive emphasis is on *fit*, whether naming a child or an illness. If a name fits, then it has direct repercussions on health. A child's name that fits makes him less vulnerable to illness. An illness name that fits correlates to sure treatment. Diagnosis only recognizes an illness. But naming an illness correctly means that most of the work of treatment is already done.

ILLNESS AND TREATMENT:
CULTURAL KNOWLEDGE

There are certain assumptions about illness and treatment that are widely distributed in Pelocok. Indeed, they are so unquestionably true in everyday usage that I understand these assumptions as cultural knowledge. Specifically, the metaphors used in everyday conversations, basic illness categories, and treatment strategies are so widely dispersed throughout Pelocok that they are largely unquestioned areas of cultural knowledge.[6]

Metaphors of Illness and Treatment

In chapter 2, we examined how cultural knowledge about bodies in relation to illness was reflected in Sasak metaphors. Here I highlight the metaphors Sasaks use when discussing illness and treatment.

Illness is an entity that *tauq* (is capable of, knows) and *meleq* (wants):

---

5. Finkler (1994b) argues that although diagnosis is supposed to be based on symptoms, medical history, and examination, she found that it is in large part based on the physician's personal experience, moral values, and stereotypes about the patient's population (184). This suggests that, in actuality, the processes of diagnosis are closer to the Sasak processes of naming than a dictionary definition of diagnosis would suggest.

6. Based on scattered conversations with Sasaks from all over the island, I suspect these assumptions are widely dispersed among Sasaks throughout Lombok—whether rural or urban. How widely distributed these assumptions actually are and whether they could justifiably be called cultural knowledge for the whole Sasak population is a question that needs exploration. Whatever the answer, it would have substantial consequences for the development of biomedical health care on Lombok.

Lamun ndeq tebebubusanne, tauqne tume penyakit jemaq.
If [the infant] is not bebubused [a red betel dot of prevention placed on its forehead] illness will be able to [know to] enter later.

Ite urut ngeno serene aditne tauq turun penyakitne.
We massage in this way so that the illness will be capable of going down.

Ndeqne meleq sugul penyakitne.
It doesn't want to go out, the illness.

Lamun cocok jampine, melet sakitne turun.
If the healing spell fits, the illness wants to go down.

Tauq and *meleq* are both verbs indicating agency. *Tauq* means to be capable of doing something. It involves agency and impetus to act. The failure to do a preventive act or the act of undergoing a treatment give illness an *opportunity* to act—to enter a person or to go down and eventually out of a person. What the illness does is not an automatic reaction to either the prevention or the treatment; if it were, the word in the sentences above would be *bauq* rather than *tauq*. The verb *bauq* is best translated as "to be possible to happen"; it is a passive rather than an active verb. It is possible to say in Sasak an illness "*tauqne sugul laguq ndeqne man bauq*" (an illness is capable of going out but it hasn't happened yet), but it would make no sense to people to say that an illness "*bauqne sugul laguq ndeqne man tauq*" (it is possible for an illness to go out but it isn't yet capable or motivated to do so).[7] Motivation and agency have logical priority for something happening with regard to illness. Like humans, spirits, and other agents, illnesses can *want* to leave or not. After a treatment, if the illness does not want to leave, another treatment must be sought. *Jampi,* secret healing words or spells, convince an illness that it wants to leave. In summary, illness is not an event that happens as the result of malfunctioning or disrupted biological processes, illness is an agent acting of its own accord in the world.

The metaphors used in speaking of treatment are *bedait* and *cocok*. *Bedait* means "to meet," such as when someone meets someone else on a road. *Cocok* means "to fit, to be right for," such as when a name is said to fit a person. When speaking of treatments, the following are common:

---

7. See the discussion of *tauq* and *bauq* in the Introduction.

Wahan dait iye jampine, sehat wah.
After the healing spell has met it [the illness] one is healthy already.

Jampine si Amaq sino ndeq cocok, ndeqne dait iye.
The healing spells of that *dukun* did not fit, they did not meet it [the illness].

Lamun cocok aran, jampine tauq bedait nyakitne wah.
If the name fits, the healing spell knows/is capable of meeting the illness already.

Lamun cocok jampine, melet sakitne turun.
If the healing spell fits, the illness wants to go down.

The connotations of each of these metaphors are slightly different. Spells that meet (*bedait*) an illness are said to solve the problem. Normally when people meet (*bedait*) they interact, they converse. What is implied in using this metaphor to describe a treatment is that two agents—the healing words and the illness—meet and interact so that the spell can convince or motivate the illness to leave the body. The *jampi* (spell, healing words) is a kind of *ilmu,* thus the words have their own agency. If the *jampi* does not meet the illness, the spell can have no effect on the illness. In order to meet, the spell must fit (*cocok*): it must be the correct one for that particular illness. As the last sentence implies, if the *jampi* is correct, the illness will want to go down and eventually out of the body. This sentence suggests that the *jampi* is less an agent than a tool chosen to fit the project at hand. Ambiguously, a *jampi* is a treatment that both has and does not have agency in convincing illness to leave bodies.

Both of these connotations are decidedly different from the ways people talk about other kinds of treatment. Indeed, I found no consistently used metaphors when people described other treatments, although the phrase *aditne pecat sehat* (quickly become well) was common:

Munne beselipme, daun kelor tekadu leq mata khaki aditne pecat sehat.
If one has the sniffles, the leaves of the kelor tree are used on the ankles [eyes of the feet] so that one quickly becomes well.

Lamun mandi leq Kaliantan, wah, wah sakitande.
If you bathe at Kaliantan, your pains [illnesses] will disappear.

Wahan sugul penyakitne, bauq iye jok doktor aditne pecat sehat.
After the illness has come out, it is possible for him to go to a doctor so that he will quickly become well.

In contrast to the ways people talk about treatment with *jampi*, here, whether the treatment is an everyday remedy, "bathing" in a potent place, or one given by a doctor, the focus is not on dealing with the illness-as-agent but on becoming well. This does not mean that these illnesses have no agency, but rather it implies that there are some forms of illness that can be treated automatically with specific remedies that fit them (such as the kelor leaves) or with potencies so powerful that all illness will disappear. When discussing treatments other than *jampi* what is significant is to "quickly become well"—in other words, with few exceptions, these treatments are to speed the healing process, rather than directly deal with the illnesses themselves. As healers repeatedly told me, what is important is the *jampi*—other treatment strategies are only aimed at quickening the healing process. This is particularly true of biomedical treatments, which were often delayed until after it was supposed that the illness had been met and made to go out of the body by a *jampi*.

These metaphors suggest that illnesses have agency that needs to be acted upon by correct healing words. The dynamic between illness-as-agent and healing words is cultural knowledge among rural Sasaks. This is not to deny that other treatments can be beneficial and used to good effect. Rather, when speaking of other treatment strategies, there is never any mention of how those treatments make the illness leave the body. This suggests that other treatments are indeed less central to Sasak ways of coping with illness.

Basic Categories: Illness and Treatment

Sasak people differentiate two categories of illness: usual illnesses (*penyakit biese*) and unusual illnesses (*penyakit ndeq biese*). The difference between the two categories is more a matter of degree than a distinct line. Usual illnesses are those that generally last less than three weeks, that respond quickly to simple treatments, that do not exhibit particularly strange symptoms, or that are chronic, lasting years. Coughs, fevers, congestions, aches, stomach pains, broken bones, fatigue, diarrhea, vomiting, weight loss, not growing fat, and swelling are some of the more common physical symptoms of usual illnesses. But if any of these drag out for weeks or months, do not improve with simple lay or specialist remedies, or are accompanied by dreams suggestive of black magic, people begin to refer to the illness as not usual. Thus Sasaks have a simple illness hierarchy leading from usual illness to unusual illness.

For the purposes of clarification, it is useful to compare this Sasak distinction with a similar distinction outlined by Laderman for rural Malays (1991, 15, 40). These Malay-Indonesian speakers also have two categories of illness: usual (Indon., *biasa*) and unusual (Indon., *luar biasa*). As with the Sasak, Malays do not draw a sharp distinction between these two categories, but understand "usual" illness to be linked to humoral imbalances and unusual illness to be that which does not respond to everyday and typical treatments. The primary difference between the Malay and the Sasak categories is that for Malays the presence of an unusual illness means that the person is not whole or balanced—he has a weakened life force, too many inner winds—which has left him open to spirit attacks. Treatment must be directed toward making the person whole and balanced again, sometimes through elaborate séances. In spite of the remarkable similarities between Sasak and Malay categorization, with this link to personhood the similarities break down.

As we have seen, the Sasak concept of personhood does not have an analogous notion of life force or inner winds that can protect individuals from harmful spirits. A Sasak's best protection is ownership of *ilmu,* but even then most persons experience vulnerabilities. Everyone is less than healthy, and everyone experiences herself as vulnerable in certain contexts. Treatment does not involve making a person whole, but rather forcing an illness or a spirit out of the person, leaving the person pretty much as she was beforehand. Treatment does not change the integrity of the person. In fact, it does not even aim at healing the ill body. The goal of treatment is to force the illness to leave the body, so that the body has the possibility of reverting to its normal state.

Basic Treatment Strategies

The essence of Sasak medicine is words. Secret, potent *ilmu* whispered or breathed onto a medical medium or directly onto an ill body for purposes of treatment are called *jampi. Jampi* are more formulaic than the small words of prevention (*kata kodeq* or *puji*). Like *puji,* all *jampi* begin with the Arabic words invoking God—*bismillah irrahman irrahhim* (In the name of Allah, most Gracious, most Merciful). Once when I had repeated a *jampi* to Papuq Isa so that she could check that I had written it down correctly, I forgot to begin with the Arabic phrase. She stopped me and told me that it was *rukun* and therefore obligatory. Never did I hear a detailed explanation as to why the phrase was essential, but I suspect that invoking Allah is crucial to the efficacy of the secret words.[8]

After invoking Allah, *jampi* consist of anywhere from two to ten lines in couplets of like-sounding, rhythmic lines. All the *jampi* I know were given to me in secret, with firm admonishments not to give them to anyone else. Thus, to illustrate the substance of *jampi* without breaking my promises, below is the *jampi* in translation from Sasak that I was given by Papuq Isa used to accompany a massage for *salah urat* (blocked or twisted fluid passages, analogous to blood vessels).

> In the name of Allah, most Gracious, most Merciful
> [Two onomatopoeic sounds repeated once, without meaning but
>   indicating abrupt stoppages]
> I make a ditch [groove or moat for the passage of fluid] quickly
> The fluid passage which is weak and constrained
> I reorganize the fluid passage so that it is normal
> Leave, I am washing you with my healing words
> Thus I treat *salah urat*.

As this example indicates, *jampi* describe the problem of the illness—in this case fluid passages that are weak and constrained—as well as the appropriate treatment—remaking the passages so that fluid flows normally.

All *jampi* conclude with the same two final lines. The first of these, "Leave, I am washing you with my healing words," is significant for three reasons. First, the illness is ordered to "leave," to go out of the body, which implies that the illness is not healed but rather made to depart.[9] Second, the illness is made to leave by being "washed," a word that brings images of mundane bathing as well as ritual bathing, implying that illness is analogous to dirt or impurity that must be washed away.[10]

---

8. This interpretation fits with Islamic theology that everything exists and works because of Allah.

9. See chapter 2 for a discussion of the metaphors of enter and go out in reference to bodies and the movements of illness.

10. One could argue that if illness is considered an impurity, making the illness leave actually does change the person as it is a cleansing of impurities. This contradicts my argument that *jampi* are to make an illness leave rather than to heal the body/person. Both interpretations fit the materials. I suggest that the emphasis on the impurity of illness slips in and out of focus for people in coping with illness episodes. Impurity

Third, the medium of the washing away of illness is words, not water; words have the power to cleanse and purify. Thus, illness in this one line becomes a multivocal entity: something that must leave, something impure, and something that is moved by words.

Then the final line of all *jampi* is "Thus I treat *name-of-illness*." It is in the description of illness and the imperative that the illness leave through the washing with words that illness is treated. The treatment is the words. Moreover, the naming of the illness in the last line of the *jampi* may itself be potent. Others have shown that for many peoples, if something can be named it can be controlled.[11] In addition, among Sasaks, in naming an illness, the *jampi* gains superiority over it and thus the potency necessary to make the illness depart.

Each *jampi* is illness-specific. While the above *jampi* is considered efficacious for any incidence of *salah urat,* it will not work on *kurang darah* (not enough blood). If an illness is treated with a *jampi* that is not perceived to be efficacious, often a different name for the illness will be sought and matched to a different *jampi*. As we have seen, Sasaks consider names of persons potent in the sense that incorrect names lead to illness, and names that fit lead to health. Likewise, the name of an illness must fit in order for treatments to work. As Amaq Mol's statement that opened this chapter says, for treatment to work, the name of the illness must fit, it must be correct.

What is the mechanism through which words meet an illness in order to force it to leave? I asked this question one day while I was listening to Papuq Isa and her daughter-in-law talk about healing patients. At first they assumed that I was asking how one knows which *jampi* to use. The daughter-in-law, Inaq Sur, replied: "You see the patient, recognize the name of the illness, and you know already which *jampi* is right" (*Gitaq si sakitne, terus te tandoqin aranne. Tauq wah jampi si kenaq*). While this was interesting in itself, I eventually got back to my original question, and after repeating it in every possible way, both the daughter-in-law and Papuq Isa burst out in roars of laughter. No, there is no path, no road, no mechanism that brings the *jampi* to meet the ill-

---

implies that the person is somehow at fault or responsible for the illness. But in most cases such a moral stance on illness seems, if not completely absent, at least silent and dark in the background. Although it is more common in cases of unusual illness, it is still rare for a person to be faulted for becoming ill. Moreover, no person is ever avoided or ostracized for being ill—just the opposite: people swarm around to keep the person company. Overall, in my opinion an interpretation of Sasak healing that foregrounds illness treatment as cleansing impurities would badly miss the mark.

11. See the literature on magic and the power of words (e.g., Tambiah 1990).

ness. If the name is correct, the words just meet it already.[12] The key is in identifying the correct name.

But for three reasons, even when the name is correct, *jampi* do not always work. First, and most important, *jampi* are secret knowledge. Thus no one's *jampi* are the same. Some people are said to have better *jampi* than others. Also, because they are mouthed or breathed rather than spoken, it is relatively easy for a person to misplace a word or forget a line, thus making the *jampi* ineffectual. Because *jampi* are effective only if expressed precisely, Sasaks acknowledge the possibility of error caused by forgetting and the resulting ineffectuality of the treatment.[13]

Second, some illnesses seem to require that the *jampi* be administered through accompanying mediums—smoking incense, sprays of water, certain foods, certain ritual prayers, chewed betel. From those I spoke with there was no clear consensus as to when an accompanying medium was absolutely necessary and what that medium should be. Indeed, some people favor certain mediums over others—Papuq Isa nearly always used chewed betel, Amaq Sunin never used betel but rather used mixtures in water, and Papuq Ali always used sprays of water—arguing that the treatment would not work otherwise.

Finally, in one case, the case of Lo Budin, there was some indication that *jampi* must be administered by someone pure, or at least superficially clean. Otherwise the *jampi* would be rendered ineffectual by the dirtiness of the person administering it. Together, these three qualifications render the business of treatment even more problematic: not only must the name of the illness be correctly identified and matched to the correct *jampi*, but the *jampi* must be perfectly recited over the correct medium (if one is necessary at all) by someone who was clean of dirt, grime, and other impurities.

Then, once a *jampi* has met an illness and made it leave—sometimes a gradual process requiring days or weeks—the symptoms must still be treated so that the person can return to normal. This is where massages, special diets, herbal teas, pills, and injections come in. These, according to rural Sasaks, are designed to help the body regain its preillness strength, to restore its normal flow of fluids, and to make a person fat.

---

12. In their response, I was reminded of Evans-Pritchard's words about the Azande: "How do Azande think their medicines work? They do not think very much about the matter" (1976, 200).

13. Forgetting secret knowledge as a recognized problem of social reproduction has been noted by a number of anthropologists, particularly in connection with the reproduction of ritual (see Barth 1975; George 1996).

Thus, the treatment of illness is really two processes. The first and most important is the correct administration of secret knowledge to make the illness leave the body. The second and lesser aspect of treatment is the administration of tactile medicines (herbs, pills, injections, massages, foods) designed to restore the weakened body to its normal state. More than once, when I questioned healers or laypersons about not administering the medicines I had seen them use for similar cases, they responded that those items were not handy at the moment, but "it doesn't matter, the *jampi* is the necessary part" (*Ndeqne mbe-mbe, jampine si usah*). In the treatment of both usual and unusual illnesses, the most important step is to name the illness correctly.

NAMING USUAL ILLNESS

For usual illness, there is typically little or no debate about a name. These are not illnesses that people tend to worry about.[14] Upon recognizing an illness in themselves or others, if they happen to know a *jampi* or other medicine for that illness, they will treat it on the spot. Whenever possible, people feeling ill will stay home, avoid working, and chat with neighbors passing the compound or go visiting themselves. To whomever they encounter, Sasaks are very likely to voice their complaints, saying that they are ill with a pained back (*sakit bongkor*), sick stomach (*sakit tian*), runny nose (*selipme*), and so forth. More likely than not, someone in their audience will start chewing betel as a precursor to saying a *jampi,* or will recommend they go seek medicine from so and so, or sometimes, if it is a very close friend, s/he will go retrieve a precious bit of bark or a bottle of healing oils and mix a healing drink for the person—after mouthing a *jampi* into the glass of liquid. Everyone—except the smallest children—has *jampi* and knows remedies for ailments. Everyone is a potential healer.

The typical naming of usual illness and dispensing of treatments is done with as little focus as hushing a crying child. Illness, like a crying child, requires attention, but both are such everyday, mundane occurrences that they cause no great excitement, and people carry on other

---

14. The exception to this is *sakit toaq,* the illness of old age. When old people start to die, everyone recognizes the name of the illness, and although some people try *jampi* to help prolong their lives, everyone realizes that ultimately there is no treatment for it. Nonetheless, this usual illness causes much heartache, worry, and grief among family and neighbors, who gather, sitting for days at a time with the old person, to see and be with them before they die.

conversations and continue with other interests, while comforting a child or preparing a herbal healing drink. In the course of visiting on any given day, I heard between three and seven complaints of illness. Early in the fieldwork, I followed up every mention of a headache, feeling of fatigue, or runny nose with extensive questions. But it was not long before I realized I was the only one pursuing the complaints with such interest. Others would nod or say something noncommittal about how ill one feels with a runny nose, and the topic of conversation would shift to the crops in the fields or the neighborhood gossip. Then, sometime later, without another word being said about the complaint, someone in the circle would turn to the person with the complaint and mention that she should wet kelor leaves and put them on the eyes of her ankles, and then her nasal congestion would be clear! There was no lack of real interest or concern regarding the ailments of others; neighbors and friends freely gave remedies for usual illness with the single mention of the complaint. Offering remedies and *jampi* is a show of goodwill and friendship. The apparent lack of interest merely reflects the low level of anxiety regarding the ailment. Naming everyday illnesses and dispensing everyday treatments is part and parcel of normal, everyday social interactions.

The complexities involved in naming usual illnesses become most clear in cases in which the same symptoms are explained with different names, and different symptoms are explained with the same names. Below are three cases of usual illness that illustrate these dynamics.

Case 1: Same Illness, Different Names

Inaq Suli was the wife of a *dukun*, the mother of eight, and lived in my compound. I was visiting with Papuq Isa one morning in August 1994, when Inaq Suli arrived with her youngest son on her hip, carrying a small basket filled with rice (half a kilogram), a circle of cotton string, a 50 Rp coin, and betel chewing materials.[15] She sat down quietly on the *barugah* (covered platform) while Papuq Isa and her neighbor gossiped about the divorce of a mutual acquaintance. Gradually, Inaq Suli entered the conversation, getting a short version of who had divorced and why. Papuq Isa reached over and opened the basket; she started to work the betel nut, leaf, and lime chalk in her *pelocok* and handed the

---

15. In total, the contents of the basket would have been worth about 350 Rp (a third of a day's average income) if Inaq Suli had had to purchase them. Everything but the coin she had assembled from the family supplies stored in bins in the attic of her hut.

coin to one of her grandchildren milling about, which he took with glee and headed off to a kiosk to buy some candy. Inaq Suli mentioned that her son was ill with diarrhea. Papuq Isa asked if he had been ill long. "No, just a few days," came the reply. I asked if Inaq Suli's husband had not treated him. "Yes but his *jampi* had not wanted to work," she answered. Papuq Isa took the boy in her lap, and noted, "*Panas tianne. Ngeno mentretne*" (His stomach is hot. That is the way with diarrhea). Then mouthing a *jampi,* she spit betel juice on his stomach and rubbed it in so that he had an orangish-red circle covering his belly. The treatment was finished. She had named the illness as one of simple diarrhea from too hot a stomach.

Then Inaq Suli mentioned that she had begun taking birth control pills five months ago and wondered whether they were affecting the boy's health. Immediately, with rare anger in her voice, Papuq Isa lectured: "The pill is what is making this boy ill. It is not necessary to drink such as that. Stop it already" (*Pilne miaq Lo iniq sakit. Ndeqne ulaq ninum si ngeno. Wahan wah*). Papuq Isa told Inaq Suli that the boy would not become well until she quit using birth control. Inaq Suli was silent. After a long pause, attention shifted to making lunch, and Inaq Suli and I left for our compound.

As soon as we were out of earshot, Inaq Suli lamented that she had only started taking the pill because she did not want more children and was afraid of dying in childbirth. She asked me if I thought she should stop taking the pill. Rather than answering, I asked about her son. Apparently, he was often sick, and lately he had gotten thinner and thinner. I noted his mild fever, swollen feet, and thin arms and thought he was probably suffering from malnutrition. I suggested that she feed the boy beans and eggs as often as possible and told her how to mix homemade rehydration therapy for the diarrhea.

Later that afternoon, Inaq Suli came by and asked if I thought the medicine of a doctor might help her son. Saying that it might, I agreed to accompany her to the clinic in Lindung—a 45-minute walk away. After exchanging initial pleasantries with the clinician, I was silent, allowing Inaq Suli to converse directly with him. She told of the boy's diarrhea and how he did not want to get fat. The clinician took the boy's blood pressure and temperature, then began collecting pills in a bag and lecturing on the importance of washing hands before handling food and boiling water. He gave her the pills explaining the dosage to give the boy and asked for 1,000 Rp (a day's wages) in payment. I paid the bill, asking him for his diagnosis. He answered in Indonesian, "Diarrhea because of dirtiness" (*Mentret karena keko-*

toranya). Just before we left Inaq Suli asked him if birth control pills could be linked to the illness. No, he said.

On this one day, only Papuq Isa's initial illness name of diarrhea due to a hot stomach attributed the illness solely to a detectable physical symptom. All the other etiologies suggested—birth control pills, malnutrition, dirtiness—called upon knowledge not specific to the boy's symptoms. Inaq Suli was obviously concerned about a possible connection between birth control pills and her son's diarrhea; she made the initial suggestion of that etiology. Papuq Isa had a long-standing disapproval of birth control pills; the new information reinforced her opinion that biomedical birth control methods were dangerous, and she morally condemned Inaq Suli and biomedicine for the illness.[16] My unspoken diagnosis of malnutrition was based not on observations of what Inaq Suli fed her children, but on a general understanding of children's diet in Pelocok; my illness name blamed the mother and the poverty of the community for the child's illness. The clinician's etiology made an assumption about the cleanliness of Inaq Suli's house and cooking techniques based on his general assumption that all rural Sasaks are ignorant of proper ways to prepare food safely. All three of these etiologies were formed by drawing on general assumptions and prejudices. Papuq Isa would never have made the connection between the child's illness and birth control pills if the mother had not suggested it. Had the child been the son of a wealthy townsperson, I should have never thought of the possibility of malnutrition, any more than the clinician would have inferred dirty living conditions. The etiologies we constructed had less to do with the boy's symptoms than with the context.

Case 2: Same Symptoms, Different Persons,
Different Names

One day in March 1994, both Amaq Mol and I awoke with dry coughs and sore throats. I was utterly exhausted and only wanted to sleep. Amaq Mol complained of aches and also slept most of the day. Neither of us ate much. Both of us had worked the day before in the cool, dry mountain fields with Amaq Sunin, La Nan, and one of the young sons.

---

16. Papuq Isa's etiology could also be read as an implied criticism of the national birth control program, whose personnel strongly urge and frequently coerce women into accepting one of four birth control methods: IUD, pill, monthly injections, or implants (Norplant).

No one else was ill. According to our expressed symptoms, Amaq Mol and I seemed to me to have the same thing.

Inaq Mol hovered over me most of the day. She would interrupt my sleep to bring me food and tea, which I had no desire to consume, and to bring in visiting neighbors, whom I had no desire to see. Conversations with these visitors followed similar patterns beginning with:

> *Visitor:* Ah, Cameron is ill.
> *Ehh, Eron sakit.*
> *Cameron:* Yes. Ill. I cough all the time and am very tired.
> *Ayo. Sakit. Ku batuk terus, lelah endah.*
> *Visitor:* Yes. You are ill with cough and tiredness.
> *Ayo. Ide sakit batuk dit lelah.*
> Or, Cough. Have you already drunk the water of a betel leaf?
> *Ooq. Batuk. Wah teninum aiq lakoq?*
> Or, Yes. [Touching my hand] You are cold. A wind has entered you [you have a cold].
> *Ayo. Nyet ide. Masuk angin ngeno.*
> Or, You don't know how to work. You are not strong like people here. Don't go to the forest [mountain fields] again. You are not capable. The result is sickness.
> *Ide ndeqne tauq begawaian. Ndeq kuat mara dengan iteh. Dendeq jok gawa malik. Ndeqne tauq ide. Sakit jarine.*

There were about a half-dozen of these well-intentioned visitors in all. Had I felt slightly less miserable, I would have been more attentive to their words and less irritated at their constant interrupting of my sleep. As it was, I paid their assorted illness names little mind. Eventually, Inaq Mol asked Papuq Isa to look at me.

She examined me by feeling the back of my neck. Saying "*tabey*" (excuse me),[17] she put her hands on my head and blew air onto my forehead twice, pausing between each to mouth a *jampi*. Then she repeated the process, this time blowing on the back of my neck. Afterward she and Inaq Mol together decided that the illness was the result of my working in the mountain fields. Calling for a dish of cooking oil,

---

17. *Tabey* (excuse me) is said whenever a healer needs to touch the head of another person, although the formality is always ignored with small children. The taboo against touching another person's head is common throughout many places in Indonesia and mainland Southeast Asia. Sasaks have no similar restrictions for touching any other part of the body among like sexes.

Papuq Isa then began to massage my arms and legs. When I asked her directly what the illness was, she named it *salah urat*—twisted or blocked fluid passages in my hands and feet. My cough, sore throat, and exhaustion were apparently due to a humoral imbalance caused by blockages in my hands and feet, in turn caused by physical labor.

In contrast, Amaq Mol received very little attention during the day, nor was he treated by Papuq Isa when she came to see me. From the frequency of his cough and the number of his complaints, I had assumed he was much more ill than myself. Early in the morning, before I had given up the struggle and had gone to bed for the day, the family gathered as usual for a morning glass of coffee. Although we both coughed, Amaq Mol was the only one to give voice to his complaints saying how everything hurt (*seleputne sakit*). Without once touching him, Amaq Sunin, the son-in-law, said he had *sakit tian*, a sick stomach. Amaq Sunin went to a corner of the house and, with his back turned to us, fumbled in a sack he pulled out of hiding for a chip of wood. He shaved bits of the *kayu putiq* (white wood) into a glass of boiled water.[18] Holding the glass, he mouthed a *jampi* onto it. Amaq Mol drank the mixture, tied a square of pink cloth around his head as he always did when he had a headache, and went to bed for the day.

This is a case of two people in the same household on the same day exhibiting, in my opinion, the same symptoms. Yet, the names people gave to the illnesses were strikingly different. Considering that I was still relatively new in the community, and household members had often expressed fears that they would get in trouble if harm should come to me, it was unsurprising that I received more attention than Amaq Mol.[19] But the names given to my illness—a cough, cold, exhaustion, twisted fluid passages—are surprisingly different from the ill stomach name given to Amaq Mol's illness.

The differences can be attributed to how I was perceived in contrast to Amaq Mol. I was considered incapable of physical labor and weak; as one woman put it all too plainly: "You don't know how to work. You are not strong like people here." Moreover, although I was not blamed, this

---

18. At another time, I watched Amaq Sunin use the *kayu putiq* in the same fashion, but he said then it was to replenish a deficit of white water/blood. In this, his treatment fits nicely with the humoral logic of correcting a humoral imbalance homeopathically. In his treatment for Amaq Mol, Sunin mentions no humoral deficit, simply implying that the white wood, together with boiled water, breath, and a *jampi*, would solve the problem of a sick stomach.

19. While Radan Suwetomo had emphasized to the family that they would have to take care of me when he placed me in their home, neither he nor any government official had cause to warn them of dire consequences should anything happen to me.

woman's verb choice of the active *tauq* (to know, to be capable of) rather than the passive *bauq* added an edge of personal culpability to my illness. In their eyes, my soft, white skin and my life as a student left me perpetually incapable of field labor, and I should have known better than to attempt it. With the exception of Papuq Isa's physical examination, this etiology pointing to overwork was based on a general perception of my personal vulnerabilities and knowledge of what I had done the previous day. A similar etiology would not fit with Amaq Mol, who had worked his entire life in the fields. He was not vulnerable to manual labor; indeed, as a person of Pelocok, Amaq Mol was by definition strong: recall the woman's words, "You are not strong like people here." Different perceptions of our personhoods prompted different interpretations of our illnesses.

In my opinion, we were both suffering from colds, as some of my visitors had suggested in the words *masuk angin*.[20] Colds are common ailments that just happen and are not attributed to any weakness or wrongdoing. These visitors named my illness based on my cough and cold skin, on my physical symptoms, rather than on my personhood. I preferred calling my illness a cold, in part because it fit most of the symptoms, but also because I was too proud to admit that I could not work in the fields without suffering from exhaustion afterward. In the end, my pride was humbled, for a "cold" was not the name that stuck; in the following days, people frequently admonished me not to work in the fields anymore.[21] The etiology that stuck linked the illness to personhood.

Amaq Sunin's name of ill stomach for Amaq Mol's illness was not based on estimations of personhood and vulnerability. *Sakit tian* is a common illness name and not associated with any of the typical vulnerabilities. Nor was Amaq Mol particularly susceptible to ill stomachs.

---

20. *Masuk angin* literally means "entered winds," implying that it is the result of a humoral imbalance of too much wind. I translate *masuk angin* as "cold" here because its symptoms and its perceived seriousness are the same as a cold in the United States. The term *masuk angin* used in naming the symptoms of colds is common throughout Malay-Indonesian Southeast Asia.

21. Ignoring the recommendations of Inaq and Amaq Mol, I continued to work in the fields, arguing that it was part of my study. Eventually I learned how to work without bloodying my hands or dropping from exhaustion. Others praised my work in the fields and seemed to enjoy my company. Inaq and Amaq Mol, until the last, preferred I did not work in part so that I would not hurt myself, but also in part to protect my status as higher than that of others, thereby protecting their own privileged status as my host family. In this way, I fear I was a disappointment, because being more quietly stubborn than they, I was determined to live in ways that distinguished myself from others as little as possible.

But unlike colds, ill stomachs are potentially serious and therefore legitimate more elaborate treatments. Amaq Sunin was a new son-in-law at the time, eager to prove that he had potent *ilmu*. As is fairly common practice among *dukun*s but uncommon among *belian*s, he gave the name without touching the patient. Moreover, the name of *sakit tian* gave Amaq Sunin an excuse to pull out a unique treatment medium— the white wood—as proof of his wisdom. In this case, I suspect that the name given to Amaq Mol's illness had less to do with his personhood or symptoms than with the motivations and knowledge of Amaq Sunin.

Case 3: Many Cases of Illness with Various Symptoms, but the Same Name

Ketemuq is the illness that results from meeting a ghost and is considered a usual, mundane sort of illness. Most adults in Pelocok know a *jampi* and various remedies for *ketemuq* and are likely to perform them on themselves while working in a field or chatting at a ritual. The treatment strategies are various, but the ones I most commonly saw were (1) putting a bit of lime chalk in the belly button of the victim after mouthing a *jampi* over it, (2) yanking on a tuft of hair while breathing a *jampi* until there was a popping sound of the scalp pulling away from the skull, and (3) being sprayed by someone else with a mouthful of water that had previously had a *jampi* mouthed over it. All of these treatments are done with little fuss. In terms of its seriousness, having *ketemuq* can be equated with having a cold in the United States. Although we might complain of the symptoms, we say, "it is just a cold," and go about our normal business.

I recorded 16 cases of *ketemuq* in Pelocok, although undoubtedly there were many more. These cases suggest trends that further investigation could prove false or true. First, two-thirds of the cases, 11, occurred to females whereas I counted only 5 instances of male *ketemuq*. This might suggest that women are perceived as more vulnerable to meeting ghosts. Second, in chapter 3, I showed how Sasaks consider the likelihood of meeting a ghost to be highest during times of rituals and ceremonies because ancestors are said to return to join in the festivities. Yet, among the cases I recorded, only 4 occurred during rituals and ceremonies. This suggests that while the common assumption that rituals are times of vulnerability is true, vulnerability to *ketemuq* in everyday life is an equally valid concern. Finally, and most interesting in terms of naming illness, is the variety of symptoms that identified the illness as *ketemuq*.

The most common expressed symptom (in 8 cases) was a sudden stomachache (*sakit tian*). People would rub their stomachs and complain that it hurt or churned (using hand signals, making circles with a fist). Nor did it matter what symptoms accompanied the stomachache—whether a fever, diarrhea, or childbirth—the name given was *ketemuq*.

For instance, I arrived about an hour late for the birth of Inaq Teli's third child. The *belian*, Papuq Isa, was asleep on a mat on the dirt floor, the wailing child swaddled beside her. Inaq Teli sat dozing on a blanketed half-coconut, propped upright by a four-foot-high stack of pillows.[22] There was a large smudge of blood across her right temple and cheek. She smiled as I entered. Sitting down in the dirt, I asked if she and the baby were healthy. She answered me, saying, "The birth was easy. The painful part is the waiting before the birth. But immediately after the baby came out, I met a dead person. Oh, my stomach hurts. Do you have anything for it? [I shook my head.] Oh, it hurts. Right after the baby came out, to meet a dead person." The *belian* had awakened by this time, picked up the wailing infant, and added as if waving aside the importance Inaq Teli was giving to her discomfort, "*Ketemuq.* I have already treated it."

Two things are striking in this instance. First, it is surprising that stomach pain immediately after giving birth should be attributed to meeting a dead person, rather than as a consequence of childbirth (i.e., normal postpartum uterine contractions). In making the impersonal statement that "the painful part is the waiting before the birth," Inaq Teli seems to be expressing a bit of common knowledge—perhaps common knowledge validated personally for her by her previous birth experiences. Stomach pain after childbirth is not part of the expected experience of childbirth, therefore the pain is attributed to another cause. Second, it is striking that Papuq Isa waves aside Inaq Teli's pain, saying in effect, "It is only *ketemuq,* and I've treated it, so be patient and it will go away." The experience of pain becomes irrelevant by naming the illness *ketemuq,* and she thereby silences any further expressions of pain. It is significant to note the difference between the experience of *ketemuq* as an uncomfortably painful stomach and the name of *ketemuq,*

---

22. The half-coconut symbolizes the open womb and functions as a place on which the woman sits balanced so that her dirty blood (*daraq siq kotor,* minor postpartum bleeding) can flow unhindered out of her body. According to tradition, women must remain in an upright, sitting position, even while sleeping, until the *belaqan api* ceremony (a smoking ceremony) given on the seventh or ninth day after birth (for comparable postpartum practices see Grace 1996; Laderman 1983).

which, because it is so common, is perceived by the nonsufferer as an unimportant illness.[23]

Although a sudden stomachache is often attributed to *ketemuq*, other perceived symptoms are also so named. Among these are sudden headaches or dizziness, aches in the back of one's neck, persistent crying (in infants), sudden shakes and shivers, numbness, a large facial rash, and uncontrolled, abnormal movements.[24] The variety of these symptoms suggests that the name of *ketemuq* is not based on perception of symptomatology. In addition, although most often *ketemuq* is associated with sudden pain, ache, or episode onset, in some cases the symptoms develop gradually. How can we understand *ketemuq* when faced with such a variety of symptoms and onset rates?

It could be that *ketemuq* is a grab-bag etiology, a residual illness name. Perhaps any complaint not easily explained is named *ketemuq*. It could be that *ketemuq* is a common illness name because it is so easily treated. As I mentioned above, every adult in Pelocok knows how to treat *ketemuq*—it is part of their personal stock of knowledge. So, naming an illness *ketemuq* allows people to do something about the suffering. They have a treatment on hand.

It could be that *ketemuq* has such a wide variety of symptoms because the name is based on an experience, a sensation of meeting a ghost, rather than on physical symptoms. Sometimes in their descriptions of their complaints, the sufferer of *ketemuq* would indicate which ghost they had met: "I met the person who died there a while ago" or "I met the dead person who was being given her death ceremony" or "I met my dead neighbor." Sometimes they had seen the person in a dream, but more often, they just knew: "It was him already." Perhaps these Sasaks occasionally have strange sensations—maybe analogous to the feeling of being watched even though one is alone—which, if followed by aches and pains, are recognized as moments of meeting ghosts.

Or it could be that *ketemuq* with its various symptoms is such a common illness because people assume themselves to be vulnerable to it. In a world filled with spirits and ghosts, perhaps feeling oneself vulnerable to *ketemuq* becomes a self-fulfilling prophecy.

---

23. This interpretation is strongly influenced by the works of Byron Good, which foreground the experience of illness for the sufferer (e.g., Good 1994).

24. The case supporting this last symptom description comes from an acute episode suffered by Inaq Nori in October 1995. The episode started at about 11:00 A.M. when she, for no apparent reason, began wailing and moaning, moving her body in unusual, apparently uncontrolled ways as friends and neighbors tried to restrain her. By midafternoon, she had quieted. One of the many names suggested for this strange episode was *ketemuq*.

Ketemuq is one instance of many in which a single illness name is used for multiple, disparate cases—evidence that supports Pool, who writes:

> I tend to conclude that there is no ideal level of cultural competence which can be revealed by eliciting the categories and classifications of 'knowledgeable' informants. Rather, there are a number of clusters of more or less indeterminate terms, which together and across many instances of communication, refer to a loose constellation of symptoms. *It is not simply a question of polysemy: one term having different but more or less fixed meanings (in the sense of a reasonable degree of consensus), the meanings are fluid and vary as the term is used in different contexts by different people, and the variations are not necessarily systematic.* (1994, 118–19; emphasis added)

PLURALITIES OF DIAGNOSIS

These three cases of usual illness exemplify the nonsystematic ways Sasaks name illness. In the first case, a single episode of illness is given multiple etiologies in the space of a few hours. In the second case, two persons within a single household suffering from the same symptoms are given multiple illness names. Both of these examples powerfully suggest that expressed physical symptoms are less important to naming illness than perceptions of the victim's vulnerabilities and overall personhood, presumptions about how the victim lives and how biomedical medications work, and the motivations of the treatment giver. In the third case, multiple episodes among a variety of persons are given the same illness name. This example strengthens the argument that physical symptomatology is not a particularly important aspect of naming illness, suggesting instead that the meanings of illness are fluid. Names for illness vary based not so much on expressed symptoms but on perceptions of personhood and vulnerability, context and presumptions, personal experiences and the available repertoire of treatments.

Thus who is doing the naming has an enormous impact on what name the illness will be given. As Leslie suggests, the first task when approaching the complexities of diagnosis is to acknowledge the range of persons doing the diagnosing (1992, 195). In Pelocok, this range includes nearly everyone.

Healing specialists—the *dukuns*, *belians*, and clinicians—tended to foreground their own expertise in making diagnoses. *Dukun*s were more likely to point to etiologies involving spirits, ancestors, *epe* (shadowy twin, soul), and black magic. *Belian*s tended to point to humoral imbalances caused by excess or want, as well as spirits and ancestors. Clinicians used technologically measurable symptoms to name an illness, usually turning, for an etiology, to poor living conditions, habits, and education. This tendency to name illness based on one's own expertise was in no way unique to healing specialists. Amaq Sunin, in the case above, pronounced Amaq Mol's cough and aches to be the result of a sick stomach, an illness for which he happened to have a rather flashy treatment. And *ketemuq*, an illness in which everyone is an expert, turns out to be a remarkably common diagnosis for widely variable symptoms. As other examples, one man tended to name every irritable child as having *taget* (surprise, shock) for which he was renowned to have a particularly good *jampi*. Another woman named every sore, twisted, sprained, or broken joint, as *polaq*, indicating a break, that she claimed to be able to treat successfully. In other words, an illness could receive a number of different names based on the expertise and experience of the people doing the naming. Even so, the names of usual illness tend to overlap. In the case of the young boy, his illness was diarrhea among all those who gave it a name; what varied were the given etiologies based on presumptions about biomedicine and living conditions. Likewise, the difference in the names of my illness as opposed to Amaq Mol's can best be explained by how we were each perceived as persons: one incapable of working and the other capable. These cases exemplify an overall tendency among Sasaks to ascribe names to an illness episode according to who is ill and what that person's vulnerabilities and weaknesses are perceived to be. These are at least as important as the symptoms exhibited.

In his discussion of cognitive models, Shore maintains that medical diagnostic models "include taxonomies and divination rites as well as metonymic and metaphoric models that *read somatic symptoms in relation to classifications of disease types*" (1996, 63; emphasis added). I sense that even the rural Sasak might think of their identifications of etiologies and diagnoses as the matching of symptoms with illness names; recall the words of Inaq Sur: "You see the patient, recognize the name of the illness, and you know already which *jampi* is right." People see naming as a matter of instantaneous recognition, particularly in cases of usual illness. But although this may be a cross-culturally pervasive medical model, my materials suggest that more goes into the naming of illness than *just* reading the somatic symptoms.

When confronted with illness in Pelocok, I looked for what was written on bodies, checking it against my own past experiences and against the descriptions in *Where There Is No Doctor* (Werner 1992). In giving a name to an illness, I foregrounded deductions based on the symptoms I perceived, but as is painfully clear, presumptions and personal motivations (as in cases 1 and 2 above, respectively) also entered into the names I gave to illness.

Sasaks use the writings on bodies as just the first step in naming illness. They understand that those writings can be deceptive: pain experienced in one part of the body does not necessarily indicate the locus of the problem. Sizing up symptoms is important to naming an illness—at least to recognizing that an illness is present—but symptoms tend to take a backseat to the patient's personhood—personal history, social relations, economic problems, ritual responsibilities, vulnerabilities—and the experience of the person doing the diagnosing, which are integral to the naming process.[25]

DREAMS AND DIVINATIONS

Dreams and divinations are two supplemental ways of naming illness. Although sometimes used in connection with everyday illnesses, normally these processes only become factors in naming unusual illnesses. Names of illness revealed in dreams and divinations have a special status. Unlike names given by people, which are considered fallible, the names revealed in dreams and divinations are thought to be unquestionably true.

Dreams

In Sasak cosmology, dreaming is a time when a living person enters the second world (*alam kedua*). The second world is a dimension of clarity and truth; concealment and uncertainty are not possible in the second world as they are in the everyday world (*alam ite,* our world). While dreaming, one can see and speak with spirits and ancestors. While dreaming, one can meet with other living people, learning from them

---

25. This argument has similarities with Jaspan's observation that in southern Sumatra, who a victim is as a social person has significant impact on the diagnostic process (1976a, 271ff.). To a lesser extent, doctors in biomedical traditions also take aspects of the social person—e.g., ethnic background, gender, economics—into account in making diagnoses (see, e.g., Brown et al. 1994; Fabrega 1980).

truths sometimes unclear in everyday interactions. While dreaming one can see the future. Ill persons and those around them use dreams as sources of etiologies, diagnoses, and prognoses.[26]

Often illness names are revealed straightforwardly through conversations in dreams. For example, one ill man dreamed of eating food at a girlfriend's house and then listening as the girlfriend told him she had just poisoned him, thus making him ill. Sometimes the illness names revealed in dreams are based on standard interpretations of certain dream symbols. For example, if one dreams one is bitten by a snake, that means one is ill with *kemalikan* from being disrespectful of a potent object or space. These standard interpretations seem to be widely dispersed common knowledge in the Pelocok community.

In cases of perplexing illness, people ask if the ill person, a relative, or a healer had dreamed anything. Once when I asked Inaq Kirnim what was her grandchild's illness, she answered, "I do not know. I have to go to sleep first. In the morning, I will know."

Divinations

Divination is "an explanatory process which helps people make decisions about the causes of and remedies for illnesses" and other misfortunes (Nuckolls 1991, 57). It is common in many places in the world.[27] Elsewhere, divination involves more or less elaborate rites that, it is generally argued, are less matters of divining than expressing issues of social disorder or anxiety in a legitimate public forum.

Sasak divination functions differently. Sasak divinations are done by women who are often, although not necessarily, *belian*s. Divinations are only done in connection with identifying an illness and its likely treatments, and, like all processes of illness naming, divinations are freely available upon request. Divinations are conducted with as little ceremony as treating a usual illness with a *jampi*. Generally, someone will suggest aloud that perhaps this or that treatment (treatments that imply particular illness names) might work for a particular ailment and urge a diviner to *cobaq* (try). The diviner will isolate a small chunk of hair on or near the crown of her head. She twists the hair tightly around her fingers and makes a fist about one inch from her scalp.

26. Dreams used as true sources of medical information in personalistic medical systems are frequently mentioned in the ethnographic literature (e.g., Pearce 1993; Roseman 1991; Tedlock 1992).
27. See, e.g., Beattie 1967; Laderman 1991; Park 1967.

Then she grasps the fist with the other hand. Looking down, she quietly but audibly says words, asking an unnamed entity if the suggested treatment will work. Then she quickly gives her hand two light and then one or two hard yanks upward, tensing her arm muscles. If there is a popping sound, the answer is presumed "yes," and sometimes will be followed up with more specific questions regarding treatment.[28] If there is no popping sound, the answer is "no," and that treatment suggestion and its illness name are abandoned immediately. The divined questions always imply a spiritual, ancestral, or potent object/person agent. While the use of divination is evidence of the anxiety surrounding an illness, turning to divinations always struck me as a shot in the dark, rather than a deliberate voicing of a social problem or concern. Sasak divination functions without moral or social baggage to seek legitimation for potential illness names.

According to Sasaks, the divining process is a way of communicating with spirits and ancestors. In the second world, the causes of illnesses are obvious: "For us here everything is blurry, but in the second world everything is clear" (*Leq iteh, selaputne keliru. Lagu leq alam kedua, tauq tegita kenaq*). Spirits and ancestors know the causes of each particular illness among the living. Sometimes they approach the living and reveal their knowledge in dreams. But through divination, the living can ask spirits and ancestors whether or not they have guessed the correct cause or name of an illness.

There are two differences between identifying illness names through dreams and through divinations. First, while anyone can have dreams that name illness, only certain women can divine. Second, dreams are frustratingly unpredictable. Often, anxious family members question the victim and each other upon waking, only to discover that no one

---

28. The only explanation I was ever given for the popping sound was that it was an affirmative answer to the diviner's question. I think the popping sound occurred when the hair was yanked so hard that it pulled the scalp away from the skull. I have tried it in vain, producing instead only a sore spot on my head. I have watched as women repeatedly divined answers, repeatedly using the same tuft of hair, yet, sometimes the scalp would pop and sometimes not. In other words, there was no pattern in the "yes" answers in the divinations. Park has argued that devices or techniques that are plausibly random are rare in the ethnographic literature (1967, 239). None of the diviners I knew, some of whom were close friends, ever admitted to manipulating the results of a divination. It is plausible that they pulled their scalps with more strength when divining answers to suggestions they thought might work. Or perhaps some diviners manipulated the results, and some did not. I was always particularly struck by a diviner's evident frustration at having all suggestions rejected in her divinations. One can remain skeptical, of course, but I usually sensed honest frustration from diviners who subjected their scalp to these tests in vain.

had had a dream suggesting a name for the illness. In contrast, divinations are man-made opportunities for learning an illness name.

To summarize, dreams and divinations are processes of naming illness that *supplement* the normal social processes discussed above with regard to usual illness and, more typically, unusual illness.

NAMING UNUSUAL ILLNESS

Unusual illness (*penyakit ndeqne biese*) are those illnesses that have curious or severe symptoms, last longer than a week or two, or do not respond to normal treatments. Precisely because they are unusual, the naming process is exponentially more complicated, although not fundamentally different from the processes already discussed. If my cough and exhaustion could generate four different illness names in the course of a day, one should not be surprised that unusual illnesses can generate dozens of illness names.

The category of unusual illness includes everything from an irritating cough that develops and lasts for weeks to severe, life-threatening stomach pain with vomiting and diarrhea that lasts for months. My notes include a dozen relatively mild cases of unusual illness and seven cases of severe, life-threatening unusual illness. Unlike usual illness episodes, it is difficult to make comparisons among unusual illness episodes. Yet the *processes* of naming unusual illnesses are the same processes used to name usual ones. Detailing multiple cases of unusual illness would add ethnographic bulk, without adding qualitatively to the point at hand. Thus, to illustrate and discuss the processes through which unusual illnesses are named, I turn to the case of Lo Budin.

Naming Lo Budin's Illness

Lo Budin was about a year old (he could not quite walk, but could sit with ease) when he became ill. The symptoms the family, neighbors, and healers noted included weight loss, coughing, coldness of feet, hotness of stomach and back, inability to cry or nurse, sleeplessness, deafness, stiffness of back and limbs, and strange movements of limbs, eyes, and mouth. This welter of symptoms stimulated people to suggest a variety of diagnoses and etiologies that led to a mélange of *jampi,* divinations, and associated treatments. What I saw and heard was a hodgepodge of creative diagnoses, etiologies, and ideas for treatment motivated by the anguish of watching an ill child. To examine whether there are identifiable commonalities in this hodgepodge of naming, I analyze some of the main illness names given for Lo Budin's sickness.

Names through Dreams

One suggestion was that Budin's name did not fit. His illness was thus a manifestation of the incongruence between his person and his name. Name incongruence is commonly considered a source for illness in young children (see also chap. 3). This etiology was revealed in the dream of Lo Budin's older stepbrother, Lo Den.

Another suggestion, also revealed in a dream to Lo Den, was that Budin's *epe* (soul/shadow) was upset by his upcoming circumcision ceremony. This is an unusual etiology, because I usually heard people say that children's various illnesses would stop once circumcised. Indeed, 13 days earlier, Papuq Junin had said that he would not worry once Lo Budin was circumcised, implying that, whatever the illness, were he circumcised it would not be as serious. As we have discussed, uncircumcised boys are commonly considered more vulnerable to illness. The dream relied on another, less common idea that a person's *epe* must be ready for a major life change, so that planning to circumcise a child before he is ready is dangerous.

There are four commonalities between these two etiologies: first, both were suggested by the half-brother; second, both were revealed in dreams; third, both utilized common knowledge about the illness vulnerabilities of young boys; and fourth, both were accepted by the family as true and acted upon. Lo Den was a young, unmarried man, in his late teens or early twenties. As his father's son he presumably had been given some potent secret knowledge, but he was not known to have any special healing *ilmu*. The illness names that Lo Den suggested used such common presumptions about childhood vulnerabilities that nearly anyone in the community could have come up with them and thus reflected his own relatively limited experience with illness. Yet, because these names were from dreams, they were immediately accepted as true by family members, regardless of how ridiculous they sounded to others.[29] Some thought the name change completely

---

29. Knowledge revealed in dreams is generally considered unquestionably true, because the knowledge comes directly from spirits or ancestors who can see things more "clearly" than people can. In this case, because a name change did not fit the illness (see note 30), people doubted that Lo Den could have dreamed such a thing. Their doubt was not that the dream was true, but that Lo Den could have had the dream at all.

unwarranted by the perceptions of the ailment.[30] The name change was an unusual suggestion given the circumstances of Lo Budin's case, but it, like the not-ready-to-be-circumcised diagnosis, drew on understandings of vulnerability. It was his perceived vulnerability as a young boy that legitimated both of these unusual diagnoses. Budin's name was changed (although I continue to use Budin for simplicity's sake), and the father announced that Budin would not join the upcoming circumcision ceremony.

A Name as Expression of Criticism

Papuq Isa, the *belian,* initially connected Lo Budin's illness to the illness of his aunt, Papuq Sari. The coincidence of them both becoming ill on the same day supported her suggestion, but the explanation pointed more to Lo Budin's social identity than to temporal coincidence. Papuq Isa voiced this etiology to me the morning after Papuq Sari's death and Lo Budin's father's socially inappropriate insistence on hosting the mortuary ceremonies. In essence, she was suggesting that the sins of the father were being paid for by the son, implying that the father's potency automatically deflected the illness from himself, and it rebounded onto his most vulnerable son.[31] This explanation blamed the father for indirectly causing the illness through behavior deemed inappropriate. Papuq Isa never mentioned an ultimate source for the illness—such as the living descendants of Papuq Sari or ancestors angry that *adat* (Indon., custom, tradition) had not been followed—but focused solely on the transgressions of the father against social, traditional, and religious norms. This etiology was promptly discarded by Papuq Junin who angrily reasserted his right and obligation to host the mortuary ceremonies, and Papuq Isa too seemed to drop it, perhaps for the sake of social harmony. But this etiology is interesting because, more than any of the others, it points a finger of blame and suggests that the illness can be understood as an expression of social dysfunction.

Illness has often been understood as a sign of immorality. Illnesses such as cancer and AIDS in the United States (e.g., Sontag 1989; Martin 1994; Farmer et al. 1996), infertility in Egypt (Inhorn 1994), or lep-

---

30. Name changes are usually decided on after a prolonged period of lethargy, lack of growth, repeated minor illness, or peculiar physical traits such as having what people remember as impenetrable skin. Many people I spoke with understood that name changes are not suggested by illness that lasts for a short period, comes on suddenly, or produces such symptoms as fever, diarrhea, and vomiting.

31. Lo Budin was the most vulnerable of Papuq Junin's immediate family, because he was by far the youngest and therefore the one with the least *ilmu.*

rosy in India (Waxler 1981) are all cases where assumptions of immoral behavior are sometimes ascribed to the ill person. Elsewhere, the "geography of blame" (Farmer 1992) is broadened, focusing not on the victim but on the sins of others. Accusations of sorcery within communities, of conspiracy from outside agencies, and of ancestor or spirit neglect are common in the literature and link specific illness episodes with wider social anxieties and problems.[32]

In Lombok, illnesses attributed to black magic, sorcery, and ancestor or spirit neglect are common. But Papuq Isa did not foreground or even mention the possibility of black magic or ancestral revenge. Instead she linked the illness directly with the father's inappropriate social behavior. Had Papuq Junin not insisted on hosting the death ceremonies, Papuq Isa might still have suggested this etiology based on the temporal coincidences in the cases. But it is significant that she did not make this connection until the morning after Papuq Junin had set the community reeling with his unilateral decision to host the ceremonies, violating normal protocol. This etiology uses the common strategy of highlighting coincidence and linking illness with personhood, Lo Budin's father. As such, the etiology uniquely and boldly accuses the most potent and socially powerful senior man in the community of a breach of tradition (*adat*) and religious law (*rukun*), which he himself claims to most strongly defend.

A Name Implicating Context

The most common etiology given for the illness involved spirits of various ilk, at first ones inhabiting the newly completed water reservoir, later ones at the originating spring for the reservoir. The newly opened reservoir was a hot topic of conversation throughout the community. Praised for making water so much more accessible, the reservoir was also the source of much consternation. One day in three the reservoir would be dry, and people complained heartily that they could not get water.[33] Many people, most notably Papuq Junin, were angry about the

---

32. The literature on these wider castings of the blame net is enormous. These are just a handful of them: Evans-Pritchard 1976; Lindenbaum 1979; Hoskins 1996; Nuckolls 1991; Pool 1994; Scheper-Hughes 1992; Schieffeln 1976; Taussig 1987; Turner 1967.

33. The reservoir changed women's behavior and social patterns literally overnight. Before it was opened, women, usually in pairs, never complained of going out to the paddy fields in search of water at the various streams. Afterward, they gathered water, washed their dishes, and bathed themselves in large, crowded groups at the cement reservoir. Moreover, although men would frequently pass the streams that women

reservoir's placement right next to the mayor's (*kepala dusun*) house, a long walk for many people in the hamlet. But most disconcerting was the prevailing sense that "everyone is dying now" and "everyone is ill now." This would be illustrated with lists of the people who had recently died—indeed, five respected old people died that month as well as a few children—and lists of the people who were currently ill. Their statements were exaggerations; in fact, only a relatively small portion of the community was recognized as ill, and the death toll, although high among prominent elders, was only slightly higher than normal.[34] But what is significant was the prevalent sense that illness and death were unusually pervasive. The reservoir was a frequently mentioned explanation for this wave of illness and death.

It is interesting that a common source did not result in common illnesses. The illness of a child with a sick mouth (*sakit dodok*) was caused by the same agent that caused Lo Budin's more serious illness. But just as we have seen that the same apparent symptoms may have different etiologies, the same etiologies can be linked with vastly different symptoms; as Inaq Mol said, "The cause is the same, the illness is different." Again, symptoms are often secondary in designating illness etiologies and diagnoses.

In a time when illness was perceived to be running rampant, in a time when the community was adjusting to a drastic new structural development, Lo Budin's illness could be blamed on context. Opinions differed on the exact agent causing all this illness. For Inaq Mol, it was the spirit (*pedam*) of the reservoir; for Amaq Las it was the *dewa* of the spring from the beginning; and for Papuq Junin and Amaq Mus it was initially the *dewa* of the reservoir and later the *dewa* of the spring.[35] For

---

bathed in, etiquette demanded that they avert their eyes as the women covered themselves with sarongs. But across the road from the reservoir, men built a *barugah*, ostensibly as a place to wait for passing trucks, but it was used as a gathering place particularly popular among young men, who would sit watching the women bathe. When the reservoir was dry, rather than going back to the streams, men and women alike complained heartily and waited for the reservoir to fill again.

34. Illness and death are everyday occurrences throughout the year in Pelocok, but during the last months of the dry season (August and September) and the last months of the wet season (February and March) there seemed to be an increase in the rates in both 1994 and 1995. During those years, those months each saw large numbers of hosted rituals, which usually marked increased cases of illness—perhaps connected biomedically to poor food storage practices. August and September, falling at the end of the dry season, also tended to be unusually hungry months, which could contribute to a weakened immune system.

35. *Dewa* and *pedam* are hierarchically related spirits, with *dewa* as spirit gods being considerably more powerful than *pedam*, one of the many kinds of ordinary spirits that haunt things and can send mild illness.

all, it was common knowledge that the water god or spirits were angry because the proper rituals asking for the water had not been done prior to completing the reservoir. According to Amaq Las, the *dewa* took such vengeance on Lo Budin because his father is one of the persons in Pelocok who is responsible for conducting such rituals. According to Papuq Isa, the *dewa* took such vengeance on Lo Budin because that same *dewa* had been neglected by Papuq Junin and others many times before and now was not easily appeased. Ultimately, this etiology explains Budin's illness by reference to past mistakes rather than a misappropriation of power; this etiology was accepted, and the father initiated numerous ceremonies at the reservoir and the spring to make up for the previous negligence and to appease the *dewa*.

This water god etiology and the Papuq Sari etiology both place importance on coinciding events—the building of a reservoir and the death of Papuq Sari. Also, both make elaborate connections between Lo Budin's personhood, his identity as his father's son, and the responsibilities of Papuq Junin as a potent man with vast amounts of secret knowledge.

Names Based on Personhood, Expertise, and Symptoms

In the midst of changing Lo Budin's name, postponing his circumcision, and carrying out ceremonies at the reservoir and spring, other illness names were suggested by a multitude of people. A frequently suggested name was *masahlah epene* (problem with his shadow/soul/twin). It is widely dispersed common knowledge that each person has a unique *epe* or personal *dewa*, which bestows talents, strength, and *ilmu*.[36] Yet, *epe*, particularly weak *epe*, like that of a very young child, can easily be insulted by social slights or shocked by sudden occurrences, and all of these sufferings are understood to be manifested on the person's body in illness. Giving the name of *masahlah epe* to Lo Budin's illness used common knowledge about *epe* and illness, and drew on his identity as a very young boy. The two *ketomuai* treatment ceremonies conducted by *dukun*s, all of the incense and smoking treatments conducted by *dukun*s, *kiayi*s, and Papuq Junin, and in part also the *mul-mul* treatment were directed at solving the problem of Lo Budin's *epe*.

---

36. I am referring here to the common understanding of Sasak anatomy discussed in conjunction with the *dukun* Amaq Deri. Because Amaq Deri always spoke about it with the word *dewa*, I used that word in chapter 2. Here, to avoid confusion with the *dewa* of the spring (water god), I use a synonym for personal *dewa*s, namely, *epe*.

These treatments involved the expertise of *dukun*s and *kiayi*s, and they gave Papuq Junin himself something he could do for his child.

The *mul-mul* treatment, suggested and initiated by Papuq Isa, is a treatment to make persons *mul* (calm, neither hot nor cold). *Mul-mul* is most commonly used as a preventive treatment the night before a boy's circumcision, so that he will be relaxed for the ritual to come. In this sense, the treatment was aimed at calming the boy's *epe* so that Lo Budin would be calm. Yet *mul* also means "neither too hot nor too cold." In this sense, the treatment was a humoral response to his hot stomach and back and his cold feet. The *mul-mul* treatment thus implied that the illness was both personalistic—based on a problem with Lo Budin's *epe*—and naturalistic—caused by a humoral imbalance. Moreover, *mul-mul* is a treatment solely within the expertise of *belian*s. By suggesting this treatment, it gave Papuq Isa something she could do for the boy.

Sundry other names for Lo Budin's illness based on perceptions of his symptoms were suggested by a multitude of people. *Sakit bantaq bembeq* (goat head sickness) was suggested by Inaq Mol based on the erratic movements of his mouth. *Sakit bongkor* (sick back) was suggested by Inaq Budin based on the hotness of his back. *Sakit muntah-mentret* (sick vomiting-diarrhea), a commonly recognized and often fatal illness among children, was suggested by a number of women. Unlike the other names, these names based on symptoms were understood to be incomplete. Corresponding treatments were thought capable of making particular ailments leave Lo Budin's body, but incapable of dealing with the agent responsible for the overall illness.

Commonalities in Naming Unusual Illness

For Sasaks, bodies are not texts to be read. In recognizing ill health and giving it a name, the interpretive work is great. The first step is to identify what is actually to be read as a sign. Names depend on what signs one selects as relevant. For example, in naming Lo Budin's illness as the result of having met the spirit of a goat, Inaq Mol selected only the wild movements of his tongue and jaw, completely ignoring the fevers, vomiting, stiffness, lack of voice, and convulsions. The selection of which signs are read depends on the key characteristics of the illness, in this instance, likeness to a goat. Thus the signs are selected in terms of the illness names one knows and remembers. In another instance, Papuq Junin remembered about an illness of children unable to cry and one man's reputed expertise in treating it. Experience, expertise, and memory shape perception of ailments and the names they are given.

Equally important to naming unusual illnesses are the understandings and perceptions of the ill person. Who the victims are as persons—their own particular histories, habits, social relations, potencies, and vulnerabilities—are primary factors in naming the illness. In the case of Lo Budin, perception of his vulnerabilities and social relationships were central to the name change, the circumcision issue, the connection with Papuq Sari's death, the reservoir and spring spirits, and the problem with his *epe*. As with usual illness, who the victim was shaped the potential names his illness was given.

A final commonality can be traced among the names for Lo Budin's illness: two of the suggested etiologies utilized coincidental contexts as primary features.[37] Had Lo Budin become ill at another time, even just a week removed from Papuq Sari's mortuary ceremonies, Papuq Isa would not have come up with the etiology that blamed the father for misconduct. Had Lo Budin become ill at another time, either significantly before or after the completion of the reservoir, that etiology would never have been suggested. The larger temporal context of his illness played an important role in its naming.

The important factors in naming Lo Budin's unusual illness were (1) experience and expertise, (2) perceptions of person and vulnerability, (3) context, and, to a lesser extent, (4) symptoms. These factors are similar to those discussed as important to naming usual illness. There are two differences. First, in the cases of usual illness, the presumptions and motivations of the person naming the illness clearly came into play, whereas in the case of Lo Budin such presumptions and motivations do not appear significant. Second, temporal context was significant to the Lo Budin case, but insignificant for cases of usual illness. These differences are merely products of the particular cases discussed. In the unusual illness of Amaq Sunin, his pride was presumed by a number of men in the community to have instigated black magic attacks, yet Amaq Sunin gave an etiology of female jealousy, which inherently boasted of his own potency and virility.[38] In his case, presumption and personal motivation definitely shaped illness names. Similarly, in February 1995, when a number of people in Pelocok were ill with the same flulike symptoms, one of the names given for this usual

---

37. This is characteristic of personalistic medicine in which coincidence is meaningful: "personalistic causality allows little room for accident or chance" (Foster 1976, 775).

38. This case is discussed in detail in Hay 1998a.

illness was that it was connected with *bau nyale:* "Said a nobleman of long ago, when there is *bau nyale,* sickness comes." *Bau nyale* is a ceremony to collect sea worms that come up on the Lombok coast once each year.[39] This case shows that, as with unusual illness, usual illness can be associated with temporal events.

As is generally recognized by medical anthropology, naming illness is a complex process. Had this ethnography not begun by asking how Sasaks cope with illness, had it forgone their experiences of vulnerability and understandings of the social person, we would have been ill-equipped to understand the processes involved in naming illness. In the ways Sasaks cope with illness, experiences of vulnerability and past illness, perceptions of person, and interpretations of illness mutually inform each other.

UNDERSTANDING THE PROCESS OF NAMING

The process of naming illness is difficult in any medical setting, but perhaps it is particularly so in a setting such as Pelocok where (1) ethnomedicine is primarily but not exclusively personalistic, (2) everyone has ethnomedical knowledge, (3) agency to act on health concerns does not have a definitive locus such as in the role of healers, but shifts from person to society to secret knowledge, (4) illness is only minimally organized into simple hierarchical distinctions between usual and unusual illness, and (5) treatment depends on finding the correct secret knowledge to meet and drive out an illness. With ethnomedical knowledge so minimally organized, rural Sasaks are left to find their own way to the illness names on which health depends.

The processes by which people come up with names for illness are not random. They draw on common and personal knowledge about

---

39. *Bau nyale* (Sas., literally, *bau*—to gather, *nyale*—worms) has a number of meanings and social implications. A myth tells of a princess who, unable to decide among many suitors, threw herself into the sea; her hair became the *nyale,* now plentiful for everyone. Traditionally, a key element of *bau nyale* was a formal courting ritual (see Ecklund 1977). Today, the courting ritual still takes place, with the encouragement and financial incentives of local government who are working to turn *bau nyale* into a profitable tourist attraction. The one I attended boasted at least 10,000 Sasaks from all over the island, who, as dawn breaks and after a night of gossiping and courting, walk out half a mile into the sea with nets and buckets to gather the *nyale.* The amount and color of the *nyale* are said to indicate the length of the rainy season and the quality of the upcoming harvest. In addition, the *nyale* themselves are used as a general illness preventive, as medicine for illness, and as fertilizer for crops.

vulnerability, context, and experience that Sasaks consider relevant to health concerns. We have identified the elements that illness names draw upon, discussed Sasak common knowledge about bodies and vulnerabilities, and offered case studies describing who is ill and the wider context of that illness; even so, which names will be given to episodes of illness are unpredictable. Even run-of-the-mill illnesses such as diarrhea can generate a host of etiologies. One could predict with reliability that for a majority of illnesses someone at some point would suggest the name of *ketemuq* (meeting a ghost), but not whether a specific case would be so named. The content and grounding of ethnographic common knowledge guarantees some commonalities among names, but they are no more than starting points in the process of naming. Out of the innumerable potential understandings, coincidences, events, and nuances, only one or a few become the salient signs connecting a name with an illness.

Which signs become salient and which do not is never a matter of logical elimination. When confronted with the anxiety of illness people do not have that luxury. In an unusual case such as Lo Budin's, the suggested names and treatments were numerous, and every kind of expertise in the community was used. These proliferating treatments were carried out practically one on top of the other: one of them might work, and it did not matter in the slightest which one it was. Naming the illness correctly was critical, but it was not an intellectual enterprise, it was a matter of life or death. Yet, in grabbing at straws, people inexplicably did not pursue some current events—no etiologies linked Lo Budin's illness to Papuq Junin's planned marriage to a second wife, the grading for pavement of the main road, or the celebration of Mohammed's birthday on the day the illness began. The urgency of needing a name for an illness necessitates the selection of some events as signs prior to having the luxury of systematic elimination of all potential signs.[40]

To explain this, we need the concept of imagination. Imagination is the ability to see significance without or before understanding it. It suggests connections between knowledge and sensation prior to finding the references of the connection.[41] Imagination is an act of casting forward "our attention to a target that is as yet unsupported by subsidiaries.

---

40. This would only be possible in an ideal scientific environment when no anxiety was attached to the illness at all. Even with all the technology available to biomedical physicians in the United States, diagnosis is often a matter of making a best guess (Hahn 1995).

41. See Langer 1957, 251; Peirce 1955, 43; Johnson 1987.

Although the lost meaning of a word is in recent memory when our imagination sallies forth, seeking to restore it, this meaning is not yet present" (Polanyi and Prosch 1975, 57). Intuition is the spontaneous guide that points out the most feasible direction for imagination to go (97). In the anxiety of coming up with a name for an illness, people are trying to keep a loved one alive. In so doing they must focus on aspects of reality that might be pertinent, automatically and without thought eliminating extraneous aspects of reality. They must intuitively select an event, coincidence, vulnerability, physical symptom, or nuance of personhood as a key sign of the illness, using it to cast forward to a name, before knowing what that name will be, or if the selected sign will make a meaningful connection between the illness and the name at all. In the plethora of names thrown out for Lo Budin's unusual illness, we see people casting forward, suggesting names and intuitively latching onto signs prior to any certainty that the names fit.

The process of naming draws on common knowledge to imaginatively project forward into the unknown. What is the unknown? The illness is unknown until it is named and successfully treated. What the name is for any given illness is also unknown. What the key signs are that will connect the correct name to the illness are unknown. The process of naming an illness is the process of imaginatively connecting these three unknowns into a meaningful, triadic relationship. As such, the process of naming can be explained, in theoretical terms, as a process of creativity.

CREATIVITY IN MEANING-MAKING

> Mostly we are unaware of creating anything new, yet both perception and action are necessarily creative. Much of modern life is organized to avoid the awareness of the fine threads of novelty connecting learned behaviors with acknowledged spontaneity. We are largely unaware of speaking, as we all do, sentences never spoken before, unaware of choreographing the acts of dressing and sitting and entering a room as depictions of self, of resculpting memory into an appropriate past.
> —MARY CATHERINE BATESON

It is a truism that people are agents constructing, creating, and composing their realities.[42] What is disturbing is the current proliferation of

---

42. For recent examples of authors foregrounding the creation or construction of

statements in anthropology that use the word *create*, but offer "neither a definition of creativity nor a systematic account of how it is achieved and what is created" (Csordas 1997, 249; exc. see Johnson 1987).

I define *creativity* as an imaginative process through which people arrive at tentative, conditional interpretations (cf. Runco 1999). This definition assumes that all knowledge is gained subjectively. In other words, everything any person knows is personalized and unique to that person's particular perceptions, motivations, prior knowledge (including cultural knowledge), and social values.[43] Therefore the knowledge (referent, focal object) is marked or shaped by the knower (agent) and how it is known (interpretant). Meaning is made in semiosis—the continual *projecting of connections* by the knower of signs with signs (Peirce 1955). The connections are not objectively "out there" to be "discovered," they must be made by someone; the knower constructs an "inner association" among signs so that the resulting meaning is motivated for the knower (Shore 1996, 332). They are made by a casting forward of imagination, seeking into the unknown for a connection, for meaning. Thus meanings or interpretations are the products of our personal continual connection making and are always personally marked. Every idea, sentence, action, or illness name is the product of creatively making meaning.

In his work on Bali, Barth looks at cultural traditions of knowledge and marks how people's interpretations will change if confronted with problems that somehow do not fit (1993). Toward the end of the monograph, he concludes:

> I take it that every performed and interpreted act will change, slightly, the meanings that are ascribed to any following choice, act, or expression within the circle of persons in which it was visible. The result is a low degree of order and a high degree of flux—a flux that comes about through small and humble steps yet may cumulatively challenge, invade, and transform the relevance of whole constructed worlds. (323)

Focused on the larger issues of change in cultural knowledge, Barth assumes a process of individual interpretive change. By adding the

---

social reality, see the collection entitled, appropriately enough, *Creativity/Anthropology* (Lavie et al. 1993; see also, e.g., Csordas 1997; Romanucci-Ross 1986).

43. An extensive outline of this theory of knowledge is unwarranted by our concerns here, but see chapter 9. The emphasis here on personal knowledge is balanced in chapter 6 by an emphasis on the social processes of shaping personal knowledge.

model of creativity as the way in which people make meanings, we can understand *how* people take those small steps generating flux as they go about the business of living within a social and cultural context.

The Sasak domain of ethnomedicine, as we have seen, has a "low degree of order" (Barth 1993, 323). That order, such as it is, constrains change—limiting resort to biomedicine—and constrains interpretations, as we shall see. The high degree of flux results from the almost free rein granted by the minimal organization of ethnomedical knowledge. Indeed, Sasaks respond to anxiety about health with a high degree of creativity because ethnomedical knowledge is distributed so widely and secretly that it encourages everyone's participation and creativity in interpreting illness.[44]

Almost free rein in the process of naming illness means that every person in Pelocok can suggest potentially correct names that are more or less creative. The suggestion that Lo Budin's name be changed—which drew on very common knowledge about young children's vulnerabilities—is not as creative, in the common sense of the word, as the suggestion that the illness was connected to Papuq Sari's death, which drew on social relationships, ideas of tradition and cosmology, and social impropriety. The Sasak materials suggest that the definition of creativity must have a caveat so that while all interpretation is creative, the interpretive product falls on a continuum.

Tacking back from the ethnographic materials to the theoretical discussion above, this caveat suggests that there are cognitive factors within the processes of making meaning that limit how signs are connected, or even whether a sign is perceived at all. The first factor is that the knower's prior knowledge constrains the extent s/he is able to imaginatively project into the unknown. We are not blank slates; rather we interpret in order to understand something unknown in terms of something known (cf. Turner 1967). The second factor is that knowledge has a tendency toward inertia (conservativeness, habit). Through repetition of connecting signs with a particular perception, say *ketemuq* with a stomachache, habits of interpretation are formed (cf. Peirce 1955, 358–59; see also Bourdieu 1977b on habitus). Thus, inherent to the process of naming illness, people rely on experience to intuit in which direction to cast their net, yet the greater that experience, the stronger the interpretive habits, and the more likely they are to inter-

---

44. Anxiety does not necessarily motivate action and creativity, but I suggest that in contexts that encourage creative problem solving as opposed to contexts that restrict possibilities, anxiety can be a strong motivator of creative interpretation (see also Runco 1999).

pret a new illness episode in ways they interpreted past episodes. All processes of interpretation do not generate equally innovative products, but then again, the purpose of interpretation is to solve a problem, be it innovatively or not.

BECAUSE ILLNESS NAMES MATTER

In naming illness, innovation is not the point. The point is to come up with a name that fits. Illness is an urgent business. But the word *creativity* in everyday parlance implies an activity that has no deadline. Painters, poets, and physicists can wait for moments of illuminating insight to solve an interpretive problem. In matters of illness, one does not have the luxury of time. Names for illness matter, and matter deeply. In biomedical settings, treatment cannot be decided upon unless there is first a plausible diagnosis. In the pluralistic medical setting of rural Lombok, words that heal will have no effect unless the illness is first correctly named. Life rides on coming up with a name.

Although all interpretation, all quests into the unknown, involve creativity in the act of making meaning, the process of naming illness is prompted by anxiety that sets it apart. Time is of the essence. People must actively pursue interpretations of illness, casting forward in many directions at once, dropping names or signs immediately when they do not connect into a meaningful triad with the illness. The point is not to be creative, the point is to creatively happen upon a successful treatment as quickly as possible.

Seeking a name is the first step to coping with the pain and anxiety of illness. The process of naming an illness is not a simple matter of categorization. It is a matter of connecting complex common knowledge, experience and expertise, presumptions and context, with perceptions of a particular person's illness. It is a matter of intuitive and imaginative leaps into the unknown while a person's suffering and death hang in the balance.

— 6 —

Winged Words

The Politics of Communication about Illness

It was the third morning that I had sat with Inaq Sarin in late June 1995. She was near term on her ninth pregnancy and lately had had some breakthrough bleeding. Inaq Sarin was very nervous—seven of her previous children had died, mostly in childbirth. She and her husband desperately wanted this child to be all right. Although her *belian* was Papuq Isa, she had consulted with the Bu Bidan at her clinic about a week previously. Bu Bidan had told her that the child was breech and that she should give birth in the hospital. Her bleeding was not enough to send her back to the clinic; she feared being forced to go to the hospital. That particular morning, Papuq Isa, who had been visiting in a distant village for the last few days, came to check on her. Inaq Sarin lay down on a mat in the dark, one-room house, while Papuq Isa's slight frame bent over her, gently feeling the stomach with her hands:

Papuq Isa [Patting the pregnant belly on the upper right side]:	This is the bottom. Definitely the bottom. Here. Here. This is the bottom.	*Tombong ini. Sat tombong ini.* [Pause]. *Ngoh. Ngoh. Tombongne si sini.*
Inaq Sarin:	The Bu Bidan said that it was in breech position.	*Ongkatne Bu Bidan, molang iye.*
Papuq Isa [Still feeling the belly with her hands]:	Hmm. Hmm. This is good. Here. The head is already at the bottom here. It wasn't [isn't?] necessary for you to go there [the clinic, the hospital]. Does this hurt	*Ngah. Ngah. Sola ini. Ngoh. Wah otakne bawaq sini. Kamu lalo kamu ini deq ulaq jok tono.* [Pause]. *Sakitne ini, ngoh? Ngoh? Ngoh? Ngoh? Kane otakne, ngoh. Ni tombongne.*

here? Here? Here? Here? Now this is the head here. This the bottom.

Inaq Sarin:	Is our child okay?	*Kenaq anak ita?*
Papuq Isa:	[Positive acknowledgment, yes.]	*Mmmm.*
Neighbor woman:	What about Inaq Mol?	*Ape Inaq Mol na?*
Papuq Isa:	Huh?	*Uh?*
Neighbor woman:	What about Inaq Mol? [Implying that she be consulted also. But Inaq Mol is not a *belian.* The neighbor's suggestion is ignored.]	*Ape Inaq geMol?*
Papuq Isa [Still feeling the belly]:	It's not breech. Wait for the baby here.	[Softly as if to herself] *Ndeqne molang.* [Louder] *Untah bayiq sini ini.*
Neighbor woman:	Is it strong?	*Kuatne no?*
Papuq Isa:	Yes.	*Oq.*

Papuq Isa coughs, gets up, walks outside to get a long sarong. Coming back, she puts it behind Inaq Sarin's back. Lifting gently on both ends of the sarong, Papuq Isa rocks the pregnant belly back and forth, a treatment said to correctly position the baby vertically in the womb. Inaq Sarin softly asks a question I don't catch. Papuq Isa does not answer immediately. She finishes the rocking, squats down and puts her hands again on Inaq Sarin's belly:

Papuq Isa:	Well. You are not breech here, do you believe me? See. Here. Here. Here your stomach is right.	*Anuh. Kamu ngat molang sini, sadu ini? Nah. Ngoh. Ngoh. Ngoh kan kamu ngeh tian sini.*
Neighbor woman:	But, if it is breech . . .	*Na, kan mun molang . . .*

Papuq Isa:	It's not breech.	[Rather sharply] *Ndeqne molang ini.*
Inaq Sarin:	It's not breech, right?	*Ndeqne molang, ngeh?*
Papuq Isa:	No, my child.	*Ndeq anangku.*

In this interaction, we see a mother deeply worried about the biomedical midwife's diagnosis. Papuq Isa examines her and finds that the baby is correctly positioned, definitely not breech. But the word of the Bu Bidan obviously carries considerable weight with Inaq Sarin and her neighbor. Inaq Sarin asks four times in a three-minute period if the child is all right—if it is positioned correctly. The neighbor repeats this question and does the unheard of, apparently suggesting getting a third opinion from Inaq Mol. Under normal circumstances, one *belian* never asks for the help of another midwife. To do so is considered an insult to her own abilities. The neighbor's suggestion is not even dignified with an answer, perhaps because of the implied slight, and also because Papuq Isa knows Inaq Mol (her daughter) to be wholly unqualified to render an opinion. In this brief interaction, we see a diagnosis disconfirmed.

We have seen how creativity is essential in processes of interpreting and coping with illness. Yet the interpretation of illness does not end with the names suggested by individuals. A name is usually discussed further, other opinions are sought. Names clear a place to land in the swarming anxiety that surrounds an unknown illness. But that landing is only tentative. Names are conditional, dependent on whether or not they are legitimated in social interactions.

POLITICS OF ILLNESS:
CRITICAL MEDICAL ANTHROPOLOGY

Critical medical anthropology (CMA) calls into question "the way in which all knowledge relating to the body, health, and illness is culturally constructed, negotiated, and renegotiated in a dynamic process through time and space" (Lock and Scheper-Hughes 1996, 43). For example, Gilbert Lewis (1993) discusses an illness in Papua New Guinea that locals did not perceive as particularly serious but missionaries and biomedical specialists defined as leprosy. The latter insisted on seclusion and treatments that drastically affected people's lives. The power of government-backed authority of biomedicine forced people to accept its judgment, although they never accepted the corresponding meanings of the disease. By emphasizing the politics of illness, the CMA approach pushes medical anthropology to understand its subject matter as no different from other arenas in which hidden agendas, large-scale politics, economic motivations, and the acceptance of one perspective as unquestionably true fundamentally affect the meanings, choices, and perspectives of people living their everyday lives.

While the CMA approach can and has been carried to extremes, even to the extent that suffering is forgotten in the midst of rhetoric (Trevathan 1997), it asks important questions about the politics of medical interactions. Most often, interactions are summarized in the author's discussion of power dynamics (e.g., Davis-Floyd and Sargent 1997), but those who have detailed the dialogues of interactions have shown that politics and authority are not imposed on interactions but rather emerge out of them in patterned ways.[1]

SOCIAL CONSTRAINTS ON INDIVIDUAL INTERPRETATION

In the last chapter, I proposed a model of individual interpretation as a creative process. But grounding that model in how Sasaks name illness, two caveats became clear: all processes of creativity do not generate equally innovative products, and anxiety fundamentally colors the processes of creativity. Yet another caveat must be added, one implied in all the discussions so far but so complex it deserved its own chapter, namely, that interpretation is constrained by social reaction. The purpose of creative processes is to make meanings; for our interests, it is to name an illness so that it can be treated. When someone comes up with an illness name it must be expressed either verbally or through performing a treatment for there to be any hope of getting rid of the illness.

Once an illness name is expressed, the locus of interpretation shifts from individual creativity to social transformation, legitimation, or constraint. Indeed, the success of creative constructions of knowledge is determined by the reactions of recipients to that knowledge. Recipients' reactions either legitimate or constrain knowledge production (Bourdieu 1977a, 1991). Legitimacy depends on the degree to which

---

1. See, e.g., Wilce 1995, 1997; Jordan 1997; Desjarlais 1992; Price 1987; West 1984.

the knowledge expressed by a given person fits with the recipients' expectations, motivations, and prior understandings of the topic. Because people desire to have their knowledge legitimated, they reformulate and/or constrain how they express themselves according to their perception of the context and their social relationship with the recipients.[2] The context in which the information is made available affects interpretation (Goodwin and Duranti 1992). Context refers to the people present at an event, the physical and temporal space, and all other aspects of the "intentional world" that are meaningful to a person in that particular situation (Shweder 1990). Because context marks interpretation, contexts differentially affect legitimation. By the same token, relationships with participants in an interaction affect legitimation. It matters whether the recipients of one's expressions are perceived as adversaries or friends, superiors or equals. For example, information presented to a student in a lecture hall is likely to be understood differently than if that same information is presented in a bar. As Luhrmann suggests: "There seem to be distinctive ways of talking, acting, and—one suspects—thinking in different situations" (1989, 8). Personal interpretation is constrained by context and by what the knower thinks others will agree with or at least listen to and not reject out of hand.[3]

In creating illness names, people must come up with names that fit with the cultural knowledge of ethnomedicine (minimal though it may

---

2. See Bourdieu 1977a; Goffman 1973. Unlike Leach (1964), I do not maintain that people *necessarily* act to gain political power or status, although certainly sociopolitical concerns motivate some people's actions. I am simply arguing that people want to have others respect and preferably agree with what they say and do. People want their expressions of knowledge to have social value.

3. Writing ethnography has its own strategies of legitimation, for example, citing others (as if consensus somehow validates a statement), quoting the native's own voice, giving extensive ethnographic detail, and making claims to language fluency and acceptance within the society studied. Critics have noted that these strategies of legitimation are problematic (e.g., see Clifford and Marcus 1986). Although these critiques are extremely important in foregrounding the processes and politics of writing, the problems they note are not necessarily ones that need "solving." Writings, like all other forms of expressed knowledge, reflect the motives of the author. Academic writers have much at stake when they show their writings to the world: months or years of work, degrees, careers, professional reputations all can be made or broken by what is printed on the page. Thus, of course, writers of ethnographies, myself included, tend to write with strategies that will make them accepted, which will entice others to agree with them and deem them correct, which will incite others to refer to their work. However, I suggest that this is how things necessarily are. There is no expression of knowledge without motivation. There is no expression of knowledge without striving for legitimation. It is the stuff of society, community, and that elusive thing we call culture.

be), that call upon one or more of the areas of illness causes (person-hood, vulnerability, context, coincidence, and perceived symptoms), and that do not otherwise violate the expectations of the people who learn of that illness name. In other words, creative processes are con-strained both at their beginning, by cultural knowledge and assump-tions that limit imagination, and at their end, by anticipation of others' reactions. Once a person does express an illness name, the interpretive work shifts to the social arena where one of three things happens. Peo-ple can take up the name and tinker with it, transforming it into a slightly different name. Or they legitimate the name by uttering words of agreement, defending it from criticism, further distributing that name as true, and/or acting upon that name by using it as the basis of a treatment. Or people denounce the name as false and attempt to con-strain its further expression. Any particular illness name could receive any or all of these reactions, depending on who hears it. Only when someone is treating him- or herself in secret are illness names not sub-ject to social interpretive processes. Otherwise, all illness names must undergo a social birth (Shore 1991).

Although speaking of legitimation in different terms, anthropolo-gists looking at medical systems have noted the processes that influence and constrain the practices of shamans and other healers.[4] They argue that social processes work to rein in a practitioner in accordance with the common knowledge of ethnomedicine in a given setting and the expectations of what healing entails. As the Sasak materials show, these processes are more complex in societies where there are few common-alities in ethnomedical knowledge and everyone's ideas must undergo processes of legitimation, not just those of healers. On the other hand, the Sasak materials also suggest that when healing knowledge is secret and widely dispersed, legitimation processes tend to be relaxed, tenta-tively legitimating many illness names simultaneously. With these underpinnings we return to the Sasak materials, looking for moments of transformation, legitimation, and constraint as people socially inter-pret illness.

INAQ SARIN AND HER
BREECH-NONBREECH BIRTH

In the dialogue at the beginning of this chapter, a *belian* assured her pregnant patient that, regardless of what the *bidan* said, the baby was

---

4. See, e.g., Schieffeln 1996; Tsing 1988.

not in breech position.[5] Papuq Isa also effectively silenced the neighbor woman's suggestions questioning her own competence by ignoring them. Inaq Sarin, the pregnant woman, was insistent on obtaining repeated assurances, but after four such assurances she, too, was silent about being breech. Was she silent because she was convinced, or had Papuq Isa constrained her from further voicing doubts?

When Papuq Isa left Inaq Sarin's side, I followed her. I spent that entire day with her, mostly helping the old woman harvest beans from her son's fields. En route to the fields, we stopped to chat with two different women in different compounds. With both women, Papuq Isa told of how she had just seen Inaq Sarin. She said that the *bidan* had insisted the baby was in breech position. Papuq Isa concluded her story both times by saying, "But that is not the way. The baby is positioned correctly. The *bidan* less than knows" (*Ndeqne ngeno. Kenaq baiyatne. Kurang tauq Bu Bidan sino*). Not only did Papuq Isa disconfirm the *bidan*'s diagnosis for Inaq Sarin, but she took that diagnosis and used it to reflect negatively on the *bidan*. By repeating the incident, Papuq Isa was using what she saw as an error to undermine any competence or authority that community members might have ascribed to her biomedical competition.

During the next two days, Inaq Sarin's behavior showed that she was confident in Papuq Isa's assessment. She did not return to the *bidan*. Nor did she seek opinions from other *belians* in the community. Papuq Isa had convinced her that her child was not breech—that the interpretation of the *bidan* was incorrect.

On the third day, toward evening, Inaq Sarin went into labor. Her husband went in search of Papuq Isa, but she had gone to a distant village.[6] He sought other *belians*—first Inaq Hapim, then Inaq Kalin. None could come.[7] In desperation, he went to get the *bidan,* who refused to deliver the child, insisting that it must be born in a hospital because it was breech. Because Inaq Sarin's only living child, a teenager, lived with the head of the village (*kepala desa*), a message was sent to him, and he borrowed the village head's truck to take everyone

---

5. The *belian* did not mention the possibility that the baby could have shifted position on its own.

6. Healers are not expected to stay put, and it often happens that one's first choice for a *belian, dukun,* or clinician is not around in times of need. At this particular time, Papuq Isa had gone to visit her daughter-in-law's mother who had just given birth to stillborn twins.

7. Delivering a child without a midwife of some sort to catch it is not considered an acceptable option.

to the hospital. Halfway between Pelocok and the hospital, the *bidan* made them stop in a village with a doctor. The doctor did an ultrasound, which showed that the baby was breech. This doctor declined to deliver the child and sent them on to the hospital in Selong.

Legitimation Processes among Rural Laypersons

Two days later, Inaq Sarin, along with her husband, assorted relatives and friends, and new infant daughter, returned to Pelocok. I was with the host of people who greeted them on their return, crowding their tiny one-room hut to hear all the details of what had happened. The confusion of voices, one talking on top of the other, make the audio recording difficult to follow. Below is an excerpt of approximately 30 seconds of interaction. I have transcribed and translated everything that was distinctly clear in that time period, even though some comments were not at all pertinent to the main conversation. For example, the fifth speaker, Inaq Bah, is interested in finding a person and has no interest in the topic of conversation, but I include her voice only to highlight the disjointedness within which everyday dialogues occur.

Amaq Senin [Inaq Sarin's husband]:	Our cost for just the machine [to turn the baby in utero]) was about 25,000 Rp.	*Ongkosne siq ite kire alat doang selai ribu.*
Amaq Mol:	So, was it breech?	*Ngo, malang ini?*
Inaq Ali:	She was breech.	*Iye malang.*
Inaq Selin:	Was she breech?	*Iye malang?*
Inaq Bah:	Inaq Sarin?	*Sarin?*
Inaq Sarin:	What?	*Eh?*
Inaq Bah:	Where is Inaq Kerim?	*Mbe Inaq Kerim?*
Inaq Selin:	Oh, she was breech.	*Oh, iye malang.*
Inaq Ali:	At the market.	*Pekan.*

Amaq Sal:	She was right, the Sasak *belian*.	*Iye tepat belian Sasak ini ngene.*
Inaq Selin:	Yes.	*Ayo.*
Amaq Mol:	On the contrary, she was wrong.	*Malah peleh iye.*
Amaq Senin [softly]:	Yeah.	*Ya.*
Amaq Mol:	It doesn't matter what the belian said, so don't.	*Ndeq ngumbe-ngumbe ongkatne belian sasak den- deq angkan.*
Papuq Sarin [Inaq Sarin's mother]:	Hey, it wasn't breech.	*Eh, ndeqne malang.*
Another woman:	It wasn't breech.	*Ndeq ne malang ini?*
Amaq Mol:	Is the feeling already calm?	*Wah teduq anganne?*
Amaq Senin:	The feeling is already calm.	*Wah teduq angan.*
Inaq Mol:	What were the names people gave for this? [How was Inaq Sarin diagnosed before?]	*Mbe teparan laeq isti paran dengan, side?*
Inaq Ali: [Three other woman talk about whether she was breech simultaneously; their voices are indistinct.]	People looked at her stomach . . .	*Dengan wah gitaq tian . . .*
Another woman:	. . . the *bidan* already knew it was breech at the seventh month.	*. . . wah tetauq siq Bu Bidan ne malang wah pituq bulan.*

At this point, the welter of voices turned again to the cost of the birth and to stillbirths of other women at the hospital. In this excerpt, two issues are at stake: whether the birth was breech and how correct the prebirth diagnoses had been.

Strangely, whether the birth was breech is not as clear as one might suppose. The husband and others understood the baby was in breech position and therefore had to go to the hospital and be turned by a machine, a procedure costing 25,000 Rp.[8] Because it was breech, the *belian* was initially praised for being right by Amaq Sal—an appraisal legitimated by Inaq Selin. Amaq Mol then stated that the *belian*, implicating but never naming Papuq Isa, was wrong—a statement legitimated by the husband. But then Amaq Mol, always a peacemaker in the community and himself the son-in-law of Papuq Isa, deflected further accusations of Papuq Isa's knowledge and skill by announcing that whatever she had said did not matter now. Inaq Sarin's mother's statement that it was not breech is curious. Why did she say this, flatly contradicting the statements only a few seconds before? She had been at the hospital and seen the machines used supposedly to turn the baby. Why did she say that it wasn't breech? It is plausible that she was implying that, whatever its previous position, the baby was *born* normally; it was not a breech birth. But considering that she made this statement after a flurry of subtle accusations questioning the *belian*'s ability, it could be that she was attempting to defend Papuq Isa.

At this point, Inaq Mol, who did not know much about the case, asked what names had been given to the position of the baby. It is here that the relative clarity of the tape breaks down because multiple women answer simultaneously. The loudness of their voices and the breakdown of any turn-taking rules (always rather lax) indicate the anxiety of opinions.[9] The women knew that this was the crux of the matter. The only clear statement to emerge toward the end of this upheaval was the woman's remark that the *bidan* had warned of the breech position for months.

In this brief interaction, we see statements legitimated and directly contradicted. But there is no authoritative voice that speaks loudly, stating without question whether the child was breech or not. No one per-

---

8. For an average household, 25,000 Rp would represent more than one-eighth their annual income. Inaq Sarin and her husband Amaq Senin were poorer than normal, owning no cows and just a small garden plot. To pay much of the cost of Inaq Sarin's hospital birth, totaling 107,500 Rp, they went into debt with family and neighbors.
9. Sasak turn-taking rules discourage interruption in any kind of formal interaction. People acknowledged that ideally one should not interrupt even in everyday interaction. But in practice, people often talk on top of one another.

son's voice is perceptibly more likely to be listened to and legitimated. In muddled conversations such as these, people attempt to negotiate reality by slipping from subject to subject before any final consensus about what happened is reached. People were interested in who was correct about the breech position—the *belian* or the *bidan;* at stake is a lifelong faith in and friendship with *belian*s like Papuq Isa. And yet, while hesitant to condemn Sasak medicine as personified by Papuq Isa, they do not hesitate to acknowledge that the *bidan* might have been right. Overall, people were less concerned with blaming or praising any one medical tradition than with describing the events.

Legitimation Processes: With the Bidan

Later that same day, I went to speak with the Bu Bidan, Rini. After exchanging pleasantries over glasses of coffee, I asked what had happened with Inaq Sarin. With Rini's radio blaring Indonesian pop music (*dangdut*) in the background, she explained in Indonesian:

Rini: Inaq Sarin she was high risk. She is almost menopausal she is so old, and has had many children. This was number eight. No, nine. Only one lives. See, Cameron, the risk was very high. The baby was breech. Many times I told her to give birth in the hospital. If it had been normal, I could have delivered it, but if it's not, it must be sent [to the hospital]. But she did not want to, Cameron. She wanted to go to B——.* What about that, Cameron?

Inaq Sarin, dia risiko tinggi. Tua sekali, hampir menopause, tua, dan anaknya banyak. Ini nomor delapan. Ndak, sembilan. Hanya satu hidup. Kan, Mbak, risiko tinggi sekali. Terus letak lintang bayinya. Berapa kali saya suruh dia beranak di ruman sakit. Kalau normal, bisa saya, tetapi kalau ndak, harus dikirim. Tetapi ndak mau dia, Mbak. Dia mau ke B——. Bagimana Mbak?

---

*B—— refers to a distant hamlet in central Lombok that is famous among rural Sasak women. It is said that a *belian* in B—— can deliver anyone, no matter how difficult the case.

Cameron:	So when she went into labor . . . ?	*Jadi waktu dia sakit tian . . . ?*
Rini:	I heard that she was beginning labor and went straight to her house. She cried, still wanting to go to B——, but I took her to my doctor [supervisor] in L——.* He used ultrasound to see how this and that were with the baby.	*Saya dengar dia mulai sakit tian, terus langsung ke rumahnya. Ngangis dia, masih mau ke B——, tapi saya agak dia ke doktor saya di L——. Terus dia makai ultrasonografi untuk melihat bagaimana itu, bagaimana itu bayinya.*
Cameron:	So how were things?	*Bagaimana, ya?*
Rini:	Yes, the baby was in breech position. Like this. She lay so, with the head here and the bottom here. [Pointing to her own upper and lower stomach.]	*Ya, bayinya itu letak lintang. Begini itu. Dia melintang begini, kepalanya disini, punggungnya disini.*
Cameron:	Oh, so . . .	*Ooo jadi . . .*
Rini:	Difficult right, that's why I sent her [to the hospital]. My doctor also couldn't do it; the point is she was sent to the hospital. There a specialist took actions but didn't have to operate. Thankfully. She was given an IV and a variety of medicines. The placenta, the older-younger sibling, was here [pointing to the bottom of her stomach],	*Sulit kan, makanya saya kirim. Pak doktor saya juge ndak bisa, pokoknya kirim ke rumah sakit. Terus, sampai sana spesialis ngasik tindakan tapi ndak sampai operasi dia. Sukurlah. Diinfus dia, dikasih obat macem. Plasentanya itu ya adik kakaknya itu disini, dia menghalangi jalan lahir.*

---

*L—— refers to a village just north of the market town. L—— boasts its own biomedical PusKesMas (sizable clinic) and has a doctor who lives there.

it was blocking the pas-
sage.*

Cameron: In front of the head?   *Didepan kepalanya?*

Rini: It's not normal for it to   *Kan ndak normal didepan*
                 be in front of the baby's   *kepala anak itu. Terus,*
                 head. Then there was a   *pendarahan banyak, gini-*
                 lot of hemorrhaging,   *gini besarnya. Tadi*
                 about so much [and she   *malam katanya lahir, di*
                 made a bowl shape by   *malam jum'at.*
                 cupping her hands
                 together].† They said it
                 was born last night, Fri-
                 day night.

At this point Rini began talking about other patients she had seen at the hospital, emphasizing how all of the women who had come from B—— had stillborn infants.

There are three important issues worth noting in this interaction. First, the context for the interaction was vastly different from the milling crowd at Inaq Sarin's house. Here, it was only Rini and I, a person she confided in as an equal and assumed to share her presumptions about the value of biomedical care. This different context is reflected structurally in the simplicity of the interaction: there are only two voices, with a minimum of interruptions, and one person is primarily the listener while the other is the speaker. It is also reflected in the lack of challenges to information. In the interactions at Inaq Sarin's

---

*Placenta in its Indonesianized form is the biomedical word, but Sasaks throughout Lombok refer to it as the younger-older sibling. Rural Sasaks treat this "sibling" with respect. It is carefully washed, as carefully as the newborn itself. Then it is wrapped in a cloth, placed in a hollowed coconut shell, and ceremoniously buried under the eaves of the newborn's house. The placenta can be dug up and used in treatments if the baby becomes ill during childhood.

The biomedical name for an abnormally implanted placenta is placenta previa. It is a associated with bleeding in the third trimester, which may account for Inaq Sarin's experiences of minor bleeding as she approached term. If the placenta is truly blocking the cervix, a cesarean section is usually performed.

†It's unclear whether Rini is saying that Inaq Sarin hemorrhaged substantially, or that in cases of placenta previa, one can hemorrhage substantially. Because it is clear from the next sentence that Rini was not present at the birth, she probably was speaking in generalities rather than about Inaq Sarin's experience.

house, statements were repeatedly challenged and contradicted. In this interaction, I made brief comments, implying agreement with whatever she said, asking for clarification at times, and generally encouraging her to talk further. Although primarily a listener, I made statements that legitimated and encouraged Rini's talk and in no way put her on the defensive.

Second, the lack of challenges allowed Rini to press her own agenda. Her narrative tells a story that was not focused on the details of what happened to Inaq Sarin. She did not mention Inaq Sarin's reaction to the ultrasound, the doctor, or her treatment at the hospital, nor did Rini feel it important to describe what actions the specialist had taken to turn the baby or what medications Inaq Sarin had been given. In Rini's worldview, Inaq Sarin's personal experience was not of interest and the quality of hospital care was not in doubt. Instead, the narrative very neatly justifies Rini. She could not deliver Inaq Sarin's child because it was high risk, her diagnosis of breech positioning was legitimated by the ultrasound, even the doctor was unqualified to deliver her, a specialist and special medications were required, and it turned out that the placenta was implanted abnormally, with all the additional risks of hemorrhaging that accompany that condition. What Rini said in this interaction showed her motivation to justify her decision not to deliver Inaq Sarin herself.

Third, in this interaction Rini subtly criticized Inaq Sarin and all like her who prefer Sasak medicine to biomedicine. Rini implied that Inaq Sarin was stupid not to realize that her pregnancy was high risk and that she should go to the hospital. In pointing out Inaq Sarin's crying—the one time Inaq Sarin's experience is important in the narrative—there is a tone of irony: Inaq Sarin does not know what is best for herself, she cries when she should be grateful for the ultrasound and the trip to the hospital. Toward the end of the conversation, Rini justified her criticism by pointing out that all those who went to midwives in B——, as Inaq Sarin wanted to do, had stillborn babies. Indeed, Rini's condescension is warranted. She probably did save the lives of Inaq Sarin and her baby, and she has reason to be frustrated at women who avoid biomedicine in favor of midwives, like those in B——, who often deliver stillborn babies.

In this interaction, statements are not constrained or contradicted, and one person's voice and opinion dominate. Because I was an encouraging recipient, her narrative gradually attained a significance that the voices in the interaction at Inaq Sarin's house never had. She did not have to defend her opinion; she was not stopped in weaving her narrative. I suggest that it was my voice—mostly silent though it was— that enabled Rini to express her interpretation of the events. Notably, her interpretation was motivated by a wish to defend her decisions and the greatness of the medical tradition to which she belonged and simultaneously to devalue the knowledge and approaches of people who choose alternatives to that medical tradition. My encouragement gave Rini the social space in which to express—and, in the act of expressing, perhaps further develop—her own interpretation of the event.

Comparing the Processes of Social Interpretation

Comparing this interaction with Rini to the interaction at Inaq Sarin's house is instructive. In one interaction expressed knowledge is uniformly legitimated by the listener, and the speaker is allowed to elaborate her own interpretation of the event. In the other interaction, the same expressed knowledge (e.g., "She was right then, the Sasak *belian*") is both legitimated ("Yes") and invalidated ("On the contrary, she was wrong"), which constrained the speaker from defending his first statement. Moreover, there are so many listeners that no one speaker attempts to elaborate an interpretation of the entire event, including Inaq Sarin's husband who had been in the midst of the event from beginning to end. I suggest that it is not just sheer numbers of recipients that make a single narrative impossible to express. While muddled voices are the norm in everyday Sasak conversations, I have witnessed numerous times when one person's voice will gain the floor while a crowd of people listen patiently. More important than numbers are the recipients' reactions—whether encouraging, legitimating, and patient, or else argumentative, constraining, and interruptive. These determine the quantity and tone of expressed knowledge.

In the aftermath of Inaq Sarin's birth, neither the *bidan* nor Papuq Isa was used for Inaq Sarin's postnatal care. A *belian* from an eastern hamlet was used instead. Rini's interpretation of success in correctly identifying Inaq Sarin's risks and getting her to the best possible place for care did not disseminate throughout the community. Although all knew that Inaq Sarin had given birth in the hospital, and that mother and child were healthy, neither the hospital nor the *bidan* was praised. Nor in the months that followed were women any more likely to go to the *bidan*. Until I left the field four months later, although some pregnant women would go to Rini for prenatal care, none went to her to deliver their children, even when told that they too were high-risk. In her postnatal actions Inaq Sarin again gave her confidence to a local midwife-healer, but notably not the same one who had held her confidence before. In a sense, Inaq Sarin voted with her feet. However, Papuq Isa's credibility was not noticeably affected. Indeed, within a month, two of Inaq Sarin's immediate neighbors used Papuq Isa to catch their babies' births, and it was Papuq Isa who six weeks later performed the *bekuris* ceremony for Inaq Sarin's newborn.[10]

FROM LEGITIMATION TO AUTHORITY

These interactions suggest that it is the recipient who determines whether authority comes into play in an interaction. In the case of Papuq Isa, before the baby's birth the authority of the *belian*'s voice emerges in the silence of the recipients (Inaq Sarin and her neighbor) after Papuq Isa answers their questions. In the interaction at Inaq Sarin's house, authority does not emerge at all. In the interaction with the *bidan,* it does.

I define *authority* as the ability to gain respectful attention or, to put a more negative cast to it, to silence conflicting voices and actions. The duration of authority can vary from a few moments in a particular interaction to the lifetime of a particular person or a particular government. Again, the burden of authority is on the recipients who choose to silence their voices and constrain their actions. When authority lasts beyond a specific interaction, I suggest that it does so through habits of legitimation.

Long experience, habits of legitimating a particular interpretation or the interpretations of a particular individual or institution, undergird durable authority. The *bidan* in Pelocok is an example of interactional authority without duration. In conversations with Rini, I was not the only one to be silent. When I sat in her clinic observing interactions, rural Sasaks, after saying what hurt or what they thought was wrong, were largely silent, regardless of what she said. Often her patients would seek me out afterward, hand me a packet of variously colored pills given to them by the *bidan,* and ask what they were for and when they should be taken. She was successful at silencing their voices

---

10. The *bekuris* ceremony is a life-cycle ritual to symbolically break the child's ties to its mother and become a person in his or her own right. Normally it is performed at the age of three or four, but the head of the hamlet (Indon., *kepala dusun*) used considerable political pressure to force Inaq Sarin and her unwilling husband to have their infant *bekuris*ed earlier to increase the number of participants in the ceremony the hamlet head was hosting.

in her presence, but their actions—not going to her exclusively, resisting her recommendations, criticizing her lack of *ilmu* behind her back—spoke loudly that her authority did not extend beyond her immediate earshot. The medical tradition she represented was not highly valued; in fact, in the seven months between the establishment of the *bidan*'s clinic and my departure from the field, because of the evident inability of her medicines to make people fat or virile, the increasing criticism of the *bidan*'s lack of *ilmu* and experience (*ndeq ne tauq*), and the increasing number of stories about deaths in clinics and hospitals, the biomedical tradition of knowledge showed few signs of gaining ground in Pelocok.[11] In contrast, although Papuq Isa was largely understood to be mistaken in her estimate of Inaq Sarin's condition, her knowledge and experience, her person and mannerisms with her patients were so highly valued within the community that even an error did not undermine her authority. She was still called to deliver babies, while the *bidan*, who had been right, was not.

In chapter 2, two types of relationships between peasant patients and healers were identified. Relationships with local healers, *belian*s and *dukun*s, are horizontal and multistranded. Relationships with outside healers, such as *bidan*s, are vertical and single-stranded. The horizontal, multistranded relationships are so strong that they can withstand errors in judgment. People's trust in local healers' skills, however misplaced by objective standards, grants them authority as healers. As long as people continue to seek out Papuq Isa and defend her even when she is mistaken, she will retain her authority. The vertical and single-stranded relationships are so brittle and full of distrust that even when the healer (*bidan*) is correct, it is not enough to build confidence in her. By not seeking her out, the villagers vote on the *bidan*'s authority with their feet.

It is during processes of social legitimation that authority can emerge. When carefully grounded in interactions, authority becomes something that can be traced by whether or not one voice speaks loudly enough to silence others.[12] When a voice speaks loudly for long enough to convince others not only that they should be silent but that the loud voice is the only possible voice describing the only possible way

---

11. See Hay 1999.

12. I am using the word *voice* metaphorically. A loud voice could also be a violent voice, threatening livelihood and life if not listened to respectfully. Sasaks gave authority to the Japanese during the years of occupation because the Japanese raped their children, stole their crops, and killed them if they dared resist. Violence adds urgency to silence. I suggest that violence need not undermine this theoretical argument about the origins of authority; but this is a question for experts on violence and beyond our scope here.

the world could be, authority becomes hegemonic. To focus on authority and the associated politics of health care with a wide-angle lens backgrounds the cares and anguish of actually coping with illness. While it is important and instructive to place these materials within a broader framework, authority's emergence and importance is within mundane, everyday processes of legitimation and constraint that enable people to cope with illness.

WHEN LEGITIMATION COUNTS:
THE CASE OF LO BUDIN

The processes of legitimation and constraint discussed above suggest issues of anxiety only just before the birth, in the initial worries expressed by Inaq Sarin to her midwife, "Is it breech?" In the interactions after the birth, although there definitely were significant things at stake for speakers (the rightness of their interpretation, the reputations of midwives), life and death were no longer immediate concerns.

If we return to the case of Lo Budin, life and death *did* ride on which expressed knowledge was legitimated and which was not. As the child's suffering increased, and the parents became more and more anxious wondering whether he would be alive or dead at the end of the day, we need to ask about anxiety's effect on the social interpretation of Lo Budin's illness. To what extent does anxiety shape processes of legitimation and constraint? What is the relationship between anxiety and authority?

The Politics of Coming Up with Names
in Everyday Conversations

The day was overcast. At midmorning I sat with about 15 other women, including Inaq Budin and Papuq Isa, on and around the front stoop of Papuq Junin's house. I had brought my tape recorder, as was my habit, putting it down in plain view for all. Toddlers and small children crowded the scene. Women sifted rice and hulled beans. Many of the women moved in and out of the conversation, in and out of the gathered group as they went off to start lunch or bathe.[13] Dogs scavenged. Doves cooed. Chickens ran between us, pecking at the scattered rice

---

13. In transcribing the tape, I have been unable to recognize all of the women's voices, and to those women I have assigned letters rather than names.

hulls and the few grains that flew onto the earth. It was in all ways a typical, noisy everyday scene, except that the child in Inaq Budin's arms was having continual, mild seizures.

Politics, at the level of legitimating some expressions and constraining others, is as evident in everyday dialogues as in presidential speeches. The conversation presented below shows these social processes in strong confirmations (e.g., "Yes" or "True"), weaker, more tentative affirmations (e.g., sounds like the English "uh-huh"), and strong rejections of expressed knowledge (e.g., "You are stupid" or "It's not possible"). The rapidity of different suggestions as well as the sustained concentration on the topic of Lo Budin are indicative of the level of anxiety about the boy's condition. Moreover, throughout this exchange, one voice does not dominate. Here is conversation marked by anxiety but lacking a single authority.

Inaq Mol and Papuq Isa were talking together in hushed tones. By their gestures toward Lo Budin, I surmised he was their subject. I pressed the *record* buttons. Gradually, as is true in most Sasak conversations except ones when secret words are being given, the whispering got louder and louder:[14]

1 **P. Isa:**	Like, uhh a chicken [pause] . . .	*Misan, e manuk . . .*
2 **I. Mol** [interrupting]:	Like chicken that is also fighting. The way a chicken moves like this and this [she jerks her arms as if making an erratic punching movement]. . . . If this was given by a chicken it is easy to treat, one only waits a little bit.	*Misan manuk si begebuk indah. Cere manuk sino sang sini, ampok si ngene-ngene. . . . Lamun iye genne te'embeng mola aris te ngowatin, sebendot unguq.*
3 **P. Isa:**	That's true.	*No.*
4 **I. Sun:**	He doesn't cry.	*Ngangis si ndeq iye.*

14. In this dialogue, the teknonymic prefaces to names of the speakers are abbreviated as follows: P. for Papuq (grandmother) and I. for Inaq (mother). Also, true conversational analysis would number each sentence and mark the speech for tone, inflection, and interruption. Such detailed analysis would not substantially forward the argument here; therefore I only number the different voices in this conversation. These numbers will be used in the discussion to refer to a particular speaking turn.

5 **I. Mol:**	Yes.	*Aoq.*

6 **I. Budin:**	He doesn't cry at all, Older Sister, right?	*Ndeq ne ngangis jamat, Inaq Kakak, ndih?*

7 **I. Mol:**	Carry him, carry him at night—this night.	*Ngendong, ngendong malin—malin iniq.*

8 **P. Isa:**	This baby he slept in my dreams. It was Friday prayer. Older men tried using twine. You see, this thing was pulled to split an areca nut in half so he could sleep.*	*Iye baiyak terus iye pedam aku nimpi ni Jum'at. Akak-akak ngobe entan inuk. Kan si ngeno nolok calan gen pedam.*

Conversation degenerated to talk about whether or not there are nuts for chewing betel. Approximately seven minutes later, the conversation returned to the subject of Lo Budin.

9 **I. Mol:**	This here [the stomach] feels as if it is rumbling.	*Ne perasaan berumbung . . .*
10 **P. Isa** [interrupting]:	. . . this is the illness that wants to be treated. [Pause] His ??? has been lost, it must be sought.†	*. . . q ne sakitne meleh teowat.* [Pause] *Iye pepri petri telangang, ne tepete.*

---

*Papuq Isa is describing a treatment in her dreams involving twine and the splitting open of an areca nut. Strings made of round thread are often used in preventing illness and are wrapped around the stomachs of pregnant women, postpartum women, and infants. I have seen cloths tied around heads to treat headaches and dizziness. The fibrous twine Papuq Isa describes was probably used around either the stomach or the head in her dream. I am aware of no other form of treatment that involves splitting an areca nut and have never witnessed a treatment like the one she describes, which occurred in her dreams. The association in the dream with the holy Friday prayer implies a spiritual causal agent.

†I do not know the Sasak words *pepri petri*. These words seem to refer to some entity that comes in pairs. The word *pereq* refers to the scrotum, and is similar enough to be distorted into *pepri* in conversations—particularly when the conversant is speaking through a mouth full of betel juice-soaked tobacco, as was Papuq Isa. If this is correct, *pepri petri* might refer to Lo Budin's scrotum and testicles, but I never noticed that these had retracted into his body. *Pepri petri* also call to mind the rhythmic pairs of words often used in *jampi,* and could therefore be words from the ancient Sasak language used now only in potent texts (*lontars*) and in ilmu.

11 [Quiet voices jumbled together.]

12 **I. Ju:** Oh, this dog, like this and this and this and this [moving her arms in a repetitive round motion], once it is finished, it feels at home and then sleeps. [Implying that the child has the illness of dogs which impels it to make strange movements, but will eventually be quieted].

Ehh, ancong si ngene ngene ngene ngene, wah buet te-isah angatne pedum.

13 [Others] Sound of affirmation.

Ummm.

14 **P. Isa:** The name is not like the way of dogs when a baby moves like this, like this. [Indicating Budin's erratic movements.]

Aran ndeq sere encong biakne si ngene, ngene.

15 **Inaq A:** You are stupid. [Talking to Inaq Ju]

Ano gebol side.

16 [Three voices talk at once.]

17 **I. Sal:** [Phrase meaning]: It may be hopeless.

Kareng due keli siwaq nggakne bilang.

18 **Inaq A:** If it is like this, right?

Munne ngeno nah?

19 **P. Isa:** What?

Eh?

20 **Inaq A:** If it is like this, right?

Munne ngeno nah?

21 [Papuq Isa coughs while other women exchange three or four sentences quietly and inarticulately.]

22 **P. Isa:** . . . fill [a container] with coconut milk to drink so that he can

. . . isa betik antan minum gen nai no iya mentan unti- keh! Iye, antan ente

		defecate. And then wait for - keh [sound meaning "well that's it"]! The coconut milk will become [will meet] blood. I am not making it come out; he will live.	*miq daraq. Aku ndeqne besugul nat hidup.*
23	**Inaq B:**	But does he want to urinate only?	*Sange meleng iye enet aja?*
24	**P. Isa:**	Last night. Last night he managed to a little. [Turning to a child] Be patient, eat this.	*Malin. Malin isti bauq ni ani-aneh ye.* [Turning to a female child] *Ahan juluq, nakan bi.*
25	**Inaq B:**	But he didn't scream last night, Inaq. Your baby?	*Podokan ndeq sorok malin, iniq. Ni bayakde?*
26	**Inaq C:**	[Words unclear. From what transpires, she must have told of a similar case in another hamlet.]	
27	**P. Isa:**	It moved like this?	*Ngini-ngini no?*
28	**Inaq C:**	One like this is like the child of Inaq Nojaq. The one with . . .	*Neh ngnih gerang anak Inaq Nojaq. Si barang...*
29	**P. Isa** [interrupting]:	When?	*Piran?*
30	**Inaq B:**	Once.	*Sekeli so.*
31	**Inaq C:**	It was the same with the child of . . .	*Baran antoqan kanak . . .* [her voice became too quiet to understand.]
32	**P. Isa:**	Amaq Kalim?	*Amaq Kalim?*
33	**Inaq C:**	No.	*Neh.*
34	**P. Isa:**	Amaq Apak?	*Amaq Apak?*

35 **Inaq C:**	Yes. He is the one to do treatments.	*Aoq. Si no baran teowat.*
36 **P. Isa:**	But did it die? The baby?	*Matiq laguq? Bayakno?*
37 **Inaq C:**	Yes. That same day he died.	*Aoq. Barang jelo iye wahan.*
38 **P. Isa:**	Was he an acquaintance of yours?	*Iye kenangbi juluq?*
39 **Inaq Ju:**	The child of whom?	*Anak saiq?*
40 **Inaq C:**	Inaq Nojaq. The smallest one.	*Inaq Nojaq. Si palen kodeqne.*
41 **Inaq Ju:**	Oh. Inaq Nojaq.	*Oq. Inaq Nojaq.*
42 **Inaq A:**	He was already big, Inaq Nojaq's baby.	*Iye wah beleq bayakne Inaq Nojaq.*
43 **P. Isa:**	True. Come here my grandchild. [Takes Lo Budin in her arms].	*Tentu, nih wayangku.*
44 **Inaq B:**	His *ketemuq* is very strange [indicating Lo Budin with her eyes].	*Aneh jamat ketemuq bebayak si iniq, si kodeq.*
45 [Child screaming.]		
46 **P. Isa:**	It will be done like this later.*	*Nih ngenetne nih bareh.*
47 [Multiple voices talking at once.]		
48 **Inaq Budin:**	. . . tomorrow, late Monday, this should be the treatment.	*. . . jamat bareh senin ape-ape nih teowat.*
49 **P. Isa:**	[Sound of noncommital affirmation.]	*Nnn.*

*Papuq Isa is evidently referring to some kind of treatment that will be administered to Lo Budin later. It is unclear from the cassette what the treatment is or what illness name it implies.

50	**I. Sal:**	Will Amaq Mol be doing a *berinjam* [treatment for the child addressed to the water spirit]?	*Nares berinjam Amaq Mol?*
51	**I. Budin:**	For two nights, he has done many things I think, Inaq.	*Iye due kelum ape-ape kenangbe Inaq.*
52	**P. Hem:**	Was he given porridge before? [Was the child given the illness-preventing rice porridge of the Bubur Puteq and Bubur Abang ceremonies that had occurred two and three months before-hand?]	*Ape iye tebubur laiq iniq?* [Her question receives no verbal response. It is likely that Inaq Budin replied with an affirmative facial gesture, but because this interaction was recorded without videotape it is impossible to be certain.]

53 [Chaotic noises and voices.]

| 54 | **P. Isa:** | Where does Inaq Ali and whomever else live? | *Embe tauqne Inaq Ali ape-ape?* |
| 55 | **Inaq B:** | Here with Inaq Acok. Close by. | *Siniq dit Inaq Acok. Pandes.* |

56 [A voice, speaking at the same time as the sentences above.]

57	**P. Korin:**	Why don't you see if she will come around here, accept money for Amaq Sirum. . . .	*Gitaq bai iye pandes seketan datan, kepeng doang gen Amaq Sirum. . . .*
58	**P. Isa** [interrupting]:	We should anyway [regardless of the cost].	*Kewe doang.*
59	**Inaq B:**	If, if you really want. . . .	*Lamun, lamun ngeh kewe. . . .*
60	**Inaq C** [interrupting]:	Okay let's go. . . .	*Bai alo. . . .*

61 **P. Isa:**	[Sound of noncommital affirmation.]	*Mmmm. Mmm.*
62 **Inaq Sopi:**	It fits that Amaq Sirum knows the path [for treatment] . . .	*Iye cocok Amaq Sirun itne tauqne langan . . .*
63 **P. Korin:**	Yes, but divine it first.	*Aoq laguq puputan si ini*
64 **I. Mol:**	Yes.	*Aoq.*
65 **I. Sahim:**	Hopefully tomorrow there will be. . . .	*Mudah-mudahan jamat aditne are. . . .*
66 **I. Mol:**	Just try.	*Coba doang.*
67 **P. Isa:**	It should be tried.	*Ankan tebayak.*
68 **Inaq A:**	In Sembalun [a distant village] everything is worked.*	*Leq Sembalun ape-ape tegawaine.*
69 **P. Korin:**	Okay. Go ahead and try.	*Aoq. Saran.*
70 **P. Isa:**	This is the baby to be looked at. Look closely. He was nobility long ago.	*Iye bayakne tegitaq. Gitaqne pandes. Iye ne ese laiq.*
71 **I. Sahim:**	He doesn't know how to [has no agency to] nurse.	*Ngusu ndeqne tauq.*
72 **I. Sal:**	It was about midnight. Like this chicken, the movement of his body resembles a chicken.	*Si mare nu jam dueolas. Mare ne manuk, si ngeno mare manuk awak sino.*
73 **P. Korin:**	Yeah.	*O.* [quietly]

Gawai—the root of *tegawaine* (Sas.)—literally means to work, but ceremonies, rituals, divinations and treatments are also referred to by the use of the word *gawai*. In this case, the speaker seems to be saying that in this other village, all suggested illness names are divined.

| 74 **Inaq Sopi:** | These [indicating the arms] are stiff, not flexible. | *Tegam gene iniq, ndeqne sosokan.* |

| 75 **P. Isa:** | Yes, yes. . . . | *Aoq. Ndih. . . .* |

There is a break in the recording while I switched cassettes. During that time, Papuq Isa did two divinations. One inquired if Amaq Sirum would know the correct treatment. One asked if the illness was from meeting the ghost of a chicken. In both divinations, the answer was no.

| 76 **I. Sopi:** | Still not yet. [Still the right treatment has not been found.] | *Ndeq man doang.* |

| 77 **[Many women]:** | Yes. Nothing is working. Yes. | *O. Nggakne. Aoq.* |

| 78 **I. Budin:** | Earlier he nursed a little. Earlier, and not for just a moment. | *Onet seket susu. Onet bejulu ndeq sebendot.* |

| 79 **P. Korin:** | Try popping [divining] for them both asking if early in the morning they were met [by a ghost]. Try, Inaq. | *Obaq bertoq si pude lamat-lamat bedaitin coba, Inaq.* |

| 80 **Inaq D:** | Oh. It's the illness *ketemuq.* | *Ooq. Ketemuqan.* |

| 81 **I. Sopi:** | It's not possible. | *Ndeqne mungkin.* |

| 82 **I. Mol:** | It couldn't have happened that way. | *Ngeno ndeqne tauq.* |

83 [Rooster crows; indistinct voices.]

| 84 **P. Korin:** | Ask through divination so he doesn't die. | *Ketoaq ngene obaq mun ndeq mati mati.* |

| 85 **I. Sahim:** | Yes. Hopefully it will be easy. | *Aoq. Mudah mola siye.* |

86	**P. Isa:**	[Sound of affirmation.]	*Mm.*

87	**Inaq D:**	Yes.	*Aoq.*

88	**P. Isa:**	It's essential to promise two malaman cere- monies.* Try it already, my child. [This is an order to Inaq Mol to do the divination, telling her what to promise.]	*Ulaq bai cocok kebai janji- janjian kamis due mala- man iniq. Coba se wah anakku, ng.* [Order to Inaq Mol].

89	**P. Korin:**	Try it my child. Try it my child.	*Cobaang anangku. Cobaang anangku.*

90	**P. Isa:**	Try it.	*Cobaang.*

91	[Quiet voices. Inaq Mol tries a divination.]		

92	**P. Korin:**	It doesn't pop.	*Ndeqne ampok-pok.*

Inaq Mol rubs her head, while the conversation continues as women suggest illness names, and potential healers and remark on the child's movements and eating. I left the gathering after about an hour when the women began departing to their respective homes to finish lunch preparations.[15]

---

*Normally malaman ceremonies mark the end of the fasting month. I never heard malaman ceremonies used as treatment other than in this instance, and it suggests how extremely serious these women consider the illness and their conviction that only divine or spiritual intervention of the highest order prompted by a rare and highly sacred ceremony, would treat the illness.

15. My presentation of this conversation is in many ways incomplete. Although some of the women—such as Inaq Budin, Papuq Isa, Inaq Mol—have names, cares, rela- tionships, and personalities that have emerged over various discussions in this ethnography, I have not provided the backgrounds of some of the named women— such as Inaq Ju, Inaq Sal, Inaq Sahim, Inaq Sopi—and other women not only lack backgrounds but names. Moreover, other factors of context are lacking such as com- plete information on the case of the other child who had apparently had a similar ill- ness or why Amaq Sirum was considered a likely person to treat this particular illness correctly. My only defense is that, though I did not know everything of relevance to this extended interaction, I strongly suspect neither did anyone else. For example, two of the women, Inaq B and C, were not from Pelocok, but rather from an unnamed hamlet to the east. They apparently had some connections of social alle- giance with Papuq Junin, but when I asked Inaq Sahim and Papuq Isa about them later, they too did not know these women.

In the half dozen divinations tried, none had an affirmative answer that day. Nor was any final conclusion reached as to what should be done next for the child. I am reminded of a diatribe about dialogue that concludes:

Q. Well, we've been at this discussion for some time now, and I'm wondering how we're going to end.

A. Dialogue doesn't so much end as reach a moment of adjournment.

Q. You mean it has no goal?

A. Dialogue, in and of itself, has no goal.

Q. What if the parties to a dialogue reached complete agreement?

A. That's certainly not going to happen between us. And if we did reach agreement, we would no longer be in dialogue, but rather speaking in unison. But there can be no permanent agreement, because there is always the possibility of further interpretation.[16] (Tedlock 1995, 284)

The conversation among the gathered women did not end so much as adjourn, leaving open-ended the possibility of further interpretation of Lo Budin's illness. But whereas dialogue in itself might not have agreement as a goal, the women use conversation with a specific goal in mind: to identify a potential treatment for the child. They are not talking for their own amusement or to strengthen social bonds, although the conversation also serves this latter function; they have gathered in this place because they were drawn by the suffering of the child, and they talk to seek an answer for his suffering. In short, anxiety is an undercurrent in this entire conversation.

Anxiety enters this conversation as it did in the interaction between Inaq Sarin and Papuq Isa at the beginning of this chapter. But whereas in that case Papuq Isa was directly questioned and her answers eventually taken as authoritative, a similar authority does not emerge to ease anxiety here. Instead, anxiety itself motivates people's attention. Although the women's conversation reproduced above occasionally meandered, as when they became concerned about finding areca nuts so that they could chew betel, they kept returning to the sufferings of the child. At times the women suggested illness names: loss of an aspect of self (line 10), constipation (line 22), a problem with his blood (line 22), madness from not eating the preventive sacred red and white por-

---

16. See Shore 1998 for a critique of this "dialogue."

ridges (line 52), the water god or another spirit (lines 50, 88), meeting with the ghost of a chicken (lines 1, 2, 72), the ghost of a dog (line 12), or a regular ghost (*ketemuq*—lines 44, 79, 80). At times they remarked on the child's behavior and symptoms (lines 4, 6, 9, 23–25, 71–72, 74, 78). At times they made associations between Lo Budin and another case (lines 26–42). At times they discuss persons who should be called in to treat the child (lines 34–35, 50, 57–62). Thus, the majority of the voices that are clear enough to understand during this extended interaction are focused on Lo Budin and not on extraneous subjects. This extended focus on a single subject is unusual in everyday group interactions in Pelocok except in cases when a particular situation or event has riveted everyone's attention as in the case of an unusual death, an enormous life-cycle ritual, or an acute or serious illness episode. The anxiety of context focuses interactions around single topics, urging people to offer suggestions.

Most suggestions are recognized by others in noncommittal ways. For example, Inaq Mol's first suggestion that the illness was given by the ghost of a chicken is greeted by Papuq Isa with "That's true" (line 3). But before committing to this illness name, focus turns to symptoms and to Papuq Isa's dream. Only much later is the chicken illness name reintroduced (line 72), and this time, while Inaq Mol is doing other divinations, she does one for the chicken suggestion. The divination, with its negative answer, rejects once and for all the chicken illness name. Until that point, the lack of negations implies that it was tentatively considered correct. Similarly, the women tentatively affirm the suggestion that Amaq Sirum, who apparently is staying with Inaq Ali at Inaq Acok's house, should be called to come and look at the boy (lines 54–57). In a place such as Pelocok where poverty is ubiquitous and often dissuades people from seeking expensive treatments, Papuq Isa's suggestion that Amaq Sirum be called regardless of his fee (line 58) attests to her high level of anxiety about Lo Budin's condition. Two women leave immediately to go find him (lines 59–60). But after they leave, a divination reveals that Amaq Sirum will not be able to treat the illness. Nonetheless, no one stops the two women. Later that afternoon Amaq Sirum does arrive and say healing spells over the child for a few coins. The rejection of the suggestion issued by the divination did not override the hope that perhaps the question about Amaq Sirum had been asked incorrectly in the divination. In the dialogue and in the developments afterward, no one stakes her reputation or the child's life on any single suggestion. Rather, they tentatively affirm that any reasonable suggestion just might work.

There are also suggestions that are not even tentatively legitimated. Inaq Ju's suggestion that the illness was connected to dogs (line 12) was tentatively affirmed by others (line 13). But when Papuq Isa rejects that suggestion (line 14), and another woman affirms Papuq Isa by degrading Inaq Ju as stupid (line 15), Inaq Ju's voice is largely constrained throughout the rest of the interaction, and no one mentions the connection with dogs again. Another example is when Papuq Korin asks for a divination to find out whether it is *ketemuq* (meeting a ghost—line 79). The next speaker (line 80) transforms the suggestion into a definitive statement that is immediately pounced upon and rejected (lines 81–82). Notably, the voices rejecting knowledge are each different—there is no one decision maker in the crowd.

Why is this important? Or perhaps I should begin with a more fundamental question: why did I include this conversation at all? Admittedly, it is not easy to follow, partly because context is sometimes missing, partly because it is an audio transcription that leaves out essential gestural communication, partly because some of the words and voices are unclear, and partly because I chose not to overedit or shorten it. As it stands though, the conversation shows that its participants also were tuning in and out of what was going on around them. The conversation is filled with non sequiturs (lines 4, 8, 12, 17, 22, 44, 52, 70, 71, 72), showing that speakers were thinking of something other than others' voices right before speaking. More completely than any other interaction in this ethnography, this one shows the disjointedness of normal social communication in Pelocok. But even so, expressed knowledge is responded to more often than not, and those responses determine whether that knowledge will be further considered or completely silenced.

Social interactions that legitimate some suggestions and constrain others are political. But these everyday politics work *without* establishing authority. Legitimated suggestions are tentative, not final, and in no way constrain people from seeking other suggestions. Even the rejection of knowledge is tentative. Likewise, no one voice claims to have the correct suggestion or the final legitimating word. In a dialogue motivated by anxiety, the processes of legitimation and constraint are very evident, but these everyday politics proceed with an air of tentativeness rather than the finality of authority.

Legitimacy and Four Illness Names

Beyond this arena of tentative social legitimation, when significant treatments are planned an authority does emerge. By significant treat-

ments, I mean those treatments that involve more than just whispering
a healing spell over the child, treatments such as name changing, consulting specialists, or conducting lengthy rituals for water spirits and
gods. Recall that in chapter 5, four main illness names were discussed,
each involving significant treatments: Lo Budin's wrong personal
name, the too-early planned circumcision, the connection with the
dead aunt, and the water god. Limiting ourselves to these four, notice
that three mutually incongruent etiologies were accepted and one was
rejected. Although each suggestion was more or less discussed prior to
acceptance or rejection, one person made the final decisions regarding
Lo Budin, namely, his father, Papuq Junin. He was given this authority
not based on his status as the boy's father, for in many matters including health care the father's voice is not necessarily final or dominant in
Pelocok. Papuq Junin's authority sprang from his status as a community
leader and a relatively wealthy, senior, potent man. He was used to having his opinions listened to, and people were used to legitimating whatever he said, at least in his presence. Thus, when illness suggestions
were made, it was Papuq Junin's legitimation or rejection that was
heeded. Why did he legitimate some illness names and reject others?

The name and circumcision etiologies were presented as dream
knowledge, thus carrying inherent validity. Apparently the discussion
following each suggestion was brief and noncontentious, for the father
changed the child's name in the middle of the night and had postponed the planned circumcision by the time of my early morning visit.
Regardless of the fact that others in the community were less certain of
the validity of the young man's dreams, the parents never questioned it,
and these etiologies were quickly accepted, acted upon, and not discussed further. With these illness names, the anxiety of trying to hit
upon the right treatment combined with the automatic legitimation of
dream knowledge so that, rather than waiting and consulting with others the next day, the father initiated name changes and ceremony post-
ponements immediately.

But the anxiety of the illness did not mean that every potential illness name was accepted. The father immediately and angrily rejected
the etiology that connected Budin's illness with the death of the aunt.
Its implied social and spiritual criticism indicated that Papuq Junin had
been wrong to insist on hosting the death ceremonies; it threw into
question Papuq Junin's status as a community leader. Concern for his
son did not override indignation. Others, however, were not so quick to
reject it, and it lingered in the gossip of the community for several days.
In these conversations the father's behavior was criticized circum-

spectly, but whether it was the cause of Budin's illness was a matter of uncertainty in conversations. After a few days this etiology drifted out of conversations altogether. Papuq Isa, who first proposed it, rejected it immediately after Papuq Junin so strongly denounced it. Papuq Junin's voice constrained the pursuit of this etiology—not only could it not be discussed in his presence, but no treatments that implied such an etiology could be undertaken. Because the ultimate goal was to keep the child alive, perhaps people dropped this etiology because pursuing it would gain nothing for the child. Perhaps they dropped it because another etiology had been suggested that did not threaten to disrupt social order as an outright accusation of Papuq Junin would have done. Together these forces not only constrained talk in Papuq Junin's presence, but made it evaporate from the general gossip.

The other, accepted etiology that helped to oust the connection with the aunt's death was the etiology of the water god. This etiology stimulated much discussion, even though it was quickly accepted, and appropriate treatments were immediately initiated. The explanatory story initially accepted was that the water god was causing Budin's illness because his father had failed to perform the necessary rituals. As the symptoms changed in response to various treatments, the explanatory story was revised. These revisions include statements that the problem was not with water spirits of the reservoir but the water god of the originating spring, that the water god was taking possession of Budin's body, and that the water god was angry about past grievances that also needed to be addressed. The revisions were made in conversations and motivated by perceived changes or lack of changes in Budin's condition. But what is interesting is that this illness name stuck. Unlike the wrong personal name, the too-early circumcision, and other assorted illness names discussed in chapter 5, the water god etiology continued to generate treatments even after past treatments for the water god had failed. Thus, not only was this illness name legitimated, it resisted delegitimation.

Resisting Delegitimation

The persistence of the water god illness name suggests that not all knowledge is open to negotiation. Some kinds of knowledge resist all attempts at contradiction, constraint, or delegitimation. Regardless of how many other illness names were considered and treated, regardless of some people's doubts including those of respected healers, regardless of the apparent failure of a variety of treatments to appease the water god, Lo Budin's parents remained convinced that the water god etiology was correct. Why should an illness name become so unquestionable?

There are a number of possible reasons for this. First, the water god etiology fit. It was timely, coinciding with the construction of a water reservoir. It was unusual and complex, thus matching the unusual symptoms and severity of the illness. It dealt with the unpredictable agents of the unseen world, thus calling to mind perpetually experienced vulnerabilities. The water god etiology was complex and timely enough to fit the case, as well as ungraspable enough to defy easy disproof by failed treatments.

Second, the water god etiology, regardless of the failure of various treatments to meet and drive out the illness, continued to be socially legitimated. Papuq Isa whispered doubts about the etiology based on the lack of successful treatments, but to my knowledge, no one else questioned it. Other illness names continued to be suggested, but as frequently people came up with a new treatment for appeasing the water god. The water god etiology stayed active in people's conversations, and thus active in their associations with the illness.

Third, it gave the people who loved this child something to hang on to. They had an illness name, and therefore the illness could be treated. With a name, they could avoid feelings of powerlessness (cf. Laderman 1991, 299). The complexities of the causal agent simply meant that the right treatment had not yet been found, but they suggested that it still could be. Hanging on to this etiology meant that they were not left in the dark without any interpretation to help them make sense of Lo Budin's strange and troubling illness. The illness name gave them understanding and hope.

In matters of life and death, the social processes of legitimation and constraint are still at work, validating some illness names and rejecting others. If less were at stake, perhaps the water god etiology would have been questioned more in social interactions. It is the combination—of a name that fit the coincidences and symptoms, continued social attention to the etiology, and the anxiety and desperation to have some bit of understanding and hope—that made processes of delegitimation jam up, that made an illness name stick.

PARTICIPATION AND SOCIAL LEGITIMATION

People who feel ill often first discuss their symptoms with family members or friends and then later go to a physician who questions, evaluates, and perhaps prescribes treatment. In the course of this exploration the "trouble" itself is transformed from vague and disconnected symptoms to a labeled condition, that is, an illness that others in the society understand to have a particular explanation and social meaning. Thus, *social negotiations turn symptoms into social facts that may have significant consequences for the individual.* (Waxler 1981, 169, emphasis added)

Malinowski, in a little-known work called "The Problem of Meaning in Primitive Language," argues that the meaning of language "lives only in the winged words passing from man to man (1948, 240). Malinowski emphasizes that meaning only arises through *participation in context.* In other words, it is inherently and necessarily social. Intersubjectivity is only possible if there is a shared participation in a particular social world.

Malinowski's approach to meaning, like that of many after him (e.g., Whorf 1956; Fish 1979), depended not only on having the same language, but on common participation in the life-worlds that give words significance. Given the context of Pelocok, with its pluralistic medical setting where everyone is a potential healer and potential illness lurks unseen at every corner, and given the context of Lo Budin's illness, the long dialogue among the women gathered around Papuq Junin's stoop is somewhat understandable. Without that context, no matter how well the words were transcribed and translated, the dialogue would not have made any sense. By *common participation* I do not mean shared experience. Although there are some bits of knowledge that are widely dispersed throughout the community, what any one person has is a unique constellation of understandings that to a greater or lesser extent differs from the constellations of others, even those in the same household. Instead, *common participation* refers to the social experience of being with someone else through the concerns of life day after day, year after year, decade after decade, of building a history—no matter how fragile and temporary—around certain events with other persons, of learning empathy and participating in others' lives. Participation provides the groundwork necessary for intersubjectivity.

Participation is engagement in interaction: a willingness to express knowledge as well as be a recipient of the knowledge of others. In expressing knowledge, what can be said or done is confined to what a person thinks others will listen to and understand without ridiculing, ostracizing, or silencing her. In being a recipient of others' knowledge, a person interprets their words and actions, and tentatively or permanently accepts or rejects them.[17] It is the recipient's reactions that legitimate knowledge. And it is the recipient's reactions, in particular the willingness to be silenced, that grant speakers authority.

The organization of Sasak ethnomedical knowledge requires social participation in order to cope with illnesses. Because medical knowledge is so widely dispersed, the participation of the community in conversations with each person making suggestions maximizes the chances of finding an illness name and a treatment that will fit a particular case. Everyone's suggestions undergo processes of social legitimation; everyone's knowledge must be attended to. Some suggestions are rejected, but the majority of suggestions are tentatively legitimated, because they are based on secret knowledge whose potency can not be judged by others. The ultimate goal in discussing illness is not to find the right illness name or legitimate the right treatment; it is to overcome the threat to someone's health. Anything that could potentially work is tentatively legitimated.

Summary

I have argued that coping with illness has an essential social component in which meaning is given a social birth—or death if it is rejected—in the social processes of interpretation. Individual interpretations of illness are insufficient by themselves to endow illness with a name; they require social legitimation. Once expressed, suggestions for names become the object of others' interpretation and are legitimated tentatively or strongly, or they are ignored, constrained, and rejected, reduc-

---

17. My argument here is little more than a summary of the work of sociolinguist C. S. Volosinov ([1929] 1973). Whereas I speak of the movement of knowledge, he speaks of this same movement in terms of signs. For Volosinov, signs are inherently marked by the individual psyche; they are a personal product. But once expressed, the sign, the enunciated word, is objectified, detached from its producer. If perceived by another psyche, "the enunciated word is subjectified in the act of responsible understanding in order to generate, sooner or later, a counter statement" (41). In his discussion of the construction of meaning, which is basic to intersubjective understanding, Volosinov uses the word *theme* to designate the significance of an utterance as uttered by a particular person for a particular person and in a particular context. In other words, a theme is shaped by its creator, directed toward a recipient, and constrained by perceptions of context (99). The theme as a whole is not reproducible because of its extreme contextual markedness, but within the theme is meaning that is reproducible—meaning is the technical equipment of the utterance (100). Meaning, in which there is an intersubjective convergence and constraint of its potentialities, is the foundation of intersubjective communication and converging understandings.

ing the speaker, however momentarily, to silence. The egalitarian distribution of ethnomedical knowledge in Pelocok means that not only can anyone suggest illness names, no one's voice is necessarily authoritative, so even the names suggested by healing experts must be socially legitimated. These social processes are conservative. While ethnomedicine in Pelocok is relatively egalitarian, while people are open to trying new ideas, and while people grasp at straws when constructing illness names, medicine is not a domain where anything goes. In order to be legitimated, illness names must make sense according to cultural knowledge (e.g., illness is nearly always personalistic and based on connections with personhood, spirits, coincidences, symptoms), and illness names must not undermine someone else's status. The interpretation of illness is a single process consisting of two moments, one of individual creativity with its tendency toward flux and the other of social legitimation with its tendency toward order.

In a society in which ethnomedical health care is fairly egalitarian because everyone has secret healing knowledge, the authority of knowledge about illness is negotiable. Even people designated as healers do not have automatic authority: the names they give an illness must be legitimated socially. However, when people from Pelocok seek biomedical health care, the processes of legitimation are far more complex.

Communication Slippages

Interactions with Biomedicine

In egalitarian knowledge systems everyone has access to knowledge, and the social processes legitimating one interpretation over another require that authority must constantly be negotiated in social interactions. In hierarchical knowledge systems, people have differential access to knowledge, and knowledge is legitimated or rejected automatically based on the knowledge and corresponding social position of the knower.[1] Biomedicine on Lombok is a hierarchical knowledge system, selectively limiting those who have access to biomedical knowledge and automatically legitimating the interpretations of physicians over those of less-trained biomedical personnel, and the interpretations of these latter over those of laypersons.[2]

As discussed in chapter 2, relations between rural Sasaks and biomedical healers are vertical and single-stranded, as opposed to the horizontal and multistranded relationships they have with ethnomedical healers. By looking at biomedicine on Lombok as a hierarchical knowledge system, we can explore what ramifications those vertical and single-stranded relationships have on communication.

---

1. The notion of hierarchy is complex, and, as Dumont has suggested, all social organization is necessarily hierarchical: "To adopt a value is to introduce hierarchy, and a certain consensus of values, a certain hierarchy of ideas, things and people, is indispensable to social life" (1980, 20). Rural Sasaks, in valuing secret healing knowledge above all other medical knowledge, legitimate it as automatically superior to all other kinds of healing knowledge including herbal, medicinal, or humoral therapies. A theoretical discussion of the notion of hierarchy is beyond the scope of this investigation. I use the words *egalitarian* and *hierarchical* in the common senses of the terms to differentiate knowledge systems based on two qualities: access to knowledge and access to authority based on that knowledge.

2. Modern ideology, according to Dumont, is based on egalitarian theory (Dumont 1980, 4). Ironically, biomedicine, which is also often called "modern medicine" and which in Indonesia is supported by a state ideology of modernity and progress, is organized by a hierarchical knowledge system.

ANTHROPOLOGICAL EXAMINATIONS OF
BIOMEDICAL CULTURE

Anthropologists have shown that biomedicine is not a cross-cultural constant: the practice of biomedicine in America is substantially different from its practice in places like France, England, and Mexico (Hunt 1992; Finkler 1991). Like other ethnomedical traditions, biomedicine is a product of a particular cultural milieu "containing culture-specific values, beliefs, and practices" (Brown et al. 1994, 98). Moreover, biomedicine constitutes specialized knowledge and skills that are selectively distributed primarily to medical students who are so transformed by the processes that they become partially alienated from society (Good and Good 1993; Helman 1994). Because of this, as well as biomedicine's tendency to be dramatically different from other ethnomedicines, communication problems are common between physicians and their patients.[3]

West (1984) argues that understanding the communication problems between biomedical personnel and laypersons is not forwarded by a Parsonian assumption of social asymmetry inherent in the roles of doctor and patient (cf. Parsons 1951). West's task is to examine whether there is an empirical basis for this asymmetry that can be revealed in sociolinguistic analysis of dialogues between doctors and patients. She found:

> In general, physicians were the ones who asked the questions, interrupted their co-parties to talk, and initiated the familiarities in these encounters. Conversely, patients generally were the question answerers, the recipients of interruption, and the ones to use formal terms of address in naming their co-participants. (West 1984, 153)

However, her general observation that patients see doctors as "nearly godlike" persons who are "not to be questioned" (99) was qualified when the doctor was female; in these interactions, patients frequently interrupted women physicians (150). She concludes that the asymmetries between doctors and patients are not so much institutionalized as negotiated in patterned ways during interactions. West's research on communication problems was conducted in the United States, where

---

3. See, e.g., Finkler 1991; Hahn 1995; Brown 1998; Haram 1991; Logan 1977; Jaspan 1976b.

doctors and patients usually speak the same language and share basic understandings of body, illness, and therapy. Communication problems are significantly greater when language and basic assumptions of medicine are not common among the participants.

BIOMEDICINE ON LOMBOK:
A STRUCTURAL OVERVIEW

Biomedicine has long been among the choices for medical care in eastern Lombok. In 1928, the first clinic was opened in Selong providing limited biomedical care for people in East Lombok (van der Kraan 1980, 134). The clinic's doctor was Radan Sudjono, a Javanese man who respected local understandings of illness and healing. To this day, among the oldest rural villagers, he is remembered for his great *ilmu* and his curative skills. Apparently he was successful precisely because he was willing to use biomedicine in conjunction with spells and other ethnomedical forms of treatment. This positive experience with biomedicine did not have a lasting impact on resort patterns.

In the last two decades, biomedical facilities have expanded dramatically throughout Lombok, so that by 1988, Lombok boasted 6 general hospitals, 49 subdistrict health centers (PusKesMas), and 160 smaller clinics. Nonetheless, Lombok's infrastructure does not compare favorably with that of other provinces in Indonesia. Inexplicably, provinces with the same approximate population as that of West Nusa Tenggara (the province of Lombok and Sumbawa) have over twice as many biomedical facilities and receive over twice as much money on a per capita basis from the national government for health expenditures (Mboi 1995, 188–98). Finding sufficient qualified personnel to staff facilities is also a problem. In 1988, Lombok's population was 2.2 million people, who were served by 197 medical doctors and 1,848 other medical personnel, only 7 of whom had bachelor's degrees (Kantor Statistic 1988). Doctors are stationed at the hospitals and the district health centers. The smaller clinics are staffed by medical personnel with minimal medical training. All medical personnel have limited access to technological equipment and supplies, and shortages of basic medicines, particularly in the smaller clinics, is not uncommon.[4] Overall, biomedicine on Lombok is geared toward supplying basic health care;

---

4. See Hay 1999 for a case when inadequate access to medications had serious repercussions.

nonetheless, Lombok continues to have among the worse health records in Indonesia.

The organization of biomedical care is complex. There is a hierarchy of facilities, ranging from the smallest, most ill-equipped village clinic to the island's largest hospital in Mataram, with the skills of personnel and available equipment generally paralleling the size of the facility. Seeking biomedical health care is hard work. If one goes to a clinic, more often than not the clinician is making rounds in other villages or in meetings with supervisors. But if one waits long enough, the clinician eventually returns and can issue medicines for such diseases as colds, the flu, anemia, parasites, and diarrhea. For more complicated conditions, one must seek more sophisticated care. If one goes to the hospital, doctors are only in residence in the morning. If one goes instead to a doctor's private practice, it is only open two or three hours in the early evening with patients treated on a first come, first served basis. Clinics that can perform basic laboratory tests are only open a few hours in the mornings. Moreover, each clinic only runs specific tests. Thus, for example, if one needs an X ray and a blood test, one would have to go to two separate clinics. The likelihood of getting through the waiting lines at one clinic, traveling to the next, and getting through the second waiting line on the same day is slim. A person usually must wait another day for any laboratory results, then take those results back to a doctor during private practice hours so that the results can be interpreted. The entire process can easily take a week or more.

While time-consuming, by urban standards biomedical care is affordable. Urban dwellers earning an average 125,000 Rp per month (1,500,000 Rp annually) could afford to pay between 6,000 and 10,000 Rp for a doctor's visit, 10,000 Rp for a day at the hospital, between 2,000 and 15,000 Rp for laboratory tests, or 20,000 Rp for a week's supply of antibiotics.[5] By rural standards, these costs were astronomical. In contrast, the costs of visits to village clinics were affordable: many visits were without charge, and others usually cost the equivalent of a day's wages (between 1,000 and 2,000 Rp).

---

5. These costs were estimated between 1993 and 1995, when the Indonesian economy was fairly strong, and the Indonesian rupiah had a fairly constant exchange rate of 2,210 Rp to the U.S. dollar. Thus a doctor's visit cost between $2.70 and $4.50, a hospital stay cost $4.50 per day, laboratory costs ranged from $0.90 to $6.80, and a week's supply of antibiotics cost $9.00.

Access to Biomedical Knowledge

Biomedical knowledge on Lombok is the exclusive domain of a selected urban elite.[6] To have access to any training in biomedicine, one must first complete elementary and middle school—an educational feat almost unheard-of for rural Sasak children (cf. Corner 1989, 192). Moreover, the programs training *bidans* or clinicians are prohibitively expensive for all but the well-to-do. Attending medical school to become a physician requires years of substantial educational expense—millions of rupiah annually—in addition to academic excellence. There is no medical school on Lombok, and, to my knowledge, none of the medical doctors on Lombok are ethnically Sasak; they are Balinese, Javanese, or Sumatran and are probably all from wealthy, well-educated, nonpeasant families.[7] In short, unlike ethnomedical knowledge, biomedical knowledge is not democratically available to all; it is the exclusive domain of the urban elite.

Organizing Biomedical Personnel

Once educated, doctors and other biomedical personnel are subject to compulsory service for a period of three years. During that time, they are assigned to a district health center or smaller clinic, most often in the rural areas where biomedical personnel are in the greatest need. Mboi (1995) describes how doctors understand and use their time during these assignments:

> Among the young doctors there are men and women of high dedication and creativity, young adults who see their service outside Jakarta as an opportunity to learn things they would never meet in medical school but which are part of Indonesia. However, there have also been those marking time, counting the days until they could return to a comfortable urban practice of their own. Good or bad, the doctors spend a considerable amount of their short

---

6. For the purposes of this discussion, I leave aside the training of traditional midwives or birth attendants (TBAs) in basic biomedical obstetrics at workshops. These *belians*, although trained in biomedical technique, tend to associate themselves with ethnomedical traditions.

7. Physicians from Flores are not necessarily from wealthy or nonpeasant families. Interestingly, people in Flores greatly value formal education (perhaps due to the strong Catholic influence on the island). It is not uncommon for peasants there to educate their children in Timor or Java (see also Corner 1989).

time getting orientated, attending district and provincial meetings, and preparing to return to 'civilisation' after their period of
work in the community centre. (190)

Thus, even during the three short years they staff health centers and
clinics, doctors have required duties that take them away from serving
people. After the required period of service, the government encourages doctors, clinicians, and *bidans* to stay on, settle in the community,
and continue to serve the medical needs of that facility. But most
return to urban areas instead.

Their desire to "return to civilization" is understandable. The living
conditions of rural areas in Indonesia are difficult to adjust to coming
from even a modest Indonesian urban life-style. Doctors, even the most
dedicated and adventurous, are used to the metropolises of Indonesia,
glittering with sophisticated hospitals, easy transportation, telephones,
computers, and air-conditioned buildings, and thus understandably
could find the dirt paths, lightless huts, and paddy fields something of
an adjustment.

Aside from the lack of creature comforts, rural areas also often lack a
community in which highly educated outsiders could feel at home. Rini,
the *bidan* in Pelocok, returned to Selong at least once a week to see her
family and friends. She did not even pray in Pelocok during the Friday
service but "went down" (Indon., *turun*), to the larger mosques in Masbagik, Pancor, or Selong where she was not the only woman worship-
ping. In Pelocok, the only two people she saw socially besides her own
maid (who was her cousin) were myself and the wife of the hamlet head.
Eager as she was to ease the suffering of people, Rini told me that when
she was in Pelocok she was often sad, that it was too quiet for her, and
that it was too frustrating to not be sought out as a healer. She looked
forward to the day when she could be a *bidan* in Selong or Mataram.

Thus, dispersing biomedical personnel into relatively rural areas is
problematic. On the one hand, the mandatory service works to minimally staff health facilities. On the other hand, it requires considerable
life-style and emotional adjustment on the part of the personnel; even
those who are excited about the challenges of serving a rural place usually find it too taxing to contemplate staying permanently.

Assumptions of Authority

Doctors, *bidans*, and other biomedical personnel assume authority with
good reason when they interact with peasants. They have, after all,

been trained in an exclusive field of knowledge, biomedicine. In addition, they often have overcome experiences of personal hardship in order to provide biomedical service to rural areas, and understandably they expect some gratitude and respect. Finally, their status as healers is sanctioned by the state. Biomedicine is the only medical tradition officially recognized as valid health care.

Biomedicine itself is associated with the goals of the state: modernization, development, urbanization, and Indonesianization (the emphasis on being Indonesian rather than on local identity). The ramifications of this status are complex,[8] but ultimately they combine to make biomedicine an exclusive and competitive medical tradition rather than an inclusive and complementary one. Biomedical personnel, by extension, are the noble knights leading the charge of development to significantly improve the health of Indonesians.

The people to whom they bring biomedicine not only have poor health, but suffer from all the disadvantages the state fights against. The very being of people like those in Pelocok goes against these national goals and corresponding accepted ideals. Rather than modern/progressive (Indon., *maju*), rural Sasaks are backward (Indon., *tertinggal*). Rather than living in civilization, they live primitively (Indon., *primitiv*), in *tradisional* villages, and lack familiarity with many of the conveniences—like electricity and indoor plumbing—deemed essential to modern life. Rather than having high school degrees, they have little or no formal education. Rather than being fluent in the national language and seeing themselves as Indonesians, they know only Sasak, have only vague ideas of what Indonesia is, and see themselves as people of Lombok (Sas., *dengan Lombok*). From the perspective of the urban, highly educated, modern biomedical expert whose job forwards development toward the national ideals, almost everything about rural Sasaks needs improving.

Admitting Biases

At this point, I need to confess that my own experiences with biomedical treatment on Lombok have colored the portrait I paint. In 1990, toward the end of preliminary fieldwork, I became ill while staying in Pelocok. Recognizing that I was seriously ill and, at that point, unable

---

8. Biomedicine is one of the symbols that the state has incorporated into its creation of a national identity as a unified, modern, developed, and progressive nation. For discussions of the complexities of this identity building, which is infused into all state activities from schools to theme parks, see, e.g., Pemberton 1994; Siegal 1986.

to communicate in Sasak, I ran back to the city of Mataram. There, over the course of two weeks, I saw four biomedical physicians, two of whom were internal medicine specialists. I was horribly weak and in excruciating pain, so, after two of these physicians diagnosed me with acute appendicitis needing immediate surgical attention, I believed them and checked into the general hospital in Mataram. Because it was already afternoon when I checked in, the doctors had left the hospital for their respites and to tend their private practices, so no doctors would be able to see me until the next morning. After I had a blood sample drawn, an orderly took me to a huge room with two cots lit by a single lightbulb hanging from the ceiling and told me the toilet was down the hall. The room and the toilet were dirty. There were no linens in the room, no nurses to check on me, no food or water that would be brought to me—all of this was the patient's responsibility. The lack of amenities and cleanliness were disconcerting but it was the view from my window that made me leave. It looked out onto a flat roof literally covered with used syringes. I paid my bill of 10,000 Rp ($4.50), checked out, and called the American consulate in Bali to see if he had any suggestions. Within hours, his physician on Bali had determined I didn't have appendicitis, and I was on a flight to Bali. There I saw two physicians who concurred that I only had kidney stones, wrote me a prescription for the pain, and within a week, I was back in Pelocok. In retrospect, this bad experience with Lombok's biomedical health care—aside from the hospital's unsterile conditions—was as much my fault as the four physicians', because I could not describe my symptoms for them in Indonesian. My four consultations were each a communication nightmare trying to find a middle ground between my all-too-basic Indonesian and the physicians' elementary English.

When I returned to Lombok in 1993, I met very competent medical doctors, many of whom had trained abroad and were fluent in English. Those whom I know best were genuinely concerned about their lack of success in reaching the rural Sasak population. They were excited about my research, hoping that it would help them better understand rural Sasaks so that they could better treat them. Their frustration at being unable to save lives and ease suffering was quite apparent in their questions to me: "Why won't the people from villages [Indon., *orang desa*] come to the hospital?" "Why do they wait so long to seek [bio]medical help?" "People from villages, they just want an injection. Why don't they understand that medicine is more complicated than that?" I sympathized, offered what answers I could, and secretly wondered why none of these physicians had ever sat down with rural Sasaks and asked them. But of course they couldn't. Their wealth, education, and high social status would have barely permitted them to "go down" to the villages and ask, and the same things would have prohibited the villagers from answering.

The Politics of Deference

Prior to incorporation within the Indonesian state, hierarchies were clear in Sasak society as in many societies throughout Indonesia. At the top of the Sasak pyramid were kings (*datu*), then came lords (*mameq*) and commoners (*dengan biese*). In this hierarchy, Sasak language levels were manipulated so that those at the top of the pyramid spoke down to those underneath, whereas those underneath had to speak up (use a higher language level) to those above. Deference to those higher up the social pyramid was also shown by keeping one's eyes down, sitting so one's head was lower, and generally not speaking unless spoken to.

The modern Indonesian state uses Indonesian, a nonhierarchical language, that, in theory, collapses social pyramids. But social hierarchies remain important to interaction on Lombok and elsewhere (see, e.g., Anderson 1990; Errington 1989). Those higher on the social pyramid can have inherited status, but more frequently status is earned by one's wealth or position. The position of doctor commands very high status, whereas the status of other lesser biomedical personnel is considerably lower. But even the most menial clinician has higher social status than peasants do. Rural Sasaks are expected to and typically do acknowledge their lower place in society by showing deference commensurate with the status of the biomedical personnel: they use more formal language (using Indonesian words whenever possible), they avoid eye contact, they do not ask questions.

AT THE HOSPITAL: ANXIETY, SILENCE, AND GIVING AUTHORITY

After all treatments for the water god had been completed, after dreams no longer warned against seeking biomedical care, and after Lo Budin's illness was said to have left his body, I was permitted to take him to the hospital with his mother for an injection so that he would quickly become fat again.

It was midmorning on September 9 before Inaq Budin, Lo Budin, and I climbed onto the truck heading south to the market town. There,

I guided her to a minivan (*bemo*) to take us the rest of the way to Selong. By this time, Lo Budin's movements were quiet and weak, but he looked dreadful, his head overlarge on his wasted infant body. The hospital lies at the entrance to Selong along the main road from the market town; Inaq Budin had never even passed by it before. As soon as we disembarked, Inaq Budin, still cradling her son, stood bewildered on the asphalt driveway leading to the imposing, cream-colored building. A sign identified it for those who read Indonesian as *Rumah Sakit Umum: LOTIM* (Public Hospital of LOTIM—an acronym for East Lombok). Seeing a little sign at the far front corner, I guided her to the emergency room.

The emergency room was a room large enough for only a single gurney. In the small antechamber patients waited their turn. For once, the prompt attention my white skin drew was a blessing. The doctor came up to us immediately, leaving his patient on the gurney and ignoring the half dozen patients still waiting. With little more than a glance at Lo Budin, the doctor diagnosed him with hydrocephalus and ordered the nurse to admit him.

Hydrocephalus is a neurological disorder in which there is excessive buildup of cerebrospinal fluid in the brain. In the United States it is usually treatable with a surgical procedure in which a shunt or tube is inserted in the brain to carry away the excess fluids to other parts of the body where they can be absorbed. Although there is a risk of infection, and the condition can leave the patient with some permanent mental retardation, there is usually a fair prognosis for a normal life. In Indonesia, as the doctor informed me, the prompt neural surgery the boy needed was only available on the island of Java or possibly Bali at a minimum cost of 3 million Rp, not including travel expenses (roughly $1,500 or 15 times the average annual household income for rural peasants). He told me flatly that the family would not be able to pay for the surgery and that the child would inevitably die without it. Then, turning to Inaq Budin, in broken Sasak the doctor said that he wanted to keep the child in the hospital to treat him and make him well again. In other words, he made a promise that the hospital was incapable of fulfilling.

He returned to his other patients and I turned to the blank, questioning eyes of Inaq Budin. As gently as I could, I translated what the doctor had said to me into Sasak. I expected astonishment. After all, although people in Pelocok know about surgery, it is commonly considered a ludicrous treatment that would only be performed by people who lack *ilmu*. Furthermore, although to the wealthy and well-traveled

Bali and Java are merely neighboring islands, to peasants these are impossibly faraway, foreign, and frightening places. Finally, the thought of paying 3 million Rp for medical treatment, when local healers cost 50,000 Rp at the very most, is an amount any peasant would balk at. But Inaq Budin did not. Her expression changed not at all, as she replied, "The important thing is to get him well."

Inaq Budin cradled her child as I filled out the admissions paper-work that she could neither read nor write answers to. The hospital was a one-story complex with tentaclelike buildings all connected by cov-ered walkways slicing through small gardens or patches of open dirt. A nurse guided us to a room, talking all the while with me. Where was I from? Why was I in Lombok? Why did I wear the clothes of a peasant?

In Pelocok, no one much notices clothes. Cheap tops and sarongs are everyday wear, and no one has more than two or three of each. Thus, before a week is out, one can know everyone's entire wardrobe, at least half of which is faded and worn. The only dress items of dis-tinction are the white headcloth of *kiayi*s during rituals, the black head-cloth of some *dukun*s, the civil servant shirt and trousers of the mayor, and, in 1995, the skirts and white blouses of the *bidan*. Otherwise, dress is not noticed, nor does it mark distinctions. But in less rural areas, clothing is very much noticed. Men wear trousers. Women wear skirts and blouses. Their clothing marks them as modern and wealthy. In this building weighted with semblances of modern medicine and nurses in their white blouses with crisp, white caps, Inaq Budin and I looked like country mice.

It was not long before a pediatrician came in to look at Lo Budin. He examined him in less than a minute and confirmed in English the hydrocephalus diagnosis, saying that it was probably congenital. Then, with Inaq Budin silently staring at the doctor while holding Lo Budin, the doctor spoke directly to me in a combination of Indonesian and English. He had seen a case like this once before. The child had been the adopted daughter of a medical doctor who, he emphasized, could afford the neural surgery. The surgery had been done in Java, and the child had healed completely. But, while that same surgery could save Lo Budin's life, the doctor assumed Lo Budin's parents would be unable to pay for it.[9] Thus, he concluded in English, "This child will die."

Then the doctor went on to complain about the problems of health care in Lombok, Inaq Budin still silently looking on. He stated that the

---

9. It is possible to have hospital fees waived with a certificate proving the patient's poverty, but the costs of medications, laboratory tests, and the use of technical equip-ment must be paid for by the patient.

province (Nusa Tenggara Barat—NTB) has the highest infant and maternal mortality rates in Indonesia, and that East Lombok's rates are the highest in NTB. He said that this was due to many factors, including economics, but that "the biggest problem is culture" ("*masahlahnya yg terbesar itu culture*"—using the English word *culture* rather than the Indonesian *kebudayaan*). He went on to cite the Muslim practice of polygamy as an example of culture causing infant mortality, arguing that with many wives, finances and attention are spread too thin and children are neglected. Saying, "The populace has little understanding" (*Masyarakat kurang pengertian*), the doctor added that that was why the Selong hospital works hard to educate people, particularly educating new parents on cleanliness. Then he went back to the issue of finances and how frustrating it was frequently not to be able to do anything for a patient because of the financial constraints of the people seeking health care. Indeed, because of his concern about the financial well-being of Inaq Budin, he said he was not even going to recommend to her that the child have surgery.

At this point, I explicitly asked the doctor to explain all that was wrong with her son to Inaq Budin in Sasak. He said: "Your child is very sick. All of the sicknesses come from his head. That is why the head is so large; it is sick. The lungs are also sick. He is sick inside. And he has convulsions. The sickness of the lungs and convulsions we can heal here." He gave no explanation of the fluid blockage in the brain, no explanation that this was probably congenital, no explanation that the lungs were filled with fluids or that the convulsions were directly caused by the neurological problems and thus couldn't be cured without surgery. All he told her was that her son was ill and that he could be healed in the hospital. Was this his idea of educating the populace about health care? Later I found out that this doctor, like nearly all of the doctors in Lombok, was not Sasak. He was from a wealthy Javanese family and seemed to speak very little Sasak. Perhaps this was the reason for his minimal explanation to Inaq Budin. But the fault was also hers. She did not ask him a single question.

The moment the doctor left, nurses in the ward called me to answer questions about the child's condition. When I said that the mother was the better person to ask, these nurses waved this suggestion aside. From their perspective, who was more interesting, another rural peasant or a white American dressed as a peasant and speaking the local language? When they finally got around to asking questions about the child rather than about me, I told them he had had convulsions for about a week, but that only now were the parents ready (Indon., *siap*) to bring him to the hospital. The head nurse asked why, and why hadn't I insisted on bringing the child earlier?[10] I answered that it was the parents' choice, and they had been busy with local healing treatments and ceremonies. They laughed loudly, and the head nurse said, "Like ghosts [Indon., *hantu*] causing the sickness?!" Irritated by their laughter, I answered seriously that it was a *dewa* (god). They laughed all the more, making derisive comments that the populace (Indon., *rakyat*) was always that way and that they had very little intelligence (*kurangne gati pengertian*). My quickly brewing anger, which I showed in typical Indonesian fashion by stubborn silence and stern expressions, seemed to prompt them to end their session of laughter and get to work doing something for the child.

Without saying a word to Inaq Budin, the nurses inserted an intravenous needle (IV) into the child's forehead and oxygen tubes up his nose. She said nothing while they were in the room, but as soon as they left Inaq Budin showered questions on me. What were the tubes and bags of fluid? Why was he hooked up to a canister (the oxygen tank)? Why couldn't she hold him? What had the doctor said? I answered her as gently and clearly as possible, leaving out of course the condescension shown by the doctor and nurses as well as (perhaps wrongly) the doctor's prognosis. I was her translator, her trusted ally in this antiseptic and foreign world. Indeed, Inaq Budin only appeared anxious when I had to leave the room, however briefly, to buy food or bags of IV fluid at the corner apothecary. Otherwise she was surprisingly calm about everything, including the strange technologies and the rudeness of the personnel who insisted on talking with me rather than with her. Nonetheless, I was surprised that after a long and sleepless night,

---

10. Why hadn't I insisted on taking Lo Budin to the hospital earlier? This is a reasonable question, for the nurse could assume that, being a foreigner, I would accept the efficacy of biomedicine. If so, to her mind, if I was a caring person at all, I should be an advocate of biomedical care for persons less familiar with it. In short, because of my assumed knowledge about biomedicine and health, I should have been responsible for disseminating that knowledge. Furthermore, she assumed that my foreignness gave me the authority to bring a child to the hospital whether or not the parents wished it. The accusations implied in the nurse's question did no more than reflect aspects of my own internal voice. Throughout my time in Pelocok but particularly in the case of Lo Budin, I was often in the paradoxical situation of having great respect for rural Sasaks and their medicine while personally believing in the superior efficacy of biomedicine for life-threatening illness. I often would try to urge people to let me take them for biomedical treatment, but, as an ethnographer without medical training myself, and without great confidence in the biomedical care available on Lombok, I felt I was not in a position to insist. Rather, I would put forward my opinion as strongly as possible, offering people health-care options, and leave it to them to decide.

instead of saying "Enough, I am taking my child home"—as I might have done given the poor quality medical care and personal abuse—Inaq Budin sent me to Pelocok to get Papuq Junin to join her. She was determined to stay in the hospital until the doctor's original promise that the boy would be well was fulfilled.

Within this first day in the hospital, who had authority and who did not was already firmly established. Inaq Budin gave the biomedical personnel authority instantly. The huge building and the immediate decisiveness of the emergency room doctor seemed to impress her into silence. It was a silence she maintained throughout all encounters with nurses, doctors, orderlies, or anyone else in a clean, pressed uniform. Her awe did not extend to other patients or cleaning women who were dressed as she was. With these people she engaged in conversation as an equal. But she was thoroughly cowed by the aura of the hospital and its personnel. True, the doctors and nurses held themselves in high esteem and ridiculed the populace for not knowing about basic hygiene and believing the illness was caused by ghosts. Their white clothing, apparent wealth, fatness, education, and position all declared their superiority. But had Inaq Budin dared to question the nurses, all of whom were townspeople of Lombok and fluent in Sasak, the authority she gave them would not have been quite as absolute. As it was, she was silent. Their voices and actions completely constrained her own.

Whereas my voice had no authority in Pelocok, except when speaking of the outside world, the moment we left the safe confines of Pelocok, Inaq Budin gradually became more and more silent, leaving me to negotiate fares with drivers and answer the nurses' questions. In interactions with doctors, I tried to indicate that the doctors should address their statements to her. But between her failure to ask any questions and my white skin, I inevitably became the main conversant. Through her silence, through turning to me for answers only after others had gone, Inaq Budin gave me authority. When we were alone, and she would question me openly and voice her fears about high hospital costs, even then, she sought my opinion although she never had in Pelocok. Here, in this strange environment, she gave authority without question.

In Inaq Budin's interactions with biomedical personnel, her silence legitimated their knowledge and actions and surrendered her son to their care. By reinforcing, through her silence, the authority biomedical personnel claimed for themselves, the social processes of interpretation that we saw in chapter 6 disappear. Through her silence and turning to me for decisions, Inaq Budin legitimated all the expressed verbal knowledge of doctors and nurses, most of which was expressed in Indonesian, which she could not understand. She also legitimated their superior status by deferring to their condescending tone and their rudeness. Through her silence, she legitimated their poor opinion of her as an ignorant peasant, acknowledging that these townspeople with all their weight, wealth, and worldliness were indeed superior to her. She surrendered all her rights as a parent to strangers whose authority she legitimated. In the hospital, she never expressed any concern even in private about whether the new illness name of hydrocephalus fit Lo Budin's illness nor uttered doubts about the ability of the hospital to treat the illness correctly. The concerns that had made Inaq Budin resistant to seeking biomedical care for so many days had disappeared. As far as she was concerned the illness was gone thanks to the healing spells and ceremonies in Pelocok. Now whatever the biomedical people thought they were doing, she understood them to be undertaking the second and lesser stage of treatment of making Lo Budin quickly well again. Perhaps it is for this reason that she legitimated the technological treatments without question. Or perhaps she legitimated the care precisely because she assumed that the superiority that the doctors and nurses claimed were reflections of true superiority.

At the Hospital: The Arts of Resistance[11]

Not all people from Pelocok were as quick to hand over the reins of authority to biomedical personnel and legitimate their treatment. But, unlike interactions in Pelocok, where the legitimacy could be outright denied (e.g., "You are stupid"), in the hospital, where a definite hierarchy of authority was presumed and largely granted by patients, resistance took less direct forms.

After that first night in the hospital, I returned to Pelocok sending others from Pelocok in my stead, including Lo Budin's half-brother, Lo Den. On September 13, on Budin's fourth day in the hospital, Lo Den returned to Pelocok. Papuq Junin had had a rough time ever since his wife and child left. He cried frequently, had lost his appetite even for chewing betel, could not sleep, and wandered around as if in a daze. He wanted them to come home desperately, but himself refused to go to Selong and retrieve them for reasons that were never made clear to me. Lo Den reported that the child had improved considerably, and had come to ask, what with mounting costs and all, whether Lo Budin

---

11. This heading is from James Scott's *Domination and the Arts of Resistance* (1990).

should be brought home. I agreed that the child should be brought home, never voicing my main reason, which was that if these procedures were only temporarily extending the boy's life, they did not justify the suffering of the parents, the distance from family and friends, and the cost. So, on September 14, I returned with Lo Den to Selong to bring the child home.

We arrived in the heat of the day during non–visitor hours, but I walked right up to the back door and knocked; the nurses who recognized me let me right in, but they wouldn't allow Den in with me. Again my white skin earned me favors denied rural Sasaks. I found the ward supervisor and told her that we'd been sent to take the child home for two reasons. First, because of the cost of treatment. Second, because if the child was going to die, it would be far better for him to die at home. The supervisor responded angrily (or perhaps defensively) that as a medical practitioner, the second reason was not viable, because it was her duty to do all within her power for the health of the child; it was "not allowed to" stop short of that even if he were going to die anyway.

While waiting for the doctor, I went in to see Inaq Budin. Lo Budin did look better, and Inaq Budin looked tired, but smiled warmly when she saw me. We talked, and I told her Papuq Junin had told me to come and bring Budin home. She said no, he wasn't well yet; they had to wait until he was well. Otherwise, the doctor wouldn't give her permission (*mbeng*) to take him home.

The doctor was not the Javanese man I'd met before, but a woman from Sumatra. Her manner was quick and her anger evident. She came in to examine the child and, with her back to us, said in Sasak, "I hear you want to take Budin home. Why do you want to take him home when he isn't well yet, Inaq?" Inaq Budin was silent, and I piped up saying it was the child's father, not the mother, who wanted the child home and told her the first reason, not wanting to say the second in front of the mother. The doctor argued that if the child stayed longer in the hospital she could indeed successfully treat all his symptoms, neglecting to mention the head full of fluid that she knew would inevitably kill him. Inaq Budin was adamant, turning to me and saying she wanted to keep him in the hospital and that her husband was wrong, so I asked the doctor to please talk with Lo Den.

Lo Den was admitted into the building, and we both went in to talk with the doctor in an office. The doctor opened the conversation by suggesting, "How about if we make everything free, medicines and all?" Thinking quickly, Lo Den replied, "Good. We are very poor [Indon., *miskin sekali*]. We don't even own a rice field. My father is sick. Sick with old age. He can't walk. But he wants to see his child, that is why he sent me to bring him home." These were bold-faced lies that he told without a blink, and I didn't contradict him. The doctor maintained her position, using Lo Den's statement in her favor to say that only the parents had the right to bring the child home, particularly now that the hospital was picking up the tab for everything. Because the mother obviously wanted to finish the treatment, the doctor argued that the father would have to come to the hospital himself to get the boy. She added that if they took the child before the doctor had agreed to discharge him, the *surat miskin* (letter of poverty) would be invalidated, and they would have to pay for everything at the hospital. The doctor countered bold-faced lies with bold-faced blackmail. Lo Den agreed, and, as we left, the doctor turned to me and said in English, "We must use a little force for the health of the baby. People here do not understand about medicine, so we have to force them."

We went and told Inaq Budin what had happened. She was angry. She was furious that Papuq Junin had wanted to take Lo Budin home before the treatment was finished, and furious that Papuq Junin had not yet come himself to Selong. But she became even angrier when Lo Den told of a Sasak medicine he had brought from Amaq Suh to give to Lo Budin, but said that he couldn't figure out how to use it because he couldn't lift Lo Budin to put the medicine where he had been told to, on the back of the boy's neck. Inaq Budin stopped him, grabbing his arm and saying loudly: "No. That was the problem before. Papuq Junin kept mixing treatments. One was not finished, and he wanted to start another one. Now we are going to wait until the doctor's medicine is finished."

THE MAKINGS OF MISCOMMUNICATION

In these interactions, knowledge that had previously been legitimated and authority that was previously granted came into question. In admitting Lo Budin into the hospital in the first place, Inaq Budin and I had legitimated biomedicine. When I came back telling the ward supervisor that he was to be discharged in part because they would fail in healing him, I was in effect delegitimating the skills and wisdom of biomedicine in general and that hospital in particular. The ward supervisor reacted not to my concern that the child be granted a humane death, but to the challenge she read in my statements. She rose to the challenge by invoking an unnamed, greater authority who, in passive voice, *would not allow treatment to stop even when death was inevitable.* She was doing her job as a medical practitioner, and I was trying to impede her from doing that job. Likewise, the initial reaction of the doctor, accusing Inaq Budin of wanting to take the boy home before he was well and implying that she would thus be impeding their attempts to treat him, was as defensive as that of the ward supervisor. Threatening to take the boy home was taken as a direct attack on their authority and their abilities in treatment.

This response is understandable given their perspective. Biomedical practitioners rightly see their skills and technologies as capable of alleviating much of the disease and suffering on Lombok. As they see it, the problem is that the populace tends to turn to them too late or ignore them altogether. While clinics may be used at any stage in seeking illness treatment, most Sasaks only go to the hospital as a very last resort, often too late for anything to be done, and so hospitals have gained the reputation of places where people die. Thus, once someone is in the hospital, and biomedical personnel are given the opportunity to help alleviate suffering, they understandably would not want to end treatment prematurely. Moreover, the ward supervisor and the doctor may well have been genuinely interested in doing what was best, in their view, for the boy. Biomedical technology could prolong his life a few days, even though he would eventually die. If they kept him long enough in the hospital, they would be able to send him home with all of his obvious symptoms—the convulsions, the coughing, the lack of appetite—temporarily removed. Thereby, in addition to helping the boy, they would be helping the reputation of the hospital as a place that could treat illness. But if he went home prematurely, he would likely die immediately, thus further injuring the fragile reputation of biomedicine. In both interactions, the authority that had formerly been assumed by the biomedical personnel came into question, and through defensive tactics—including attempts at making Inaq Budin and I feel wrongheaded for impeding treatment—they regained their legitimation when I put the decision in Lo Den's hands.

The interaction between Lo Den and the doctor would have been comical if there were less at stake. The doctor was quick to offer free treatment. She never bothered to find out about the family's financial situation, but merely assumed that because they were peasants, they were dirt-poor.[12] While she might have offered the free treatment out

---

12. In fact, Lo Budin's father was one of the wealthiest in the area, with considerable land and livestock holdings. Within two months after Budin's illness, Papuq Junin hosted four major rituals at his house, which he later boasted to me cost him

of true concern for Lo Budin or an interest in an unusual case, a less charitable motive might have been to establish hospital authority and not let a child that was still ill leave. Indeed, her final warning, that they would have to pay for everything if the boy was taken home prematurely, suggests that this last was at least part of her motivation. She uses money to legitimate biomedicine after an attempted resistance, a threat to take the child home. She did not recognize Lo Den's responses as another kind of resistance to her authority. His description of their poverty matched her own stereotypes. The sympathy he tried to gain by describing Papuq Junin's weakness, played into her attempts to keep Lo Budin in the hospital. She never realized he was lying. With his lies, Lo Den successfully manipulated authority. By lying, he resisted playing into the authority of biomedical personnel and instead manipulated it—caught up in its own insecurities and weighted down with its own stereotypes—to get free care. Unlike Inaq Budin, Lo Den resisted biomedical personnel, manipulating them in social interaction to legitimate his lies. For Lo Den, the interaction was a game that he described later with uproarious laughter.[13] For the doctor, it was a matter of such seriousness that, without first consulting any supervisors, she committed herself to battling the hospital bureaucracy to give Lo Budin free care. The doctor and Lo Den appear to be communicating, but in fact they were talking past each other. The doctor failed to communicate that the boy's life was at stake; Lo Den failed to communicate that the boy's life was not (according to him) at stake. In focusing on money, they failed to communicate about the real issue, which was how much medical help staying in the hospital would be to the boy.

RESISTING RESISTANCE TO BIOMEDICAL CARE

The final act of resistance came, surprisingly, from Inaq Budin: she resisted the stated will of her husband to bring Lo Budin home and

---

7,000,000 rupiah. This was not a poor man, and even without my financial aid—which they had—the hospital expenses would not become burdensome for a number of weeks. Indeed, the surgical operation that the boy needed would not have been financially impossible for this particular family. But the cognitive hurdles of traveling to another island and accepting surgery as a treatment were too high to be overcome.
13. For Lo Den, the treatment of the hospital was merely a way of speeding his brother's recovery, it was not saving the boy's life. The illness had already been made to leave the body by the ethnomedical treatments in Pelocok. He saw the treatments in the hospital as a more elaborate form of "getting an injection so he will quickly become fat." Lo Den could make a game of this interaction and try to manipulate free care precisely because nothing was at stake for him.

even blamed her husband for his flawed strategy in seeking multiple treatments for their son. Once before, she had voiced disagreement with Papuq Junin when he had wanted me to take Lo Budin to a doctor. Then she had argued that all Sasak medicines had to be tried before turning to doctors—establishing a clear hierarchy of resort that she herself had undermined in the early days of Lo Budin's illness when she had taken him to a clinic for an injection. On September 1, biomedicine was the last possible option. Now she legitimated biomedicine, rejected a Sasak treatment, and condemned her husband for wanting to mix treatments.

Whereas anxiety beforehand had made Inaq Budin legitimate multiple treatments simultaneously, grabbing for any straw that might work, now anxiety combined with the reassurances by people to whom she had given authority made her change strategies. Anxiety combined with authority gave her a space of hope, and she would not resist the authority that made that hope possible.

ANXIETY AND AUTHORITY

Looking at these interactions regarding Lo Budin, from everyday conversations like those discussed in chapter 6 to encounters at the hospital, we can ask how anxiety affects the social processes of legitimation and constraint. What is the relationship between anxiety and authority? This case suggests possible (although far from definitive) answers:

- Anxiety encourages the rapid generation of interpretations: it focuses interactions on a particular topic providing contexts where processes of creativity in generating illness names as well as legitimation or constraint processes selecting among those names occur within relatively short spaces of time.[14]
- Anxiety tends to make people hesitant to finally reject any expressed knowledge that might shed light on the situation.
- Anxiety does not necessarily lead to authority: people in urgent situations do not necessarily give ideas or persons authority.

---

14. Although Lo Budin may be the only study of the relationship between anxiety and subsequent interpretations of illness (both personal and social) discussed in the Sasak materials, it supports recent work by psychologists that anxiety motivates or encourages the generation of ideas directed at solving the initial anxiety-provoking problem (see, e.g., Luu et al. 1998; Runco 1999).

- Anxiety does not necessarily overwhelm other concerns—such as pride, social status, and cost—in the interpretation of expressed knowledge.
- Anxiety, on the other hand, can make people give unquestioned authority to and store their faith in a particular idea, person, or institution.

Unfortunately, this list does not give us hard-and-fast rules for how anxiety affects social interpretation or how it relates to authority. What it does suggest is that anxiety makes normal processes of legitimation and constraint more intense and unpredictable. Obviously, a sense of anxiety is variable among persons and over time. In the case of Lo Budin, even his parents waxed and waned in their degree of anxiety in accordance to how they perceived his condition at the moment. Their variable sense of anxiety was evident in their actions: postponing all treatments one day to fulfill extraneous ceremonial obligations, and frantically giving treatment after treatment the next. The Sasak materials suggest that when the sense of anxiety is low, people are more likely to question suggestions, to let other concerns enter into their interpretations, and to avoid giving authority in everyday interactions. But when the sense of anxiety is high, an illness name becomes unquestionable, to such an extent that a wife will lash out against her husband to legitimate the same medical tradition she had beforehand strongly avoided. When authority is linked to a highly urgent and anxious situation, that authority tends to be irrevocable precisely because questioning it would ruin the space of hope and control provided by that interpretation or that person/institution.

HIERARCHY AND MISCOMMUNICATION

Inaq Budin sought biomedicine to treat the child's symptoms because to her way of thinking the illness was gone. When the doctors promised that they could treat the boy's symptoms, healing the sickness in his lungs and stopping his convulsions, she believed them and kept him in the hospital giving the doctors authority to treat her son. The sad irony is that while Inaq Budin and the doctors were both talking about symptoms, she did not understand that however much the doctors treated the symptoms, without surgery to treat the disease, the boy would soon die. For Inaq Budin the symptoms were just the residue the illness had left behind, and for the doctors the symptoms were the expression of a disease that continued to threaten the boy's life. While talking about the same thing, they were unable to communicate.

The communication problems between the biomedical people and people from Pelocok have much in common with the pattern West (1984) found in interactions between doctors and their patients in the United States. The doctors were the ones who initiated interaction and did almost all of the talking; their nurses were the ones who asked questions. Neither Inaq Budin nor Lo Den asked questions of any of the biomedical personnel, and they both used the most formal, honorific language they could the few times they did speak. My presence during these interactions shaped them somewhat, because the doctors and nurses generally directed their talk and questions to me, and I asked questions in turn. But Inaq Budin never followed my example, she never asked questions even when she clearly did not understand. Unlike in West's findings, in these few examples there was no interrupting by any participant. The doctors had no cause to interrupt Inaq Budin who was almost always silent, but even in the interaction between the female doctor and Lo Den, there were no interruptions by either party. The lack of interruptions and questions could be interpreted as a sign that the people from Pelocok understood what was being told to them. But in Inaq Budin's barrage of questions to me whenever biomedical personnel left the room, we see that it wasn't so. Communication failed because the knowledge expressed by biomedical personnel was not open to normal processes of legitimation in communication.

Among rural Sasaks, processes of social interpretation work to legitimate some ideas and reject others because everyone can speak, everyone participates. As we have seen, their relationships with each other are horizontal, which they show by using the same language level, talking loudly, interrupting often, and generally acting casually. Conversations among those who have horizontal relations with each other are conducive to asking questions, and conducive to communication.

Rural Sasaks do not have daily experience with negotiating conversations with people who have vertical relations to them. For rural Sasaks, interacting with people of higher social status means that they must pay attention to the words they use, where they look, and how they sit. Rural Sasaks show their deference in interactions with biomedical personnel—everyone from the *bidan* in Pelocok to the physicians in Selong—by looking down, keeping their heads at a lower level, using the most formal level of language they know, not asking questions, agreeing to whatever the other says, and being silent. From the perspective of the rural Sasaks, their deference shows that they know (*tauq*) the good manners expected in interactions with those higher up. They do recognize the superior technology biomedicine can offer and understand that it behooves them to show respect in order to get treatment. Rural Sasaks acknowledge that biomedicine often has superior therapies for healing symptoms; biomedicine has the injections and pills that can make a person quickly get fat again. But they do not recognize that biomedicine is superior at healing illness. Without the potency of *ilmu,* biomedical knowledge can not, from their perspectives, meet illnesses and make them leave bodies. Their deference bows to what they recognize as higher social status and state-supported authority, but not to the authority of biomedicine as an overall superior kind of medical knowledge. Showing deference in conversation disallows expression of doubt, rejection, or even approval because those higher in vertical relationships do not need their inherently superior knowledge approved by those lower down. In vertical relationships, rural Sasaks have no process whereby they can check to see if they understand what is told to them.

From the other side, people trained in biomedicine often do not realize that they are not understood. Long trained in a national ideology that teaches the unquestionable value of the new and modern, they are prejudiced against those people and ideas they consider backward, primitive, and traditional. Doctors, nurses, and other biomedical personnel are acquainted with many medical ideas held by rural Sasaks including the potency of spells and etiologies pointing toward ghosts and gods. At issue is not a lack of knowledge about their patients' ideas, but the belief that those ideas are valueless. They do not realize that at the root of those ideas is an understanding of *ilmu* that renders biomedicine useless for treating illnesses and good only for treating symptoms. Doctors complain that peasants come to them too late in the course of their disease, but do not understand that biomedicine is not seen as efficacious for anything but quickly getting fat *after* suffering from an illness. Because of their vertical nature, interactions with rural Sasaks do not challenge these prejudices or give any indication that the biomedical people might be missing something in their understanding of ethnomedicine. Doctors, nurses, and clinicians, who are used to urban life and interacting daily with people socially above and below them, are more experienced at negotiating hierarchical relationships while communicating in conversations. In their interactions with rural Sasaks, biomedical personnel could easily interpret the Sasaks' silence as agreement, understanding, and acknowledgment of the superiority of biomedicine. They do not seem to realize that silence can indicate miscommunication.

In short, the vertical relations between biomedical personnel and rural Sasaks so structure interactions as to hinder communication. Combine this with a mutual lack of fluency in each other's languages as well as fundamentally different ideologies and medical knowledge, and one can understand why communication often slips between rural Sasaks and their biomedical healers.

Denouement

Epitaph for Lo Budin

Lo Budin remained in the hospital for 10 days. During all the interactions Inaq Budin had with doctors and nurses over the course of those 10 days, no one managed to communicate to her that although the symptoms were disappearing, the killing disease remained. When he was discharged, Inaq Budin brought him home, smiling and happy. She was confident that now all would be well with her son.

Lo Budin returned from the hospital alert, fatter, with clear breathing and no more erratic movements. Everyone was hopeful; I hid my pessimism. The second day after he returned, on September 21, I went to see him and was disheartened to see that his condition had worsened. He did not appear nearly as bad as he had in the past, and he still nursed, but he was limp and listless as I held him in my arms. His father told of how he had washed a sacred potent text (*lontar*) and said a healing spell over his son in the night. Amaq Deri, the *dukun,* was coming later to do more treatments, but Papuq Junin and Inaq Budin both radiated smiles, assuring me that Lo Budin's condition was just a temporary relapse, and soon he would be fine. I did my best to smile in response to their hopes and asked what the doctor had told them when Lo Budin was released.

Papuq Junin [*who had never gone to the hospital or talked with the doctors*]: The doctor said that he was sick because when he was born the midwife was not industrious at cleaning his belly button. One must use lots of soap and only once it's clean to cover it with *borok* [mixture of turmeric and lime chalk]. His head is still sick. The doctor said to use Sasak medicine.

Inaq Budin [*as if she were not contradicting her husband*]: The doctor said it was given to him by someone. Only Sasak medicine can cure his head.

Cameron: What Sasak medicine?

Papuq Junin: The spring water from before. I've already ordered someone to go get it again. Earlier when Uncle Mol did it, it didn't work because he was not clean.

Amaq Mol [*laughing*]: That day I didn't bathe at all.

Everyone then joined in the laughter.

The words of the doctor, whatever they might have actually been, were understood as an accusation of unclean birthing practices and a recommendation for treatment against black magic. Both etiologies were ignored, as they returned to the water god etiology, while taking care to wash sacred texts and see a new *dukun* as well. The illness name of the water god stuck in spite of treatment failure. Other excuses were made for the failure (e.g., the religious leader's lack of cleanliness) rather than abandoning the long-accepted illness name and perhaps admitting to themselves they didn't know the name of the illness.

I said goodbye to the smiling parents and gently handed them their son.

Lo Budin died the next morning.

— 8 —

Time to Remember

The old woman was dying. She lay on a mat on the dirt floor surrounded by the loved ones who had kept vigil with her since her collapse a few days before. Various treatments had been tried, but her primary illness, as everyone said, was old age. Neighbors, friends, and family sat with her, waiting out her illness, fearing she would die. Each time she seemed to be at the point of death, too weary to even breathe, someone, a child or grandchild, would hastily kneel next to her head and demand in a very loud voice, "*Ingat! Ingat!*" Remember! Remember! Sometimes the pleas went on to specifics—remember your self, remember your grandchildren and great-grandchildren, and do not leave them. But often, the words just were a continued imperative of "Remember!" After a week of hanging on, the old woman died. She could no longer remember.

This desperate plea to remember occurred at every deathbed. Someone always urged the dying person to remember. Even if we could know the content of what a dying person remembers, it would not explain why he should remember at the moment of death. This suggests that for Sasaks, *when* one remembers is more important than *what* one remembers.

Remembering as a Cultural Act

The considerable psychological literature explicating the sociocultural influences on the content and reproduction of memory has not expanded into detailed explorations of sociocultural influences on the *act of remembering*.[1] But ethnography has, and so I use the familiar Mela-

---

1. The core works exploring memory include Bartlett 1995; Halbwachs 1980; Neisser 1982; Neisser and Fivush 1994; Connerton 1989; Rubin 1995.

nesian case of the Kaluli *gisalo* as a point of departure into remembering.[2]

In Kaluli society, "every death is caused by a witch" (Schieffelin 1976, 78). These witches, or more accurately shadow creatures, live within living people, often without their knowledge. These creatures, as incarnations of "implacable evil," creep out at night, causing deaths (101). The *gisalo* is a ceremony hosted by grievers. Their guests perform and, through songs naming places in the landscape, evoke memories of the dead in the hosts. The emotional anguish these memories unleash is brought to closure as the hosts transform it into anger and burn the performers (their guests) with torches. This is understood as retaliation against the shadow creatures that caused the death and resolves the imbalance in social reciprocity initiated by the loss.

The *gisalo* ceremony highlights four things important for our discussion here. First, the *gisalo* is a socially organized time for remembering. The ceremony formally designates a temporal space as one needing memories. Second, the *gisalo* foregrounds the connection between memory and emotion. Memories are affectively marked, and the emotions they evoke stimulate action. Third, the *gisalo* motivates memories in culturally prescribed ways. The mnemonic tools of the songs fit the cultural importance placed on the landscapes in which events occur. Finally, in the *gisalo*, memories are stimulated for a purpose. The Kaluli bring the past into the present for the future purposes of having grief and social tension resolved.

The title of this book, *Remembering to Live*, demands an explanation. How is it that one must remember in order to live? By exploring in the Sasak materials each of the four issues raised by the *gisalo*, we can understand the act of remembering as simultaneously a personal and a cultural process of dealing with anxiety.

THE SOCIOCULTURAL ORGANIZATION OF TEMPORAL CONTEXTS

The reminder to remember, given on the threshold of death, is not in the context of a formal ceremony like the *gisalo*. Ethnographies about rituals, particularly those surrounding death, have often emphasized the importance of memories to the ritual's success (see, e.g., Battaglia

---

2. For this insight into the importance of remembering in Kaluli rituals, I am indebted to Munn's (1995) careful analysis. Following Munn, I use Feld's (1982) transcription of *gisalo* for the name of the ceremony rather than Schieffeln's (1976) transcription of *gisaro*.

1990). However, the necessity of remembering when vulnerable or ill and the reminder to remember given on the threshold of death do not occur in the context of a formal ceremony. Without such a ritual context, is it possible to argue that the personal act of remembering is socially constituted? What is it about living that for Sasaks necessitates remembering? What is it about the time of death that designates it as in need of memories?

As we have seen, Sasaks consciously emphasize two kinds of memories: the recitation of memorized knowledge (*ilmu*) and the memory of self within one's social world. In rural Lombok, the fragility of human life is a palpable aspect of everyday life. Sasaks perceive the world as full of dangers. There are dangerous months of the year, and dangerous periods in the life cycle. It is dangerous to be alone, but also hazardous to be with others who could secretly cause harm. There are dangerous places in the landscape teeming with spirits and witches, but even one's own house can be dangerous, overflowing with the powers of objects that have not been properly tended. Dangers also haunt one's sleep, for people and spirits met in dreams are believed to cause bodily harm. Dangers loom at every turn. But the most serious danger is forgetting, for in forgetting one dies. Through remembering, one can keep all dangers at bay. Any time one experiences the anxiety of vulnerability, one needs to remember. The need to remember is not organized into a formal ceremony; it is an everyday imperative.

Sasaks believe in the power of words. Words and thoughts act directly on reality. Their *ilmu*, be it in the form of small words to ward off harm or in the form of spells to treat illness, has efficacy in the world whenever it is remembered. It can both prevent and treat illness. *Ilmu* is the most powerful weapon that rural Sasaks have against the uncertainties of their lives. Therefore any time a Sasak person experiences himself as vulnerable is a time when he needs to remember. Those moments of vulnerability are understood as brief opportunities to act by remembering. Similarly, when experiencing illness, Sasaks remember *ilmu* to make the illnesses leave their bodies. When illnesses are unusual and particularly grave like Lo Budin's, the search for someone who can remember the correct *ilmu* to treat that particular illness becomes urgent. People seek the right *ilmu* before the window of opportunity is closed. Throughout their lives, whether ill or merely less than healthy, Sasaks rely on *ilmu* to carry them through. Remembering *ilmu* enables them to be able to (*tauq*) continue to live. It is their primary source of agency in an uncertain, dangerous world.

Remembering *ilmu* is not the same as remembering at the moment of death. At the moment of death, the importance of *ilmu* loses its prominence, for *ilmu* can not stop death. Only responses to the imperative of "Remember!" can stop death. At the moment of death, when the order to remember is accompanied by specifics, the dying person is told to remember self and those important to him or her. This call to remember is not an effort to remind the dying to remember the living kindly in the afterlife. It is an effort to keep the dying person alive. What is remembered is not *ilmu* but personhood, the dying one's self and social relationships. The moment of death is the only time in their lives Sasaks are ever called on to remember themselves and those important to them.

In spite of being reminded to remember, the vast majority of those at the threshold of death do die. However, in two cases during my time in Pelocok, the person did not. In the case of a drunken man (see chap. 3) and the case of a women having an acute episode of disorientation, these people were understood to be at the threshold of death because they could not remember (*ndeqne tauq ingat*), and, if they couldn't be made to remember, they would inevitably die. People keeping vigil with them broke down in sobs, deeply afraid that the ill people would die, and urgently reminded them to remember. When they lived, their ability to remember was praised for keeping them alive.

These two cases suggest that the call to remember self within social relationships is a call to perpetuate the continuity of self in this life. It is a call to remember in order to live. The act of remembering self within a social world has agency over death.

There is a gap of time between no longer remembering and death; this is the moment when people say both "she is incapable of remembering" (*ndeqne tauq ingat*) and "now she is dying" (*kane mati iye*). Dying and being incapable of remembering are one and the same thing. It is these moments that resound with "Remember!" No Sasak dies without being reminded to remember. Sasaks recognize these temporal spaces as their final opportunities to prevent death.

It is the act of remembering—be it *ilmu* or self—that saves the day. For the Kaluli, memories are needed in contexts lacking personal emotive closure as well as unresolved social tension. In contrast, for Sasaks, remembering is needed in any context perceived as potentially harmful. This need to remember is not organized in ritual, but it is nonetheless a socioculturally organized temporal context, a widely recognized moment of opportunity to prevent harm in everyday life. The act of remembering is not just a personal, private endeavor. Society gives it value and designates temporal contexts for when one must remember.

Emotions and Remembering

Since Bartlett's groundbreaking work in the psychology of memory, it has been clear that memories are associated with emotions. Memory and emotion walk hand in hand, but how are they related? In the Kaluli *gisalo*, songs are considered good if the listeners start weeping and become angry. These emotional responses are the signs that the performance has evoked memories of the dead. But in the Sasak materials, memories do not evoke manifest emotions. Even in the cases of the drunk man and the disoriented woman, although remembering was said to have kept them from dying, whatever memories they apparently had were not expressed in obvious affective ways. The Sasak materials suggest that emotions are not just a response to memories, but actually can motivate the act of remembering.

We can take a lead from cognitive anthropologists studying motivation.[3] To grossly summarize these writers, action is organized by socioculturally available knowledge, symbols, or models of appropriate conduct.[4] The motivation to act depends upon the extent to which cultural knowledge (symbols, models) is internalized and made compelling. In other words, knowledge must matter for people to be willing to act upon it. The conviction Sasaks have that the act of remembering is efficacious in the world could be described as a widely, perhaps universally distributed model for action among rural Sasaks. They remember in order to cope with vulnerability, to treat illness, and to ward off death. But how is remembering made compelling?

Times of vulnerability, illness, and death are weighty moments. They matter tremendously to the people involved. They are moments with potential consequences that could irreparably change their world. They are thus fraught with anxiety. Psychologists have suggested that because anxiety so constrains cognition by directing it toward the anticipation of a harm or threat, anxiety may be particularly important for compelling action (Luu et al. 1998). As we have seen, Sasaks' most potent agent for action is remembering. Confidence in the potency of remembering organizes Sasak anxiety, enabling them to act upon the dangers they perceive. But remembering is a personal activity. To others, a person's secret *ilmu* and heart—her knowledge and deep social

---

3. See, e.g., D'Andrade and Strauss 1992; Strauss and Quinn 1997; Holland and Quinn 1987; Obeyesekere 1990; Nuckolls 1996.
4. As discussed in the Introduction, I prefer the term *knowledge*, although others prefer to use *symbols* or *models* to designate basically the same thing—widely dispersed understandings that are used in making interpretations and acting in the world.

attachments—are hidden, and others are unable to remember for her, unable to even assist her with anything more than the word *remember.* Remembering has to be done for oneself. In recognizing someone approaching death, anxiety drives one to want to act. And so at every moment of death, Sasaks feel compelled to order the dying person to remember. I am not arguing that the Sasak emphasis on remembering at times of crisis is uniformly internalized by all Sasaks. The imperative of remembering is, however, the only model for action Sasaks have to cope with anxiety.

Casey has suggested, "In remembering, we come back to the things that matter" (1987, xii). For Sasaks, the idiom of remembering focuses them on the two things that matter most in their world, their secret *ilmu* and their social relationships. Anxiety stimulates the need to remember. Anxiety combines with the sociocultural emphasis on the importance of remembering to motivate action during times of perceived danger, especially times of illness and death.

MNEMONICS

If one must remember for oneself, how, when someone else is dying, can one person compel another to remember? For the Kaluli in the *gisalo,* the mnemonic devices for stimulating memory are publicly available images of landscape given in songs. But for Sasaks the only mnemonic device is the word *remember* (*ingat*). No one is specifically named. No specific images are indicated. The study of mnemonics has shown that persons most successful at remembering things accurately do so through associating what needs to be remembered—for example, words in a text—to something familiar such as the buildings on the street where one lives (e.g., Bartlett 1995; Carruthers 1990). Given this, and given the emotions songs evoke in the *gisalo,* using landscape imagery appears to be a very effective mnemonic device for the Kaluli. But such an evocative device is not an option for Sasaks.

It is not an option for Sasaks because *ilmu* is passed from one generation to the next in secrecy, in whispered words in the middle of the night so no one will overhear. This mode of transmitting *ilmu* affects both its accuracy and its value. The importance of secrecy means that there is no way to check if one has memorized *ilmu* correctly. Incorrectly memorized *ilmu* has no potency. Sasaks themselves recognize this problem but *ilmu* cannot just be written down. Even as more rural Sasaks learn to write, *ilmu* must enter a person to be potent. The knowledge must be in their being, in their stomachs, in their hearts. Words on a page do not do the trick. In a world without presumed Cartesian duality, knowledge and remembering are intimately bound up with hearts, stomachs, experience, and illness. It is a person's being—her body, her definition of self in relation to a dangerous world, and her potency to act in that world—that changes with memorized *ilmu.*

In addition, Sasaks speak constantly of not knowing the hearts of others. Hearts (Indon., *hati*) symbolize hidden emotions, intentions, and a memorized body of *ilmu.* Sasaks' distrust of others' appearance and actions leaves them always on guard against the offensive capacity of *ilmu,* its curses and black magic. Because of secrecy, a person never knows what *ilmu* someone else has, and because of the hiddenness of hearts, a person never knows which social relationships someone else truly values. The self, defined in terms of secret knowledge and hidden emotional ties to others, is unknowable to someone else, even one's own children. At the moment of death when it is considered essential that a dying person remember, there is no mnemonic image or name that can be used because no one else can guess what specific memories must be remembered. And so, the reminder is left vague and mnemonically weak. Anxious relatives and friends can do no more to bring a person away from the brink of death than to ask them to remember. The same cultural understandings and values that undergird the potency Sasaks give to the act of remembering make them impotent to evoke remembering when it is needed most.

THE PURPOSE OF REMEMBERING

Thus far we have explored how certain temporal contexts are socially recognized as ones needing memories, how experiences of anxiety motivate the act of remembering, and how the mnemonics for reminding others to remember are culturally prescribed. We have only one aspect of remembering left to explore: can the nature of remembering itself offer cross-culturally salient insights into why at the moment of death Sasaks rely on the idiom of remembering? What is it about remembering, which is necessarily a reaching into the past, that is considered crucial for the present and future? The *gisalo* for the Kaluli uses memories to resolve personal and social problems of unbalanced reciprocity. It draws upon the past to motivate actions in the present that will resolve the tension. Remembering for the Sasaks is not used to motivate action. Remembering is itself the crucial action. How can this be? To answer this, we must turn to a more philosophical understanding of remembering.

In his discussion of the temporality of action, David Carr argues that time is experienced in events that have temporal thickness (1986, 24).[5] In other words, time is experienced in relation to our emotive reactions to the events that take up time.[6] Our experience of time is not marked by the ticking of a clock. Fifteen minutes seem endless if one is bored, but they can fly by if one is engaged in a project or excited by an event. For Sasaks standing vigil with an ill person, the anxiety-filled moments toward death fly by. Casey remarks, "Reminders are expressly designed to draw us back from the edge of oblivion by directing us to that which we might otherwise forget" (1987, 90). In drawing attention away from the swiftly moving present leading to the ultimate oblivion of death, reminders to remember can be understood as an attempt to slow time. They divert attention away from death and into the safety of the past, and they do so for a purpose.

Returning to Carr's argument, actions within temporal events have goals motivating them and moving them forward in time. These goals are not reached by abstract notions of causality. Imagine a patient on a surgeon's table. An observer might expect one of two outcomes: either the patient recovers or dies. Then one could say that the recovery or death was caused by the surgeon's skills. But this does not portray the surgeon's experience of what happens. The surgeon's experience of the future of her patient is one she affects. She does not experience an expectation, or even less a representation of the future, as she cuts with the scalpel. She experiences an awareness of her effect on the life of the person on her table. "In a significant sense," argues Carr, "when we are absorbed in an action the focus or direction of our attention, the center of our concern, lies not in the present [or the past] but in the future . . . on the work to be done" (1986, 39). All action connects the past with the future, because action is situated within the horizon of past and future; it is meaningful only within that horizon as a note in a musical score is meaningful only in relation to the ones preceding and following it. From the point of view of the actors, the uncertain future

---

5. Philosophers have long been interested in the study of time, or more specifically, the human experience of and action within time (see, e.g., Bergson 1950; Heidegger 1996; Hegel 1977; Husserl 1970; Schutz 1970; Casey 1987). An extensive review of this literature is not warranted by our concerns here nor is a detailed development of Carr's persuasive argument about time. I refer interested readers to the original authors.

6. See also Halbwachs 1980, 88–127.

depends on their ability to connect it with the past. It depends on their actions.

For Sasaks also, the outcome of a moment of death is not predetermined. If a dying person can act, if she can draw her past into the present, she can affect her future and continue to live. The work she must do is to connect past experiences of self and beloved others with the present in order to live in the future. Anthropologists and other scholars have shown that there is not one self but many selves.[7] People continually reconstruct themselves with respect to present context and past experiences. But scholars have also shown that this multiplicity does not diminish the psychological importance of an illusion of wholeness (Ewing 1990). As Hallowell notes: "If I cannot remember, or recall at will, experiences of an hour ago, or yesterday, or last year that I readily identify as my experiences, I cannot maintain an awareness of self-continuity in time" (1955, 94). A sense of self depends upon a string of memories.[8]

But what if one can no longer remember? Then the continuity of self disappears and with it one's identity, one's orientation in the world. In such a state of disorientation, from the Sasak perspective, one has no defenses against the world's dangers. One has no means of potent agency, no means of acting upon the future. And in such a state, a person inevitably dies. One must remember in order to live.

Thus, I suggest that the emphasis on remembering at the moment of death is not simply the outcome of an arbitrary sociocultural model for action. The nature of remembering connects times, the past and the present, in order to affect the future. Sasaks remind dying people to remember in order to stimulate in them a sense of wholeness, connecting their past selves with their present and, in so doing, divert the direction of events away from death and toward a lived future. The future depends on the actions people take, including their ability to slow time by stringing together a past and connecting it to the needs of the present.

CONCLUSION

I have used four questions gathered from analysis of the Kaluli *gisalo* and related them to the Sasak materials in order to understand why

---

7. See, e.g., M. Rosaldo 1980; Ewing 1990; Kondo 1990; Desjarlais 2000.
8. See, e.g., Casey 1987, 290; Ewing 1990, 269–71; Barclay 1995.

remembering is so essential to continuing to live. In so doing, I have attempted to show that the content of memory is not all that is worth studying. In the Sasak materials, secrecy makes studying the content of people's memories futile. Sasaks themselves do not know which memories can be evoked in others. They know only that in certain contexts *one must remember.*

Here we have looked at the act of seeking memories, the act of remembering itself. Remembering is not merely a private, personal endeavor. Remembering is also socioculturally designated as necessary in certain ritual contexts and in moments of everyday life. Remembering does not just stimulate emotion, but can be stimulated by emotions. Anxiety is a compelling motivator for action. In societies like that of Sasaks in which knowledge and thoughts are efficacious, remembering itself is a potent action. Thus socially recognized contexts combine with experiences of anxiety to motivate the act of remembering. Mnemonics can stimulate remembering, although in the Sasak case, the cultural emphasis on secrecy severely limits their options. Finally, the nature of remembering is itself purposeful, not only because it can stimulate action, but because remembering is action even without being undergirded by a cultural conviction in the potency of words and thoughts. Remembering halts time and connects the past to the present in order to affect the future. The act of remembering is not about revisiting the past. Remembering is about impacting the future. To borrow Munn's phrase, "remembering is a relational process," one that connects what matters, what has sociocultural and emotional value, with time (1995, 83). What is remembered may be, as in the Sasak case, less important than the timing of when one remembers. For if remembering is itself a potent action engaging with and acting upon the world, remembering at crucial times is the only thing that will keep a person alive. One must remember in order to continue to live.

— 9 —

Illness at the Intersection of
Anxiety and Knowledge

How do Sasaks cope with the fragility of their lives? They cope by remembering themselves, those around them, and *ilmu*. In order to find and understand this answer, we have delved into people's bodies, anxieties, economics, metaphors, agencies, relationships, creativities, interactions, and authorities within a complex setting of pluralistic medicine. The undergirding thread was the understanding of life as movement. One can study movement by tracing people creating, distributing, and legitimating the knowledge they need to respond to their concerns. Throughout the book, theory has been explored and utilized to forward our understanding of rural Sasaks. Here I cull the theoretical arguments from the chapters and synthesize them. In so doing, I will suggest some perhaps unexpected directions for studying health, emotion, and the relationship between person and culture.

THE ORGANIZATION OF MEDICAL KNOWLEDGE

Illness starts with health. Illness is only recognized in comparison with what a person experiences as normal. For this reason, examinations of illness must begin before anyone is actually ill. They must start with people's experiences of what is normal. For rural Sasaks, normal is perpetually being less than healthy, not necessarily because they feel ill, but because their bodies are not as fat, strong, virile, and wealthy as they imagine urban people's bodies to be. In other words, health is understood in terms that have little to do with actual health and much to do with imaginings of nonpeasant lives. By taking their experience of being less than healthy seriously, and by examining the different ways they understand bodies, I was in a position to see that rural Sasaks live with daily anxieties about potential dangers. These vulnerabilities then shape their sense of self, agency, and relationships with others. Vulnerabilities and personhood shape later interpretations of their illnesses, which in turn influence their vulnerabilities and personhood. Sasaks change in response to the vulnerabilities and illnesses they experience. All of these processes are integral to understanding health, illness, and medicine among Sasaks. Indeed, I suspect that they are integral to understanding illness and health care among most peoples. Essential aspects of health care occur in the absence of actual illness.

We must cast our net wider. Casting our net wider also brings new insights into examinations of medical pluralism. Medical pluralism consists of multiple medical traditions within the same setting. These are established through the distribution of medical knowledge. Examining how medical knowledge is distributed and to whom it is distributed entails looking beyond the topic of health to understand how people conceptualize knowledge as well as the structures or relationships through which knowledge is distributed. Among rural Sasaks, medical knowledge (*ilmu*) is considered inherently potent and is distributed only to others with whom one has multiple social and economic ties. *Ilmu* is distributed horizontally, that is, to others within one's own social network, usually along kinship lines, and only to other peasants. The result of this pattern of knowledge distribution is that over time it becomes widely distributed and maintains a strong truth-value because it is secured by other vital social interests.

The secrecy with which *ilmu* is distributed adds further complexity. Every rural Sasak has *ilmu,* but no one knows what *ilmu* someone else has nor how potent it is. Thus when confronted with illness, although *dukun*s and *belian*s were assumed to have a greater quantity of healing *ilmu,* they were not assumed to necessarily have the right *ilmu* for that particular illness. Thus, Sasak ethnomedicine is an egalitarian knowledge system in which everyone has access to knowledge and all interpretations must be legitimated in social interaction, including that of health specialists. Healing authority is renegotiated, to a lesser or greater extent, for every ailment.

In contrast, biomedical knowledge on Lombok is conceptualized by its proponents as the only correct way of understanding illness, legitimated not only politically but also by the greatness of the international biomedical tradition. This knowledge is not secret, but it is complicated and therefore only distributed to those who are well-educated and, at least in Indonesia, wealthy. It is primarily distributed in formal educational settings, from teacher to pupil. When it is distributed informally, it is in the setting of a consultation, and the knowledge is passed from biomedical personnel to patient in vertical, downward lines rather than horizontal ones. Biomedical knowledge was hardly distributed at all within the community of Pelocok. The *bidan* was a nonpeasant outsider who resisted becoming involved with the people of Pelocok on anything other than medical grounds. When she distributed medical knowledge down to her patients, it was the only interest she shared with them. The brittleness of the social relations along which the knowledge was distributed limited its range of distribution as well as its truth-value. The *bidan* can not be faulted for this, for she was only reproducing in Pelocok the manner in which biomedical knowledge is distributed throughout Lombok. As a result biomedical knowledge has a different kind of knowledge organization from the rural Sasaks' egalitarian one. Biomedical knowledge is hierarchical: people have differential access to knowledge, and knowledge is legitimated automatically based on the social position and authority of the knower.

By casting the net wider and exploring how medical knowledge is distributed within a community, medical pluralism and the relationships within it can be explained without complexities such as measuring quality, familiarity, or efficacy. Moreover, by looking at medical traditions *as they emerge* out of the distribution of knowledge rather than at the traditions as fixed entities, we need not bound our inquiries into spheres of expertise. We can trace the movement of knowledge and in so doing follow the ontological realities of people making relationships and authorities as they cope with their health problems in everyday interactions and formal consultations.

An added benefit of this approach is its potential for cross-cultural comparison. From the Sasak materials two patterns of distributing medical knowledge emerge: egalitarian and hierarchical. These patterns allow for comparison. For example, one could compare biomedical patterns of distributing knowledge on Lombok with those in the United States to understand if and to what extent the patterns vary and whether those variations influence people's resort strategies. Or one could find another ethnographic setting in which the medical pluralism could be characterized by egalitarian and hierarchical medical traditions, then compare to what extent the relationships between the traditions and the results on people's health are similar to those on Lombok. Such comparisons could enrich our understandings of the relationships between people and health care worldwide.

People's health is shaped by the processes that organize medical knowledge. In exploring those processes, as we cast our nets wider and look at areas other than illness and medicine, we develop understandings that better fit with the complex and sometimes nonorderly realities of people trying to cope with their health concerns.

Personal and Cultural Knowledge

This ethnography examines process in two ways. One way is by tacking back and forth between macro and micro—or cultural and personal— levels of analysis. This shows the connections as well as the disjointedness between the two levels, suggesting substantial intracultural variation with family resemblances. The chapters on anatomy and vulnerability in particular show that simple nods to a notion of shared culture would misrepresent what the actual processes of distributing knowledge look like. The three major traditions for understanding the body and the seven common arenas of vulnerability could be understood as cultural models widely dispersed throughout Pelocok. But these models are my abstractions—one drawn from three experts and the other distilled from accumulated data. On both occasions, as soon as the models are sketched out, individual voices and actions give the lie to them, reminding me:

> While [cultural models] like these contain some truth, they also squeeze the life out of the reality of a people by treating human action as if it proceeded from a simple activation of unilateral cultural models. Instead, as we have seen, real life often involves the problematical and always partial resolution of dilemmas proposed by the existence of competing models, or models that are incompatible with key experiences. (Shore 1996, 302–3)[1]

Sasaks do not struggle cognitively with how to reconcile incompatible models; their concerns are pragmatic, and they grasp onto previous knowledge or imaginatively venture out to create knowledge that seems to fit in some way and at a particular moment with the problem at hand.

I found it more helpful to think in terms of knowledge distribution than in terms of models. The most widely distributed bits of knowledge—like those evidenced in metaphor usage—are cultural knowl-

---

1. This disjunction between model and experience, discussed here in cognitive terms, is not new to anthropologists. In slightly different terms, the problem is the same as the connection between form and process (Bateson 1979), structure and change (e.g., Leach 1964), or ideal and real patterns of behavior (Weber 1947).

edge, known (although not necessarily accepted as true) by all. The least widely distributed bits of knowledge—like Papuq Alus's experience of herself as vulnerable to illness after her son left for Malaysia— are personal knowledge, expressed to others in conversations or actions, but still unique to a particular individual. Between these two extremes is common knowledge, bits of knowledge distributed to a greater or lesser extent within pockets of a community. Thus, any particular person's constellation of knowledge at any given time is a unique combination of a few internalized cultural assumptions about reality, many bits and pieces of common knowledge that she has interpreted to be meaningful for her, and a huge amount of experiences, perceptions, concerns, and understandings that are essentially personal knowledge.

This way of understanding the distribution of knowledge fits nicely with what we know of the biology of knowledge. Neurology shows that the brain is not a filing cabinet or a computer somehow storing an accumulation of knowledge.[2] Instead, thought seems to be the result of a kind of chemical semiosis: one stimulus triggering connections with different cells, which in turn trigger synapses with other cells, often causing structural changes in the neurons in the process. Over time and through repetition, habits of these connections form, limiting the possibilities of new connections as neural dendrites stop branching out in new directions. The more habitualized and unwavering the connections, one can suppose, the more static and unquestionable the thought that they result in. This suggests two things: first, that cultural and, to a lesser extent, common knowledge, once internalized and inscribed in neural pathways, are highly stable; second, that each person's perceptions and habits of neural semiosis make all interpretation initially personal and unique.

These two insights from neurology are suggestive for the problem that has long plagued anthropologists: how are we to explain the analytical gap between culture and cultural stability on the one hand and persons in constant flux as they confront the new contexts of everyday living on the other? Chapters 5 and 6 offer ways to start exploring this question through this ethnography's second method of studying process, namely, in the microdynamics of verbal communication.

Ontologically, persons make meanings through a process I call creativity. The results of creativity are the subjective, unique interpretations, understandings, suggestions, and ideas of a particular person.

---

2. See P. S. Churchland 1986; P. M. Churchland 1995.

These interpretations may be either tentative and partial or habitual and perceived as complete. But this personal knowledge has no effect on anyone else until it is expressed, thereby initiating a second process of social meaning-making or interpretation that I refer to as processes of legitimation and constraint. Without social legitimation, personal knowledge has no impact. Without undergoing social processes in which expressed knowledge is legitimated and taken up by other individuals to be personally interpreted, it has no social reality. Once it has social reality, it is common knowledge, more or less widely distributed.

The continual and sequential processes of creativity and legitimation described in detail in chapters 5 and 6 can be expressed as a dialogic model of epistemology:[3] *dialogic* because the processes are of interpretation, and *epistemology* because we are looking at how knowledge is known rather than at the content of knowledge itself. I suggest a dialogic model can explain three different levels of analysis. At an individual level, persons interpret their perceptions (including other people's expressions) by making more or less creative connections among those perceptions and previous knowledge. Even at this level, processes of internal legitimation or rejection occur; some ideas run so counter to other habituated, unquestioned personal or cultural knowledge that these ideas are rejected out of hand. At the level of intersubjectivity, once personal knowledge is expressed or objectified, it goes through social processes of legitimation in which recipients begin their own personal creative interpretations of that knowledge while seeing if those interpretations can tentatively be legitimated or whether they must be rejected or constrained outright.

At the third level of analysis, this dialogic model can explain the gap between person and culture. A person engages other persons through participation in the social processes of interpreting knowledge. So where or what is culture in all this? Mannheim and Tedlock argue that "cultures are continuously produced, reproduced and revised in dia-

---

3. The processes of creativity and legitimation are dualistic processes and as such are not new to anthropologists. Shore talks about meanings as twice born, once individually and once socially (1991). Obeyesekere talks about meanings as having a double hermeneutic, both personal and cultural (1990). My one dissatisfaction with all of these, and to some extent with my own analysis as well, is that they focus on the two sides rather than the one coin. What are the processes through which interpretations become at once social and individual? Dualistic processes automatically trigger a dialectic mode of analysis, but because the processes are driven by interpretation, they are not dialectic, they are dialogic. So is there a way to model them that does not involve constantly shifting lenses from telephoto individual to wide-angle social? This is what the dialogic model I propose here is trying to do.

logues among their members" (1995, 2) and that "the shared worlds that emerge from dialogues are in a continuous state of creation and recreation, negotiation and renegotiation" (3). In short, they understand culture to be the continually revised product of intersubjective dialogue. While this understanding resonates with much of my argument, it clashes with other aspects of it. First, there is not much if any fluctuation, renegotiation, or revision of rural Sasak metaphor usage, notions of *ilmu,* or understandings of how illness is made to leave bodies. This cultural knowledge is widely distributed among rural Sasaks, but—and this is my second objection—it is not shared. My understanding of the verb *to share* implies that that which is shared be distributed in equal portion with equal ownership by all. While environment and ways of life may be shared, the verb *to share* sits uneasily in the realms of interpretation. Shared knowledge or shared worlds would be identical or highly similar interpretations incorporated basically unaltered into different persons. The early chapters of the book, which outline the extreme variation among community members, even household members, about basic health ideas, suggest that they have little knowledge that is truly shared. Moreover, there are no mechanisms, neurological or sociological, that could explain how knowledge and perceptions could be so equally distributed and adopted.

Instead I suggest that culture emerges not from dialogue itself, but from the processes of legitimation within dialogue. When knowledge is given even tentative social legitimation, that bit of knowledge, in personally variant interpretations, becomes common among the participants in that particular interaction. If those participants express a version of that knowledge again in dialogues with others, and if it is again legitimated, the distribution of the knowledge spreads. The more it is legitimated, the wider its distribution, and the less tentative and more habitual it becomes. Eventually, one could conceive of it becoming so widely distributed and unquestioningly accepted as true that it becomes cultural knowledge. In other words, I am equating cultural knowledge with hegemonic knowledge—it is that which has become unquestionable.

In the Sasak materials, we watched this process in the naming of Lo Budin's illness as one connected with the water god. It began as a tentative illness name and was legitimated and acted upon. As more and more people talked about the water god as the possible cause and suggested treatments for it, the tentativeness of the name gradually melted into certainty. Indeed, for the parents at least, the water god name became an unquestioned and unquestionable fact, overriding all other possible names. While I am not suggesting that the water god name of Lo Budin's illness became cultural knowledge within Pelocok, it did become common knowledge, and had the child not died (and had the knowledge been given more opportunities to circulate and be legitimated) it might have become a widely distributed, undisputable fact. As I understand it then, culture is those interpretations of reality that are so obviously true that they no longer need legitimation in communications.

This dialogic model is not far from Peircean semiosis, but whereas for Peirce, the process was all in the mind, in this model, as soon as an idea is expressed, it triggers interpretations by others in a constant social semiosis, a constant dialogue of person with person. In this model also, unlike Peirce's, dialogues have an end, a stopping point when meaning no longer matters.

Wovon man nicht sprechan kann, darueber muss man schwiegen.
Of what we cannot speak, we must be silent. (Wittgenstein 1998)

According to Dennis Tedlock, dialogues do not end but only adjourn (1995, 284). Yet I have seen the spaces where dialogue ends, where interpretation and participation halt, before that of which one cannot speak. I have seen spaces of silence. And this brings me to the third and final major theoretical point of this ethnography, which is that the dialogical model of epistemology—the seeking of knowledge through social interaction—is both motivated by and stops before emotional reactions to the things that matter.

THE THINGS THAT MATTER

Ultimately, the things that matter are not illness names or legitimated knowledge. Ultimately, the things that matter are the things of value: the things that resonate deeply, the things that are unquestionable, the things that bring forth strong emotional responses. It is before these values that intellectual approaches are reduced to silence. Others have sought ways to break this silence, to combine analysis of knowledge and emotions, mind and heart, words and experience. These analyses resort to complex ideas of embodiment, aesthetics, and concerns to bridge the gap between knowledge and emotion.[4] My own work has

---

4. See, e.g., Csordas 1990, 1994; Desjarlais 1992; Hollan and Wellencamp 1994; Laderman 1991; M. Rosaldo 1980; Wikan 1990.

benefited tremendously from these endeavors. In the hopes of further forwarding discussion through which the spaces of silence can be incorporated into our analyses without flattening their significance, I sketch a way of synthesizing the dialogic model outlined above with the things that matter.

Simply put, things that matter are those things (objects, ideas, people) that people value—things that, when threatened, cause people to react emotionally with fear or anxiety. While these negative affective responses can lead to depressed activity or psychological disorders, anxiety also can motivate problem-solving activity. Anxiety can stimulate action to solve the problem that caused it in the first place (cf. Chodorow 1999, 35ff.). Problem solving is a creative activity, requiring people to make interpretations drawing from their own constellations of knowledge, personal preferences, perceptions, and memories. As those interpretations are expressed, people decide which suggestions are worth trying. Anxiety about health can be the prime motivator in seeking knowledge to alleviate the health concern. This is particularly true among Sasaks. As we have seen, their distribution of ethnomedical knowledge sets up an environment particularly encouraging of people to remember or seek medical knowledge. Indeed, Sasaks respond to anxiety about health, whether vulnerabilities or illnesses, with a high degree of creativity because ethnomedical knowledge is distributed so widely and secretly that it encourages everyone's participation and creativity in interpreting illness. Therefore anxiety about health fosters creativity in seeking illness names and dialogue to get those names legitimized. Anxiety also plays a key role in stimulating the need to remember *ilmu* and the need to remind the dying to remember. Of course, one can seek medical knowledge without experiencing anxiety, and anxiety about health need not necessarily lead to the seeking of medical knowledge. But I suggest that if we are to understand how the people who experience illness cope with those experiences, we must look at the intersection of anxiety and the pursuit of knowledge. At this intersection, we can trace the affectively motivated processes of how people cope with the concerns and problems of their lives. Affect begins or motivates the pursuit of medical knowledge.

It also marks the end of dialogue. For the emotional investment in the things that ultimately matter, the things of ultimate value, is too great to be questioned. The specifics of what has ultimate value in any given community will vary, but we can seek those values through common ethnographic methods. Indeed, anthropologists already do this by answering questions such as What are the essential characteristics that make an Inuit an Inuit?[5] For what will the Ilongot take up arms?[6] What is at stake for poor Haitians when they answer questions of "How are you?" with "I'm fighting with life"?[7] These are questions anthropologists excel at. They are questions about the central elements of a culture: those aspects of a culture, those bits of cultural knowledge, that define reality and one's life within it.

For Sasaks, the knowledge that they are always less than healthy and that they may not live long enough to see someone again fundamentally defines their reality, making health something of ultimate value. Correspondingly, Sasaks have two other ultimate values that enable them to cope with problems of health, namely, the potency of remembering *ilmu* and the potency of remembering self and social relationships. These three values are absolutely essential and unquestionable. When any of these three is threatened, the resulting anxiety motivates reactions that are greeted not with legitimation processes, but with silence.

Perhaps this can best be exemplified by the case of Inaq Marni.[8] She and her family were against the *bidan* delivering her children. But after the stillbirth of Inaq Marni's first twin and Inaq Marni's physical deterioration, she went to the clinic to seek help in the second delivery. As her husband said, "*Embe, embe kanakne. Pokokne inaqne hidup*" (Whatever happens to the children, what is important is that their mother lives). Life was more valuable than medical consistency, and they were ready to try almost anything to keep her alive. But after the stillbirth of the second twin, when the *bidan* recommended that they go to the hospital because she could do nothing more to save Inaq Marni's life, Inaq Marni insisted that she wanted to die in her own home. The ultimate value of life was superseded by the value of being within one's social world. And when she died, the primary reason given for her death was that the *belian* in charge of the majority of her labor either did not know or had failed to remember the correct potent *ilmu*. *Ilmu*, not biomedical knowledge, was understood as the only medical knowledge that could have prevented Inaq Marni's death. In the anxious words of the husband, we hear the silence of his dread that she would die and his willingness to agree to anything to prevent that. For Inaq Marni, the concept of dying outside one's social world, with no one to remind one to remember, was so unfathomable it could only be greeted with silence

---

5. Briggs 1998.
6. M. Rosaldo 1980; R. Rosaldo 1980.
7. Farmer 1992, 47.
8. For a more detailed examination of Inaq Marni's death, see Hay 1999.

and refusal. And for the community, the idea that biomedicine should have been able to prevent her death never entered their minds; it would have betrayed their absolute faith in the potency of *ilmu*. These are ultimate values as revealed by the sacrifices people are willing to make for them.

As such they are areas of silence where normal processes of social dialogue do not go. Facing the death of a loved one, no one questions the choice of seeking biomedical care, or any possible care that might help. Deciding to die at home rather than seek further treatment goes unquestioned by all but the biomedical outsider. While the potency of a particular healer's *ilmu* is questioned, the potency of *ilmu* itself is never doubted. Before these spaces of ultimate value, dialogic processes of legitimation stop, and there is silence. In effect, in constantly interpreting, people generate knowledge that generates change in their lives and thoughts, all for the purpose of stasis. All for the purpose of protecting that which is unquestionable, where angels fear to tread. In the end, stasis—as the ultimate value of keeping a person alive—depends upon processes of creativity and legitimation that change the world in order to keep it the same. And those processes are only stopped when they challenge the other ultimate values of self within a community and the potency of *ilmu*.

— • —

Anxiety prompts the search for knowledge and marks when that search must stop. Anxiety is the motivator encouraging people to seek ways to cope. Knowledge is the tool of coping. But it is a tool that people must creatively fashion and socially legitimate. It is in those processes of legitimation that people make authorities, which can both ease and complicate the seeking of knowledge. Some authorities do not have lasting consequences; some become so habitual that they fundamentally shape social interactions, which can have lasting repercussions on people's health.

Illness is a rich landscape for studying how anxiety and knowledge intersect. Health matters. Health concerns automatically stimulate anxiety in patients and their loved ones. Whether as experiences of vulnerability or of illness, health concerns trigger anxieties that initiate the coping processes of seeking knowledge. Moreover, health concerns are ones that must be dealt with in a timely manner. They can not be put off indefinitely. The dynamics of anxiety and knowledge occur and can be traced within a relatively discrete period of time. But most important, as I said above, is that health matters. Examining the dynamics of anxiety weighing on the processes of seeking to alleviate vulnerabilities, name illnesses, and legitimate treatments is not just a cognitive exercise for exploring person-culture relationships; it is an exploration into why people die and how they have the courage to face very fragile lives with laughter.

Epilogue

The Irony of Knowledge

The illnesses and deaths of tomorrow are partially anticipated in Pelocok: people are aware that they are less than healthy, that they may die before they meet someone again, that they are vulnerable to a host of potential ills. When vulnerabilities are experienced or illness enters, the rush to prevent and to treat them attests to both anxiety and hope. Nonetheless, the health statistics cited in chapter 1 imply that Sasak methods of coping with illness do not work.

THE TRAGEDY OF RURAL SASAK ETHNOMEDICINE

People in Pelocok suffering from mild episodes of usual or unusual illnesses almost always recover, as do some people suffering from severe episodes of usual illness or unusual illness. Nonetheless, as we have seen, death is a not infrequent consequence of illness. Pelocok is a pluralistic medical setting where there are many options for resort including a biomedical option. Why then do so many illness episodes end in death?

Ironically, the answer is *ilmu,* the cornerstone of Sasak cultural knowledge enabling them to cope with illness. Precisely that which rural Sasaks believe gives them the most understanding of, strength against, and agency to treat illness is what inhibits advances in prevention, ethnomedical treatments, and optimal use of biomedical facilities. Because *ilmu* is potent against both natural and personal causal agents, it can prevent illnesses, and it alone (in the form of *jampi*) is seen as capable of driving out illness. Because *ilmu* is secret, knowledge is not openly communicated and therefore can not be challenged by others.

Alland (1970) hypothesizes that bad or faulty medical theories, such as theories that diseases can be cured through magic, inhibit the development of more effective therapies (156). From a scientific perspective, the potency of *ilmu* to affect illness is a faulty medical theory: words are not agents, magically capable of preventing and treating illness. Nonetheless, *ilmu* is the core aspect of Sasak ethnomedicine. *Ilmu* is so unquestioned that situations in which it fails are excused by supposed human error. If a person becomes ill despite practicing preventive measures including *puji*, Sasaks say that he or she must have forgotten (*lupaq*) some words or actions. Similarly, if a *jampi* fails to heal an illness, people do not question the efficacy of *ilmu* in general; they question either the fit of that particular *jampi* to the particular illness or the correctness of how it was performed. The efficacy of *ilmu* against illness is not subject to question. Moreover, because *ilmu* is understood to be the *only* force capable of meeting an illness and making it leave the body, other strategies for coping with illness—such as resorting to biomedical care—are understood to be unnecessary and potentially detrimental.

The secrecy of *ilmu* further inhibits the development of a more efficacious approach to medicine. Everyone in Pelocok has secret spells to prevent or treat illness. Some of this *ilmu* is gained through the whispered gifts of others, some through dreams. In either case, there is no venue for checking it at a later time. There is no mechanism for limiting or validating *ilmu*. It proliferates in all directions. Thus if one person's healing spell for a particular illness name does not work, that does not mean that another person's spell will also fail. Moreover, because *ilmu* is secret, there is no communication among healers. *Dukun*s do not share their healing knowledge and experience with other *dukun*s; *belian*s do not share theirs with other *belian*s. While some healers will distribute their *ilmu* and experience to select others, usually family members, there is no forum for the public accumulation of knowledge regarding illness.

Belief in *ilmu* also causes particular peculiarities in the relations between rural Sasaks and Lombok's biomedical health care. As noted, because only *ilmu* is deemed capable of making an illness leave a body, rural Sasaks seek biomedical care—if they seek it at all—only to "quickly get well again." That is, they seek technologies to quickly treat the symptoms *after* the illness is presumed to be successfully treated. This means that resort to biomedicine is delayed, sometimes to the point where biomedical intervention can no longer save a patient, as in the case of Inaq Marni's death in childbirth. Such delays are frustrating for the biomedical personnel whose skills and technologies are ignored until it is too late for them to be useful. Their frustration feeds stereotypes about the backwardness and lack of understanding of peasants. Moreover, biomedical healers on Lombok, like the ethnomedical healers, depend on the value of esoteric knowledge for their own status in the community. Frustration, stereotypes, and desire to protect social status combine to make nonpeasant people like the *bidan* in Pelocok unlikely to disperse much biomedical knowledge to peasants. Moreover, whatever knowledge she offers is communicated along vertical, downward, single-stranded channels because biomedical personnel are nonpeasants with the power of the state behind them who share only a single interest with peasants, that of health care. Thus, a vicious circle is perpetuated whereby biomedical knowledge is deemed less trustworthy by rural Sasaks who therefore continue to resort to the well-trusted *ilmu* of friends and healers, delaying or avoiding any resort to biomedical care.

The tragedy of Sasak ethnomedicine is that the value it places on its healing knowledge (*ilmu*) and the processes through which that knowledge is distributed inhibit improvements in health care. Because of their *ilmu,* rural Sasaks can neither develop a method of testing and refining ethnomedical treatments nor fully utilize the life-saving potential of biomedical treatments.

SASAK ETHNOMEDICINE: A POSITIVE PERSPECTIVE

This is not to imply that Sasak ethnomedicine is useless. It does have many attributes that make objective sense. Because knowledge about prevention and treatment is widely dispersed, people know how to treat illnesses themselves and can participate relatively equally in processes of social legitimation. This relative equality means that relationships with ethnomedical healers are horizontal relationships that encourage mutual communication. In contrast, because rural Sasaks do not have access to biomedical personnel's knowledge and must show deference to them, interactions with them are vertical, which inhibits communication. The ethnomedical focus on the person and the importance of community emphasizes a more holistic approach to medicine, encouraging family to stay close to ill persons giving psychological and social support. This is very different from the biomedical tradition on Lombok, which concentrates exclusively on the physiological body, shooing family out of treatment rooms and disregarding the psychosomatic component that has been recognized elsewhere as a very important part of healing.[1] Finally, the herbal, massage, and bone-setting treatments of Sasak ethnomedical traditions are often beneficiary. Broken hands, painful muscles, stomachaches, colds, and headaches are among the ailments that respond quickly to Sasak treatments. For other sicknesses and ailments, it is difficult to judge the role of ethnomedical efficacy. These attributes of Sasak ethnomedicine show evidence of its potential for positive effect on health.

While rural Sasak approaches to health care often fail to prevent death, it is not necessarily maladaptive ecologically. Theirs is a peasant economy based on access to land. As discussed in chapter 1, land is quite limited. Many households in Pelocok can barely subsist on their landholdings, and just to the north of Pelocok, a large group of people abandoned their homes altogether to seek more land opportunities through Indonesia's transmigration program. This land shortage is further taxed by fertility rates. While many young couples use birth control and plan to limit the sizes of their families, the reproductive life histories I gathered for women in Pelocok showed high rates of fertility, which would translate into ever smaller portions of inheritable land. Alland (1970) suggests that disease can provide societies with a means of limiting their population to numbers supportable by the environment: "Disease and death upset all people to some degree, but disease at least provides some external source of population control" (132). In short, to the extent that rural Sasak medical practices are less efficacious, they may function to limit the number of landless poor in an already precarious economic environment.

Aside from this functionalist perspective, it is important to keep in mind that the ultimate goal of rural Sasak approaches to health is not, I suggest, preventing death. In America, people are uncomfortable around death and seek to avoid it at any cost, and as a consequence death is hidden behind the closed doors of hospitals and nursing homes (Turner 1995). But elsewhere in the world, people have a day-to-day acquaintance with death. Certainly, rural Sasaks seek health care to prevent the deaths of loved ones, but death is not to be avoided at any cost. Taking people out of their homes, away from their loved ones, was a cost most were not willing to pay. There were many cases when I would offer to take people with life-threatening illnesses to seek bio-

---

1. The literature on this topic shows that social support or a social network contributes to the maintenance of health, the reduction of anxiety, and the healing of sickness (see, e.g., Csordas and Kleinman 1996; Finkler 1994a; House 1988).

medical care, and they would refuse or delay departure for days or weeks. Challenging the potency of *ilmu* was another potential cost of seeking biomedical care, one that people were unwilling even to contemplate. *Ilmu* enables them to cope with illnesses—to prevent, name, and treat them—without having wealth, formal education, technologies, or transportation to town. It gives them confidence in their potency against the unknown. The costs of potentially saving a life by rejecting deep-seated Sasak values were too great.

REMEMBERING TO LIVE AND RETURNING TO LAUGHTER

The tragic face of health care comes to the fore in this ethnography. But the sometimes tragic consequences of how people in Pelocok cope with illness do not overpower most people's ability to laugh and get on with life. Despite the tenuousness of life, Pelocok is not a dour place. The reason is again people's unquestioning belief in the potency of *ilmu*. *Ilmu* makes people capable (*tauq*) of surviving; it gives them agency and pride in a dangerous world beset with ghosts and gods, poverty and hunger, prejudice and condescension.

When Inaq Nori suddenly became ill, people rushed to her side. She had gone to market feeling fine, but when she returned she went into a kind of convulsive, hysterical behavior. She could neither sit nor stand, but lay wailing in pain, sometimes panting with exhaustion, sometimes in a frenzy to scoot outdoors on her back. In the first two hours, no less than seven different people treated her for different named illnesses. Neighbors said healing spells over her. *Dukun*s and a *belian* came and treated her. Inaq Nori herself panted out that she had met a ghost, implying that she was ill with *ketemuq*. Her father, a *dukun*, arrived later and diagnosed her as ill with *bebabasan*, an illness caused by a certain kind of spirit, and this was the illness name that was finally legitimated. Having *ilmu*—knowing spells—gave each of them something to do in the face of Inaq Nori's acute episode. The *bidan* came and gave Inaq Nori a sedative and an injection of vitamin B, even though the *bidan* admitted later that she did not know what was wrong and that all of Inaq Nori's vital signs had appeared normal. All through the day, Inaq Nori's sisters and mother held her, wept, and told her to remember. As long as she remembered, she would live.

Inaq Nori did remember, and as quickly as it started, her illness left her. The next day Inaq Nori was weak but fine. Nor did she worry about a recurrence, saying that whether or not the illness came back, the *ilmu* of people in Pelocok was strong enough (*kuat ilmu dengan iteh*) to make it leave again. Moreover, she added, "I know how to remember" (*Tauq aku ingat*). *Ilmu* and remembering counter the anxiety caused by even the strangest of illnesses. They give rural Sasaks agency in a world filled with dangers, and they provide courage to live fragile lives with laughter.

After the scare of her illness, Inaq Nori, her family, and their neighbors all resumed their lives. Her sudden illness became a distant memory until my videotape, shown on my last night in Pelocok, reminded them of it. And they responded to the visual memory with laughter.

Glossary

This glossary includes only those words or phrases cited frequently in the text. The language or languages to which the word belongs are indicated as Sasak (Sas.), Indonesian (Indon.), and Arabic (Ar.). For those words highlighted by an asterisk (*), the Sasak meaning is different from its counterpart in other languages, and only the Sasak meaning is given. The interested reader is directed to Echols and Shadily 1989 for comparisons with Indonesian.

adat (Indon.)	tradition, custom
aiq (Sas.)	water, blood, fluids
bakat (Sas.)	to burn, to be burned
barugah (Sas.)	large covered platform used for social gatherings
bauq (Sas.)	to have some action be possible in a passive sense
begawai (Sas.)	a ritual conducted in accordance with recognized traditions or "words of the ancestors" in the community
belian (Sas.)	midwife-healer, always female
benung (Sas.)	hot, warm (in relation to health, hotness is taken as a sign of illness)
bidan (Sas.)*	a biomedically trained midwife
coba (Sas., Indon.)	to try; the attempts or tests of black magic curses
cocok (Sas., Indon.)	to fit; in relation to health, illness names must "fit" the particular illness in order for associated treatments to work
cukup (Sas., Indon.)	enough, an adequate supply; in relation to health, implies healthy

dalem (Sas.)*	inside, the insides of a body, the heart; can refer to someone's intentions or motivations
dareq (Sas.)	blood; similar to the Indonesian *darah*
dewa (Sas.)*	soul, gods, animate but unseen entities, often animistic
dukun (Sas.)*	shaman, always male
epe (Sas.)	soul, spirit, a person's shadowy twin
hati (Sas., Indon.)	literally, liver; connotations similar to those for *heart* for English speakers
ilmu (Sas.)*	secret, potent knowledge, including *jampi* and *puji.*
ingat (Indon.)	remember
jampi (Sas., Indon.)	treatment spell or the act of performing a spell (to *jampi*); *jampi* is both the singular and plural noun form
jinn (Sas., Indon., Ar.)	spirits recognized by Islam; among Sasaks, jinn are considered largely impish and mischievous spirits, who dwell primarily on the volcano but travel and can be found anywhere on the island.
kemalikan (Sas.)	illness resulting from coming in contact with potent objects or auras
kepala dusun (Indon.)	government position of mayor or head of a hamlet
ketemuq (Sas.)	illness resulting from meeting a ghost or spirit
ketomuai (Sas.)	kind of treatment ceremony that calls on spirits to be involved in making the illness leave the patient; only performed by *dukun*s, who may be assisted by *kiayi*s
kiayi (Sas.)*	religious leader, Muslim, who must know local ritual traditions and also how to recite the Qur'an
kotor (Indon.)	dirty, impure
kurang (Sas., Indon.)	not enough; a less than adequate supply; in relation to health, *kurang* implies less than healthy
lekaq (Sas.)	to walk, move, flow
luge (Sas.)	dirty, impure
maju (Indon.)	progress, development, modernity
malik (Sas.)	taboo, very potent

mul (Sas.)	neither hot nor cold; neither anxious or disturbed, but relaxed; in relation to health, when a body is *mul* it is healthy
ndeq ku bani (Sas.)	a phrase meaning "I am not brave"
nyet (Sas.)	cold, clammy; in relation to health, coldness is taken as a sign of illness
panas (Indon.)	hot, warm; in relation to health, hotness is taken as a sign of illness
puji (Sas.)	"small words," a form of *ilmu* used to prevent harm
sakit (Sas., Indon.)	ill, not healthy
selaq (Sas.)	a witch, always female
semangat (Indon.)	life force animating a person
suci (Sas., Indon., Ar.)	pure, clean
sugul (Sas.)	to exit, leave, go out of
taget (Sas.)	to be surprised; an illness resulting from being surprised, shocked; similar to the Indonesian *kaget*
tauq (Sas.)	to be capable of doing something with agency; to know
tertinggal (Indon.)	left-behind; backward
tiak (Sas.)	rising; similar to the Indonesian *naik*
tume (Sas.)	to enter, go into
turun (Sas., Indon.)*	to go down
urat (Sas.)	channels for fluid in the body, similar to blood vessels

References

Ali, A. Y., ed. 1989. *The Holy Qur'an*. Brentwood, MD: Amana Corporation.

Alland, Alexander, Jr. 1970. *Adaptation in Cultural Evolution: An Approach to Medical Anthropology*. New York: Columbia University Press.

Anderson, Benedict R. O'G. 1990. *Language and Power*. Ithaca: Cornell University Press.

Appadurai, Arjun. 1986. Theory in Anthropology: Center and Periphery. *Comparative Studies in Society and History* 28 (2): 356–74.

Atkinson, Jane Monnig. 1989. *The Art and Politics of Wana Shamanship*. Berkeley: University of California Press.

———. 1996. Quizzing the Sphinx: Reflections on Mortality in Central Sulawesi. In *Fantasizing the Feminine in Indonesia*, L. Sears, ed., 163–90. Durham: Duke University Press.

Attinasi, John, and Paul Friedrich. 1995. Dialogic Breakthrough: Catalysis and Synthesis in Life-Changing Dialogue. In *The Dialogic Emergence of Culture*, D. Tedlock and B. Mannheim, eds., 33–53. Urbana: University of Illinois Press.

Bakhtin, M. M. 1986. *Speech Genres and Other Late Essays*. Austin: University of Texas Press.

Barbee, Evelyn L. 1986. Biomedical Resistance to Ethnomedicine in Botswana. *Social Science and Medicine* 22 (1): 75–80.

Barclay, Craig R. 1995. Autobiographical Remembering: Narrative Constraints on Objectified Selves. In *Remembering Our Past*, David Rubin, ed., 94–125. Cambridge: Cambridge University Press.

Barth, Fredrik. 1975. *Ritual and Knowledge among the Baktaman of New Guinea*. New Haven: Yale University Press.

———. 1987. *Cosmologies in the Making*. Cambridge: Cambridge University Press.

———. 1990. The Guru and the Conjurer: Transactions in Knowledge and the Shaping of Culture in Southeast Asia and Melanesia. *Man* 25:460–653.

———. 1993. *Balinese Worlds*. Chicago: University of Chicago Press.

Bartlett, Frederic C. [1932] 1995. *Remembering: A Study in Experimental and Social Psychology*. With an introduction by Walter Kintsch. Cambridge: Cambridge University Press.

Bateson, Gregory. 1979. *Mind and Nature*. New York: E. P. Dutton.

———. 1982. Bali: The Value System of a Steady State. In *Steps to an Ecology of Mind*, 107–27. Northvale, NJ: Jason Aronson.

Bateson, Gregory, and Margaret Mead. 1942. *The Balinese Character*. New York: New York Academy of Sciences.

Bateson, Mary Catherine. 1994. *Peripheral Visions*. New York: HarperCollins.

Battaglia, Debborah. 1990. *On the Bones of the Serpent*. Chicago: University of Chicago Press.

Beattie, John. 1967. Divination in Bunyoro, Uganda. In *Magic, Witchcraft, and Curing*. J. Middleton, ed., 211–31. Garden City, NY: Natural History Press.

Belo, Jane. 1960. *Trance in Bali*. New York: Columbia University Press.

Berger, Peter L., and Thomas Luckmann. 1966. *The Social Construction of Reality*. New York: Anchor.

Bergson, Henri. 1950. *Matter and Memory*. New York: Macmillan.

Birdwhistell, Ray L. 1970. *Kinesics and Context*. Philadephia: University of Pennsylvania Press.

Bohannan, Laura (Elenore Smith Bowen). 1964. *Return to Laughter*. New York: Anchor.

Borofsky, Robert. 1987. *Making History*. Cambridge: Cambridge University Press.

Bosworth, C. E., E. van Donzel, B. Lewis, and C. H. Pellat, eds. 1986. *The Encyclopedia of Islam*, vol. 3. Leiden: E. J. Brill.

Bourdieu, Pierre. 1977a. The Economics of Linguistic Exchanges. *Social Science Information* 16 (6): 645–58.

———. 1977b. *Outline of a Theory of Practice*. Cambridge: Cambridge University Press.

———. 1991. *Language and Symbolic Power*. Cambridge: Harvard University Press.

Briggs, Jean L. 1998. *Inuit Morality Play*. New Haven: Yale University Press.

Brodwin, Paul. 1996. *Medicine and Morality in Haiti*. Cambridge: Cambridge University Press.

Brown, Peter J. 1998. Preface. In *Understanding and Applying Medical Anthropology*, P. Brown, ed. Mountainview, CA: Mayfield.

Brown, Peter J., Bruce Ballard, and Jessica Gregg. 1994. Culture, Ethnicity, and the Practice of Medicine. In *Human Behavior: An Introduction for Medical Students*, 2d ed., A. Stoudemire, ed., 84–104. Philadelphia: J. B. Lippincott.

Brown, Peter J., Marcia C. Inhorn, and Daniel J. Smith. 1996. Disease, Ecology, and Human Behavior. In *Medical Anthropology*, rev. ed., C. Sargent and T. Johnson, eds., 183–218. Westport: Praeger.

Brown, Peter J., and Melvin Konner. 1987. An Anthropological Perspective on Obesity. *Annals of the New York Academy of Sciences* 499:29–46.

Carr, David. 1986. *Time, Narrative, and History*. Bloomington: Indiana University Press.

Carr, John E., and Peter P. Vitaliano. 1985. The Theoretical Implications of Converging Research on Depression and the Culture-Bound Syndromes.

In *Culture and Depression*, A. Kleinman and B. Good, eds., 244–67. Berkeley: University of California Press.

Carruthers, Mary. 1990. *The Book of Memory*. Cambridge: Cambridge University Press.

Casey, Edward S. 1987. *Remembering: A Phenomenological Study*. Bloomington: Indiana University Press.

Cederroth, Sven. 1981. *The Spell of the Ancestors and the Power of Mekkah*. Göteborg, Sweden: Acta Universitatis Gothoburgensis.

Chodorow, Nancy. 1999. *The Power of Feelings*. New Haven: Yale University Press.

Churchland, Patricia Smith. 1986. *Neurophilosophy*. Cambridge: MIT Press.

Churchland, Paul M. 1995. *The Engine of Reason, the Seat of the Soul*. Cambridge: MIT Press.

Clifford, James. 1986. On Ethnographic Allegory. In *Writing Culture*, J. Clifford and G. Marcus, eds., 98–121. Berkeley: University of California Press.

Clifford, James, and George E. Marcus, eds. 1986. *Writing Culture*. Berkeley: University of California Press.

Colson, Anthony Clarke. 1971. *The Prevention of Illness in a Malay Village*. Winston-Salem: Wake Forest University Press.

Comaroff, Jean. 1981. Healing and Cultural Transformation: The Case of the Tswana of Southern Africa. *Social Science and Medicine* 15B:367–78.

Conklin, Beth A., and Lynn M. Morgan. 1996. Babies, Bodies, and the Production of Personhood in North America and a Native Amazonian Society. *Ethos* 24 (4): 657–94.

Connerton, Paul. 1989. *How Societies Remember*. Cambridge: Cambridge University Press.

Connor, Linda, Patsy Asch, and Timothy Asch. 1986. *Jero Tapakan: Balinese Healer*. Cambridge: Cambridge University Press.

Cool, Capt. W. 1896. *De Lombok Expeditie*. Batavia.

Corner, Lorraine. 1989. East and West Nusa Tenggara: Isolation and Poverty. In *Unity and Diversity: Regional Economic Development in Indonesia since 1970*, H. Hill, ed., 178–206. Oxford: Oxford University Press.

Cosminsky, Sheila, and Mary Scrimshaw. 1980. Medical Pluralism on a Guatemalan Plantation. *Social Science and Medicine* 14B:267–78.

Crick, Malcolm R. 1982. Anthropology of Knowledge. *Annual Review of Anthropology* 11:287–313.

Csordas, Thomas. 1990. Embodiment as a Paradigm for Anthropology. *Ethos* 18:5–47.

———. 1994. The Body as Representation and Being in the World. In *Embodiment and Experience*. T. Csordas, ed., 1–23. London: Cambridge University Press.

———. 1997. *Language, Charisma, and Creativity*. Berkeley: University of California Press.

Csordas, Thomas, and Arthur Kleinman. 1996. The Therapeutic Process. In *Medical Anthropology*, rev. ed. C. Sargent and T. Johnson, eds., 3–20. Westport, CT: Praeger.

Dalton, George. 1961. Economic Theory and Primitive Society. *American Anthropologist* 63:1–25.

D'Andrade, Roy G. 1992. Schemas and Motivation. In *Human Motives and Cultural Models*. R. D'Andrade and C. Strauss, eds., 23–44. Cambridge: Cambridge University Press.

D'Andrade, Roy G., and Claudia Strauss, eds. 1992. *Human Motives and Cultural Models*. Cambridge: Cambridge University Press.

Davis-Floyd, Robbie E., and Carolyn F. Sargent, eds. 1997. *Childbirth and Authoritative Knowledge*. Berkeley: University of California Press.

Desjarlais, Robert R. 1992. *Body and Emotion: The Aesthetics of Illness and Healing in the Nepal Himalayas*. Philadephia: University of Pennsylvania Press.

———. 1996. Presence. In *The Performance of Healing*, C. Laderman and M. Roseman, eds., 143–64. New York: Routledge.

———. 2000. The Makings of Personhood in a Shelter for People Considered Homeless and Mentally Ill. *Ethos* 27 (4): 466–89.

Dentan, Robert Knox. 1988. Ambiguity, Synecdoche and Affect in Semai Medicine. *Social Science and Medicine* 27 (8): 857–77.

Dettwyler, Katerine A. 1994. *Dancing Skeletons*. Prospect Heights, IL: Waveland.

Diamond, Jared. 1997. Mr. Wallace's Line. *Discover* (August): 76–83.

Dinas Kesehatan. 1993. *Profil Kesehatan Nusa Tenggara Barat*. Departemen Kesehatan, Provinsi Nusa Tenggara Barat. Mataram.

———. 1994. *Data Upaya Kesehatan PusKesMas, Nusa Tenggara Barat*. Departemen Kesehatan, Provinsi Nusa Tenggara Barat. Mataram.

DuBois, Cora. 1944. *The People of Alor*, vols. 1–2. New York: Harper and Brothers.

Dumont, Louis. 1980. *Homo Hierarchicus*. Chicago: University of Chicago Press.

Duranti, Allessandro, and Charles Goodwin. 1992. *Rethinking Context*. Cambridge: Cambridge University Press.

Echols, John M., and Hassan Shadily. 1989. *An Indonesian-English Dictionary*, 3d ed. Ithaca: Cornell University Press.

Ecklund, Judith Louise. 1977. Marriage, Seaworms, and Song: Ritualized Responses to Cultural Change in Sasak Life. Ph.D. diss., Cornell University.

Endicott, K. M. 1979. *Batek Negrito Religion*. Oxford: Clarendon.

Errington, Shelly. 1989. *Meaning and Power in a Southeast Asian Realm*. Princeton: Princeton University Press.

Evans-Pritchard, E. E. 1969. *The Nuer*. New York: Oxford University Press.

———. 1976. *Witchcraft, Oracles, and Magic among the Azande*, abridged ed. Oxford: Clarendon.

Ewing, Katherine P. 1990. The Illusion of Wholeness: Culture, Self, and the Experience of Inconsistency. *Ethos* 18 (3): 251–78.

Fabrega, Horacio, Jr. 1980. *Disease and Social Behavior: An Interdisciplinary Perspective*. Cambridge: MIT Press.

Fabrega, Horacio, Jr., and D. B. Silver. 1973. *Illness and Shamanistic Curing in Zinacantan*. Stanford: Stanford University Press.

Farmer, Paul. 1992. *AIDS and Accusation: Haiti and the Geography of Blame.* Berkeley: University of California Press.

Farmer, Paul, Margaret Connors, and Janie Simmons, eds. 1996. *Women, Poverty, and AIDs.* Monroe, ME: Common Courage.

Feld, Steven. 1982. *Sound and Sentiment.* Philadelphia: University of Pennsylvania Press.

Ferzacca, Steve. 1996. In This Pocket of the Universe: Healing the Modern in a Central Javanese City. Ph.D. diss., University of Wisconsin-Madison.

Finkler, Kaja. 1991. *Physicians at Work, Patients in Pain: Biomedical Practice and Patient Response in Mexico.* Boulder: Westview.

———. 1994a. *Women in Pain: Gender and Morbidity in Mexico.* Philadelphia: University of Pennsylvania Press.

———. 1994b. Sacred Healing and Biomedicine Compared. *Medical Anthropology Quarterly* 8 (2): 178–97.

Firth, Raymond. 1956. *Elements of Social Organization.* London: Watts.

———. 1967. *Tikopia Ritual and Belief.* Boston: Beacon.

Fish, Stanley. 1979. Normal Circumstances, Literal Language, Direct Speech Acts, the Ordinary, the Everyday, the Obvious, What Goes without Saying, and Other Special Cases. In *Interpretive Social Science, A Reader,* P. Rabinow and W. Sullivan, eds., 243–66. Berkeley: University of California Press.

Foster, George M. 1976. Disease Etiologies in Non-Western Medical Systems. *American Anthropologist* 78:773–82.

———. 1994. *Hippocrate's Latin American Legacy: Humoral Medicine in the New World.* Langhorne, PA: Gordon and Breach.

Foucault, Michel. 1965. *Madness and Civilization: A History of Insanity in the Age of Reason.* New York: Random House.

———. 1972. *The Archaeology of Knowledge.* New York: Pantheon Books.

———. 1977. *Discipline and Punish: The Birth of the Prison.* New York: Random House.

———. 1978. *The History of Sexuality,* vol. 1. New York: Random House.

———. 1980. *Power/Knowledge: Selected Interviews and Other Writings.* New York: Pantheon.

Fraser, Gertrude Jacinta. 1998. *African American Midwifery in the South.* Cambridge: Harvard University Press.

Freud, Sigmund. 1959. *Inhibitions, Symptoms, and Anxiety.* New York: W. W. Norton.

Garro, Linda C. 1982. Introduction: The Ethnography of Health Care Decisions. *Social Science and Medicine* 16:1451–52.

———. 1986. Intracultural Variation in Folk Medical Knowledge: A Comparison between Curers and Noncurers. *American Anthropologist* 88: 351–70.

Geertz, Clifford. 1960. *The Religion of Java.* Chicago: University of Chicago Press.

———. 1963. *Agricultural Involution.* Berkeley: University of California Press.

———. 1965. *The Social History of an Indonesian Town.* Cambridge: MIT Press.

———. 1968. *Islam Observed.* Chicago: University of Chicago Press.

———. 1973. *The Interpretation of Cultures.* New York: Basic.

————. 1980. *Negara: The Theatre State in Nineteenth-Century Bali.* Princeton: Princeton University Press.

————. 1983. *Local Knowledge.* New York: Basic.

Geertz, Hildred. 1961. *The Javanese Family.* New York: Free Press.

Geertz, Hildred, and Clifford Geertz. 1964. Teknonymy in Bali: Parenthood, Age-grading, and Genealogical Amnesia. *Journal of the Royal Anthropological Institute* 94 (2): 94–108.

George, Kenneth M. 1996. *Showing Signs of Violence.* Berkeley: University of California Press.

Gerdin, Ingela. 1982. *The Unknown Balinese.* Göteborg, Sweden: Acta Universitatis Gothoburgensis.

Goffman, Erving. [1959] 1973. *The Presentation of Self in Everyday Life.* Woodstock, NY: Overlook.

Good, Byron J. 1994. *Medicine, Rationality, and Experience: An Anthropological Perspective.* Cambridge: Cambridge University Press.

Good, Byron J., and Mary-Jo DelVecchio Good. 1993. "Learning Medicine": The Constructing of Medical Knowledge at Harvard Medical School. In *Knowledge, Power, and Practice,* S. Lindenbaum and M. Lock, eds., 81–107. Berkeley: University of California Press.

Good, Byron J., Mary-Jo DelVecchio Good, and Robert Moradi. 1985. The Interpretation of Iranian Depressive Illness and Dysphoric Affect. In *Culture and Depression,* A. Kleinman and B. Good, eds., 369–428. Berkeley: University of California Press.

Good, Mary-Jo DelVecchio. 1980. Of Blood and Babies: The Relationship of Popular Islamic Physiology to Fertility. *Social Science and Medicine* 14B:147–56.

Good, Mary-Jo DelVecchio, Paul E. Brodwin, Byron J. Good, and Arthur Kleinman, eds. 1992. *Pain as Human Experience: An Anthropological Perspective.* Berkeley: University of California Press.

Goodwin, Charles, and Alessandro Duranti. 1992. Rethinking Context: an Introduction. In *Rethinking Context,* A. Duranti and C. Goodwin, eds., 1–42. Cambridge: Cambridge University Press.

Goris, R. 1936. Aanteekeningen over Oost-Lombok. *Tijdschrift voor Taal-, Land-, en Volkenkunde van Nederlands Indie* 76 (2): 196–248.

Gorlinski, Gini. 1997. "Why Should We Understand? It Is the Language of the Spirits!": Singing and the Ethic of Academic Analysis in a Kalimantan Community. Paper presented at the Indonesia Conference, Arizona State University, Tempe, June 13–15.

Graaf, H. J. de. 1941. Lombok in de 17e Eeuw. *Djawa* 21 (6): 335–73.

Grace, J. 1996. Healers and Modern Health Services: Antenatal, Birthing, and Postpartum Care in Rural East Lombok, Indonesia. In *Maternity and Reproductive Health in Asian Societies,* P. L. Rice and L. Manderson, eds., 145–67. Amsterdam: Harwood Academic.

Hahn, Robert A. 1995. *Sickness and Healing: An Anthropological Perspective.* New Haven: Yale University Press.

Halbwachs, Maurice. 1980. *The Collective Memory.* New York: Harper and Row.

Hall, Edward T. 1973. *The Silent Language.* New York: Anchor.

Hallowell, A. Irving. 1955. *Culture and Experience.* Philadelphia: University of Pennsylvania Press.

Haram, Liv. 1991. Tswana Medicine in Interaction with Biomedicine. *Social Science and Medicine* 33 (2): 167–75.

Harnish, David D. 1985. Musical Traditions of the Lombok Balinese. M.A. thesis, University of Hawaii.

Hay, M. Cameron. 1992. Tight-rope Walker or Dramatis Personae? An Exploration into Balinese Reality. Paper presented at Graduate Student Symposium, Emory University, February.

———. 1997. "They Are Not Muslims": Religious Intolerance in Indonesia. Paper presented at the annual AAA meetings, Washington, DC, November.

———. 1998a. Poison, Black Magic, and Other Hazards of Sex: The Paradox of Male Reproductive Strategies in Lombok, Indonesia. Paper given at the Male Gender and Health Conference, Emory University, Atlanta, November.

———. 1998b. Remembering to Live: Coping with Health Concerns on Lombok. Ph.D. diss., Emory University.

———. 1999. Dying Mothers: Maternal Mortality in Rural Indonesia. *Medical Anthropology* 18 (3): 243–79.

Hefner, Robert W. 1985. *Hindu Javanese.* Princeton: Princeton University Press.

Hegel, Georg W. F. 1977. *Phenomenology of Spirit.* Oxford: Clarendon.

Heggenhougan, H. K. 1980. Bomohs, Doctors, and Sinsehs—Medical Pluralism in Malaysia. *Social Science and Medicine* 14B:235–44.

Heidegger, Martin. 1996. *Being and Time.* Albany: State University of New York Press.

Heider, Karl. 1991. *Landscapes of Emotion: Three Maps of Emotion Terms in Indonesia.* New York: Cambridge University Press.

Helman, Cecil G. 1994. *Culture, Health, and Illness,* 3d ed. Oxford: Butterworth-Heinemann.

Hidajat. 1972. *Kehidupan Sosiokulturil Masjarakat Sasak di Lombok.* Bandung, Indonesia: Universitas Negeri Padjadjaran.

Hobart, Angela, Urs Ramseyer, and Albert Leeman. 1996. *The Peoples of Bali.* Oxford: Blackwell.

Hobart, Mark. 1985. Anthropos through the Looking-Glass. In *Reason and Morality,* J. Overing, ed., 104–34. New York: Tavistock.

Hollan, Douglas W., and Jane C. Wellenkamp. 1994. *Contentment and Suffering.* New York: Columbia University Press.

Holland, Dorothy, and Naomi Quinn, eds. 1987. *Cultural Models in Language and Thought.* Cambridge: Cambridge University Press.

Hooykaas, C. 1941. Indrukken van een Reis over Lombok. *De Locomotief* (June).

Hoskins, Janet. 1996. From Diagnosis to Performance: Medical Practice and the Politics of Exchange in Kodi, West Sumba. In *The Performance of Healing,* C. Laderman and M. Roseman, eds., 271–90. New York: Routledge.

House, James. 1988. Social Relationships and Health. *Science* 241:540–45.

Hughes, Charles. 1963. Public Health in Non-Literate Societies. In *Man's*

Image in Medicine and Anthropology, I. Galdston, ed. New York: International Universities.

Hunt, G. J. 1992. Social and Cultural Aspects of Health, Illness, and Treatment. In *Review of General Psychiatry,* 3d ed., H. Goldman, ed. Norwalk: Appleton and Lange.

Hunter, Cynthia L. 1996. Women as "Good Citizens": Maternal and Child Health in a Sasak Village. In *Maternity and Reproductive Health in Asian Societies,* P. L. Rice and L. Manderson, eds., 169–90. Amsterdam: Harwood.

Husserl, Edmund. 1970. *The Crisis of European Sciences and Transcendental Phenomenology.* Evanston: Northwestern University Press.

Inhorn, Marcia. 1994. *Quest for Conception.* Philadelphia: University of Pennsylvania Press.

Iskandar, M. B., B. Utomo, T. Hull, N. G. Dharmaputra, and Y. Azwar. 1996. *Unraveling the Mysteries of Maternal Death in West Java: Reexamining the Witnesses.* Djakarta: University of Indonesia Press.

Jaspan, M. A. 1976a. Health and Illth in Highland South Sumatra. In *Social Anthropology and Medicine,* J. B. Loudon, ed., 259–84. New York: Academic Press.

———. 1976b. The Social Organization of Indigenous and Modern Medical Practices in Southwest Sumatra. In *Asian Medical Systems: A Comparative Study,* C. Leslie, ed., 227–42. Berkeley: University of California Press.

Johnson, Allen W., and Timothy Earle. 1987. *The Evolution of Human Societies.* Stanford: Stanford University Press.

Johnson, Mark. 1987. *The Body in the Mind.* Chicago: University of Chicago Press.

Jordan, Brigitte. 1997. Authoritative Knowledge and Its Construction. In Childbirth and Authoritative Knowledge, R. Davis-Floyd and C. Sargent, eds., 55–79. Berkeley: University of California Press.

Judd, Mary Poo-Mooi. 1980. The Sociology of Rural Poverty in Lombok, Indonesia. Ph.D. diss., University of California.

Kano, Hiroyoshi. 1994. Landless Peasant Households in Indonesia. In *Approaching Suharto's Indonesia from the Margins,* T. Shiraishi, ed. Ithaca: Cornell Southeast Asia Program.

Kantor Statistic Provinsi NTB. 1988. *Nusa Tenggara Barat dalam Angka.* Mataram: Kantor Statistic.

Keane, Webb. 1997. *Signs of Recognition.* Berkeley: University of California Press.

Kearney, Michael. 1996. *Reconceptualizing the Peasantry.* Boulder: Westview.

Keeler, Ward. 1987. *Javanese Shadow Plays, Javanese Selves.* Princeton: Princeton University Press.

Keesing, Roger M. 1982. *Kwaio Religion.* New York: Columbia University Press.

Kendon, Adam. 1990. *Conducting Interaction.* Cambridge: Cambridge University Press.

Kipp, Rita Smith. 1993. *Dissociated Identities.* Ann Arbor: University of Michigan Press.

Kirmayer, Laurence J. 1992. The Body's Insistence on Meaning: Metaphor as

Presentation and Representation in Illness Experience. *Medical Anthropology Quarterly* 6 (4): 323–46.

Kleinman, Arthur. 1973. Medicine's Symbolic Reality: On a Central Problem in the Philosophy of Medicine. *Inquiry* 16:206–13.

———. 1980. *Patients and Healers in the Context of Culture*. Berkeley: University of California Press.

Kleinman, Arthur, and Byron Good, eds. 1985. *Culture and Depression*. Berkeley: University of California Press.

Kleinman, Arthur, and Joan Kleinman. 1985. Somatization: The Interconnections in Chinese Society among Culture, Depressive Experiences, and the Meanings of Pain. In *Culture and Depression*, A. Kleinman and B. Good, eds., 429–90. Berkeley: University of California Press.

Kondo, Dorinne K. 1990. *Crafting Selves*. Chicago: University of Chicago Press.

Krulfeld, Ruth. 1966. Fatalism in Indonesia: A Comparison of Socio-religious Types on Lombok. *Anthropological Quarterly* 39 (3): 180–90.

———. 1974. The Village Economies of the Sasak of Lombok: A Comparison of Three Indonesian Peasant Communities. Ph.D. diss., Yale.

Kuipers, Joel C. 1990. *Power in Performance*. Philadelphia: University of Pennsylvania Press.

Laderman, Carol. 1983. *Wives and Midwives*. Berkeley: University of California Press.

———. 1991. *Taming the Wind of Desire*. Berkeley: University of California Press.

———. 1992. Malay Medicine, Malay Person. In *Anthropological Approaches to the Study of Ethnomedicine,* Mark Nichter, ed. Amsterdam: Gordon and Breach Science Publishers.

Lakoff, George. 1987. *Women, Fire and Dangerous Things*. Chicago: University of Chicago Press.

Lakoff, George, and Mark Johnson. 1980. *Metaphors We Live By*. Chicago: University of Chicago Press.

Landy, David. 1977. Prevention of Illness and Social Control. In *Culture, Disease, and Healing*, D. Landy, ed., 231–32. New York: Macmillan.

Langer, Susanne K. 1957. *Philosophy in a New Key*. Cambridge: Harvard University Press.

Lansing, J. Stephen. 1991. *Priests and Programmers*. Princeton: Princeton University Press.

Last, Murray. 1981. The Importance of Knowing about Not Knowing. *Social Science and Medicine* 15B:387–92.

Latour, Bruno, and Steve Woolgar. 1986. *Laboratory Life*. Princeton: Princeton University Press.

Laughlin, William S. 1963. Primitive Theory of Medicine: Empirical Knowledge. In *Man's Image in Medicine and Anthropology*, I. Galdston, ed., 116–40. New York: International Universities.

Lavie, Smadar, Kirin Narayan, and Renato Rosaldo, eds. 1993. *Creativity/ Anthropology*. Ithaca: Cornell University Press.

Leach, E. R. 1964. *Political Systems of Highland Burma*. Boston: Beacon.

Leslie, Charles M. 1977. Pluralism and Integration in the Indian and Chinese Medical Systems. In *Culture, Disease, and Healing: Studies in Medical Anthropology*, D. Landy, ed., 511–17. New York: Macmillan.

———. 1980. Medical Pluralism in World Perspective. *Social Science and Medicine* 14B:191–95.

———. 1992. Interpretations of Illness: Syncretism in Modern Ayurveda. In *Paths to Asian Medical Knowledge*, C. Leslie and A. Young, eds., 177–208. Berkeley: University of California Press.

Leslie, Charles, and Allan Young. 1992. Introduction. In *Paths to Asian Medical Knowledge*, C. Leslie and A. Young, eds., 1–18. Berkeley: University of California Press.

Lévi-Strauss, Claude. 1963. The Sorcerer and His Magic. In *Structural Anthropology*, 167–85. New York: Basic.

Lewis, Gilbert. 1993. Double Standards of Treatment Evaluation. In *Knowledge, Power, and Practice*, S. Lindenbaum and M. Lock, eds., 189–218. Berkeley: University of California Press.

Lieban, Richard W. 1967. *Cebuano Sorcery: Malign Magic in the Philippines*. Berkeley: University of California Press.

———. 1973. Medical Anthropology. In *A Handbook of Social and Cultural Anthropology*, J. Honigmann, ed., 1031–71. Chicago: Rand McNally.

———. 1992. From Illness to Symbol and Symbol to Illness. *Social Science and Medicine* 35 (2): 183–88.

Liefrinck, F. A. 1927. *Bali en Lombok*. Amsterdam: J. H. de Bussy.

Lindenbaum, Shirley. 1979. *Kuru Sorcery: Disease and Danger in the New Guinea Highlands*. Mountain View, CA: Mayfield.

Lindenbaum, Shirley, and Margaret Lock. 1993. Preface. In *Knowledge, Power, and Practice*, S. Lindenbaum and M. Lock, eds., ix–xv. Berkeley: University of California Press.

Lindstrom, Lamont. 1990. *Knowledge and Power*. Washington, DC: Smithsonian Institute.

Lock, Margaret, and Patricia A. Kaufert. 1998. *Pragmatic Women and Body Politics*. Cambridge: Cambridge University Press.

Lock, Margaret, and Nancy Scheper-Hughes. 1996. A Critical-Interpretive Approach in Medical Anthropology: Rituals and Routines of Discipline and Dissent. In *Medical Anthropology: Contemporary Theory and Method*, rev. ed., C. Sargent and T. Johnson, eds., 41–70. Westport, CT: Praeger.

Logan, Michael H. 1977. Humoral Medicine in Guatemala and Peasant Acceptance of Modern Medicine. In *Culture, Disease, and Healing: Studies in Medical Anthropology*, D. Landy, ed., 487–95. New York: Macmillan.

Luhrmann, T. M. 1989. *Persuasions of the Witch's Craft*. Cambridge: Harvard University Press.

Luu, Phan, Don M. Tucker, and Douglas Derryberry. 1998. Anxiety and the Motivational Basis of Working Memory. *Cognitive Therapy and Research* 22 (6): 577–94.

Mageo, Jeannette Marie. 1995. The Reconfiguring Self. *American Anthropologist* 97 (2): 282–96.

Malinowski, Bronislaw. 1948. *Magic, Science and Religion and Other Essays*, R. Redfield, ed. Boston: Beacon.

Mannheim, Bruce, and Dennis Tedlock. 1995. Introduction. In *The Dialogic*

Emergence of Culture, D. Tedlock and B. Mannheim, eds., 1–32. Urbana: University of Illinois Press.

Marsella, Anthony J., Norman Sartorius, Assen Jablensky, and Fred R. Renton. 1985. Cross-Cultural Studies of Depressive Disorders: An Overview. In *Culture and Depression*, A. Kleinman and B. Good, eds., 299–324. Berkeley: University of California Press.

Martin, Emily. 1994. *Flexible Bodies*. Boston: Beacon.

Marx, Karl. 1977. *Capital*, vol. 1. New York: Random House.

Massard, Josiane. 1988. Doctoring by Go-Between: Aspects of Health Care for Malay Children. *Social Science and Medicine* 27 (8): 789–98.

Mauss, Marcel. 1975. *A General Theory of Magic*. New York: W. W. Norton.

———. 1985. A Category of the Human Mind: The Notion of Person, the Notion of Self. W. D. Halls, trans. In *The Category of the Person*, M. Carrithers, S. Collins, and S. Lukes, eds., 1–25. Cambridge: Cambridge University Press.

Mboi, Nafsiah. 1995. Health and Poverty: A Look at Eastern Indonesia. In *Indonesia Assessment 1995: Development in Eastern Indonesia*, C. Barlow and J. Hardjono, eds., 175–97. Singapore: Institute of South East Asian Studies.

Munn, Nancy. 1986. *The Fame of Gawa*. Cambridge: Cambridge University Press.

———. 1995. An Essay on the Symbolic Construction of Memory in the Kaluli Gisalo. In *Cosmos and Society in Oceania*, D. de Coppet and A. Iteanu, eds., 83–104. Oxford: Berg.

Nichter, Mark. 1992. Of Ticks, Kings, Spirits, and the Promise of Vaccines. In *Paths to Asian Medical Knowledge*, C. Leslie and A. Young, ed., 224–56. Berkeley: University of California Press.

———. 1996. Vaccinations in the Third World: A Consideration of Community Demand. In *Anthropology and International Health*, Mark Nichter and Mimi Nichter, eds. Amsterdam: Gordon and Breach.

Neisser, Ulric, ed. 1982. *Memory Observed*. San Francisco: W. H. Freeman.

Neisser, Ulric, and R. Fivush, eds. 1994. *The Remembering Self*. Cambridge: Cambridge University Press.

Nuckolls, Charles. 1991. Deciding How to Decide: Possession Mediumship in Jalari Divination. *Medical Anthropology* 13:57–82.

———. 1996. *The Cultural Dialectics of Knowledge and Desire*. Madison: University of Wisconsin Press.

Obeyesekere, Gananath. 1983. *Medusa's Hair*. Chicago: University of Chicago Press.

———. 1990. *The Work of Culture*. Chicago: University of Chicago Press.

Ohnuki-Tierney, Emiko. 1984. *Illness and Culture in Contemporary Japan*. Cambridge: Cambridge University Press.

Olesen, Virginia, Leonard Schatzman, Nellie Droes, Diane Hatton, and Nan Chico. 1990. The Mundane Ailment and the Physical Self: Analysis of the Social Psychology of Health and Illness. *Social Science and Medicine* 30 (4): 449–55.

Ortner, Sherry. 1984. Theory in Anthropology since the Sixties. *Comparative Studies in Society and History* 26:126–66.

Park, George K. 1967. Divination and Its Social Contexts. In *Magic, Witchcraft, and Curing,* J. Middleton, ed., 233–54. Garden City, NY: Natural History Press.

Parsons, Talcott. 1951. *The Social System.* New York: Free Press.

Paul, Robert A. 1989. What Does Anybody Want? Desire, Purpose and the Acting Subject in the Study of Culture. Paper presented to the Society for Cultural Anthropology Meetings, Washington, DC, May.

Peacock, James. 1987. *Rites of Modernization.* Chicago: University of Chicago Press.

Pearce, Tola Olu. 1993. Lay Medical Knowledge in an African Context. In *Knowledge, Power, and Practice,* S. Lindenbaum and M. Lock, eds., 150–65. Berkeley: University of California Press.

Peirce, Charles Sanders. 1955. *Philosophical Writings of Peirce,* J. Buchler, ed. New York: Dover.

Peletz, Michael G. 1996. *Reason and Passion: Representations of Gender in a Malay Society.* Berkeley: University of California Press.

Pemberton, John. 1994. *On the Subject of "Java."* Ithaca: Cornell University Press.

Polak, Andrew. 1978. Traditie en tweespalt in een Sasakse boerengemeenschap (Lombok, Indonesia). Ph.D. diss., Rijksuniversiteit te Utrecht.

Polanyi, Michael. 1958. *Personal Knowledge.* Chicago: University of Chicago Press.

Polanyi, Michael, and Harry Prosch. 1975. *Meaning.* Chicago: University of Chicago Press.

Pollock, Donald. 1996. Personhood and Illness among the Kulina. *Medical Anthropology Quarterly* 10 (3): 319–41.

Pool, Robert. 1994. *Dialogue and the Interpretation of Illness.* Oxford/Providence: Berg.

Price, Laurie. 1987. Ecuadorian Illness Stories: Cultural Knowledge in Natural Discourse. In *Cultural Models in Language and Thought,* D. Holland and N. Quinn, eds., 313–42. Cambridge: Cambridge University Press.

Quinn, Naomi, and Dorothy Holland. 1987. Culture and Cognition. In *Cultural Models in Language and Thought,* D. Holland and N. Quinn, eds., 3–42. Cambridge: Cambridge University Press.

Rachman, S. 1998. *Anxiety.* Ann Arbor, MI: Taylor and Francis.

Romanucci-Ross, Lola. 1986. Creativity in Illness: Methodological Linkages to the Logic and Language of Science in Folk Pursuit of Health in Central Italy. *Social Science and Medicine* 23 (1): 1–7.

Rosaldo, Michelle. 1980. *Knowledge and Passion.* Cambridge: Cambridge University Press.

Rosaldo, Renato. 1980. *Ilongot Headhunting, 1883–1974: A Study in History and Society.* Stanford: Stanford University Press.

———. 1989. *Culture and Truth.* Boston: Beacon.

Roseman, Marina. 1991. *Healing Sounds from the Malaysian Rainforest.* Berkeley: University of California Press.

———. 1996. Of Selves and Souls, Bodies and Persons, Individuals and Societies: A Commentary on Donald Pollock's "Personhood and Illness among the Kulina." *Medical Anthropology Quarterly* 10 (3): 342–46.

Rubin, David, ed. 1995. *Remembering Our Past*. Cambridge: Cambridge University Press.

Runco, Mark A. 1999. Tension, Adaptability, and Creativity. In *Affect, Creative Experience, and Psychological Adjustment*, Sandra Russ, ed., 165–94. Ann Arbor, MI: Taylor and Francis.

Saltonstall, Robin. 1993. Healthy Bodies, Social Bodies: Men's and Women's Concepts and Practices of Health in Everyday Life. *Social Science and Medicine* 36 (1): 7–14.

Scheper-Hughes, Nancy. 1992. *Death without Weeping*. Berkeley: University of California Press.

Schieffeln, Edward L. 1976. *The Sorrow of the Lonely and the Burning of the Dancers*. New York: St. Martin's Press.

———. 1985. The Cultural Analysis of Depressive Affect: An Example from New Guinea. In *Culture and Depression*, A. Kleinman and B. Good, eds., 101–33. Berkeley: University of California Press.

———. 1996. On Failure and Performance: Throwing the Medium out of the Seance. In *The Performance of Healing*, C. Laderman and M. Roseman, eds., 59–90. New York: Routledge.

Schneider, David. 1984. *A Critique of the Study of Kinship*. Ann Arbor: University of Michigan Press.

Schutz, Alfred. 1970. *On Phenomenology and Social Relations*. Chicago: University of Chicago Press.

Scott, James C. 1976. *The Moral Economy of the Peasant*. New Haven: Yale University Press.

———. 1985. *Weapons of the Weak*. New Haven: Yale University Press.

———. 1990. *Domination and the Arts of Resistance*. New Haven: Yale University Press.

Sears, Laurie J. 1996. *Shadows of Empire*. Durham, NC: Duke University Press.

Shore, Bradd. 1982. *Sala'iula: A Samoan Mystery*. New York: Columbia University Press.

———. 1991. Twice-Born, Once Conceived: Meaning Construction and Cultural Cognition. *American Anthropologist* 93 (1): 9–27.

———. 1996. *Culture in Mind: Cognition, Culture, and the Problem of Meaning*. New York: Oxford University Press.

———. 1997. *What Culture Means, How Culture Means*. Worcester, MA: Heinz Werner Institute.

———. 1998. A Dialogue on Dialogue. *Journal of Linguistic Anthropology* 7 (2): 1–11.

Shweder, Richard A. 1985. Menstrual Pollution, Soul Loss, and the Comparative Study of Emotions. In *Culture and Depression*, A. Kleinman and B. Good, eds., 182–215. Berkeley: University of California Press.

———. 1990. Cultural Psychology—What Is It? In *Cultural Psychology*, J. Stigler, R. Shweder, and G. Herdt, eds., 1–46. Cambridge: Cambridge University Press.

Siegal, James. 1978. Curing Rites, Dreams, and Domestic Politics in a Sumatran Society. *Glyph* 3:18–31.

———. 1986. *Solo in the New Order*. Princeton: Princeton University Press.

Singer, Merrill. 1990. Reinventing Medical Anthropology: Toward a Critical Realignment. *Social Science and Medicine* 30 (2): 179–87.

Sontag, Susan. 1990. *Illness as Metaphor and AIDS and Its Metaphors*. New York: Anchor.

Spiro, Melford. 1987. Collective Representations and Mental Representations in Religious Symbol Systems. In *Culture and Human Nature*, B. Kilborne and L. L. Langness, eds., 161–84. Chicago: University of Chicago Press.

Steedly, Mary Margaret. 1993. *Hanging without a Rope*. Princeton: Princeton University Press.

Strauss, Claudia, and Naomi Quinn. 1997. *A Cognitive Theory of Cultural Meaning*. Cambridge: Cambridge University Press.

Tambiah, Stanley J. 1968. The Magical Power of Words. *Man* 3 (2): 175–208.

———. 1990. *Magic, Science, Religion, and the Scope of Rationality*. Cambridge: Cambridge University Press.

Taussig, Michael T. 1987. *Shamanism, Colonialism, and the Wild Man: A Study in Terror and Healing*. Chicago: University of Chicago Press.

———. 1992. *The Nervous System*. New York: Routledge.

Tedlock, Barbara. 1987. An Interpretive Solution to the Problem of Humoral Medicine in Latin America. *Social Science and Medicine* 24 (12): 1069–83.

———. 1992. Zuni and Quinche Dream Sharing and Interpreting. In *Dreaming*, B. Tedlock, ed., 105–31. Sante Fe: School of American Research Press.

Tedlock, Dennis. 1995. Interpretation, Participation, and the Role of Narrative in Dialogical Anthropology. In *The Dialogic Emergence of Culture*, D. Tedlock and B. Mannheim, eds., 253–88. Urbana: University of Illinois Press.

Tedlock, Dennis, and Bruce Mannheim, eds. 1995. *The Dialogic Emergence of Culture*. Urbana: University of Illinois Press.

Toth, Andrew. 1978. Record Reviews: Panji in Lombok. *Ethnomusicology* 22 (2): 370–75.

———. 1979. Record Reviews: Panji in Lombok II. *Ethnomusicology* 23 (2): 354–57.

Traube, Elizabeth G. 1986. *Cosmology and Social Life*. Chicago: University of Chicago Press.

Trevathan, Wenda. 1997. An Evolutionary Perspective on Authoritative Knowledge about Birth. In *Childbirth and Authoritative Knowledge*, R. Davis-Floyd and C. Sargent, eds., 80–90. Berkeley: University of California Press.

Tsing, Anna Lowenhaupt. 1988. Healing Boundaries in South Kalimantan. *Social Science and Medicine* 27 (8): 829–39.

———. 1993. *In the Realm of the Diamond Queen*. Princeton: Princeton University Press.

Turner, Bryan. 1995. *Medical Power and Social Knowledge*. London: Sage.

Turner, Victor. 1967. *Forest of Symbols*. Ithaca: Cornell University Press.

———. 1969. *The Ritual Process*. Ithaca: Cornell University Press.

Tylor, Sir Edward Burnett. 1958. *Primitive Culture*, vol. 2. New York: Harper and Row.

United Nations. 1994. *United Nations Statistical Yearbook for Asia and the Pacific*. New York: United Nations.

U.S. Department of Statistics. 1993. *Statistical Abstract of the United States for 1993*. Washington, DC: Department of Statistics.

van der Geest, Sjaak. 1991. Marketplace Conversations in Cameroon: How and Why Popular Medical Knowledge Comes into Being. *Culture, Medicine, and Psychiatry* 15 (1): 69–90.

van der Kraan, Alfons. 1980. *Lombok: Conquest, Colonization and Underdevelopment, 1870–1940*. Singapore: Asian Studies Association of Australia.

Van Gennep, Arnold. 1960. *Rites of Passage*. Chicago: University of Chicago Press.

van Leur, J. C. 1976. *Indonesian Trade and Society*. The Hague: W. van Hoeve.

Vaughan, Megan. 1991. *Curing Their Ills: Colonial Power and African Illness*. Stanford: Stanford University Press.

Vlekke, Bernard H. M. 1943. *Nusatara*. Cambridge: Harvard University Press.

Vogelsang, A. W. L. 1922. Eenige Aanteekeningen betreffende de Sasaks op Lombok. *Koloniaal Tijdschrift* 11:260–306.

Volosinov, V. N. [1929] 1986. *Marxism and the Philosophy of Language*. Trans. L. Matejka and I. R. Titunik. Cambridge: Harvard University Press.

Walens, Stanley. 1981. *Feasting with Cannibals*. Princeton: Princeton University Press.

Wallace, Alfred Russell. 1922. *The Malay Archipelago*. London: Macmillan.

Waxler, Nancy. 1981. Learning to be a Leper. In *Social Contexts of Health, Illness, and Patient Care*, E. Mishler, ed., 169–94. Cambridge: Cambridge University Press.

Weber, Max. 1947. *The Theory of Social and Economic Organization*. New York: Free Press.

Werner, D. 1992. *Where There Is No Doctor*. Rev. ed. Palo Alto: Hesperian Foundation.

West, Candace. 1984. *Routine Complications: Troubles with Talk between Doctors and Patients*. Bloomington: Indiana University Press.

Whorf, Benjamin. 1956. *Language Thought and Reality: Selected Writings of Benjamin Lee Whorf*, J. B. Carroll, ed. Cambridge: MIT Press.

Wikan, U. 1990. *Managing Turbulent Hearts*. Chicago: University of Chicago Press.

———. 1996. The Nun's Story: Reflections on an Age-Old, Postmodern Dilemma. *American Anthropologist* 98 (2): 279–89.

Wilce, James M., Jr. 1995. "I Can't Tell You All My Troubles": Conflict, Resistance, and Metacommunication in Bangladeshi Illness Interactions. *American Ethnologist* 22 (4): 927–50.

———. 1997. Discourse, Power, and the Diagnosis of Weakness: Encountering Practitioners in Bangladesh. *Medical Anthropology Quarterly* 11 (3): 352–74.

Williamson, David Forrest. 1984. Household Buffering of Seasonal Food-

Availability in a Crisis-Prone Area of Lombok, Indonesia: Implications for Timely Warning and Intervention Systems. Ph.D. diss., Cornell University.

Willis, Paul. 1977. *Learning to Labor.* New York: Columbia University Press.

Winterson, Jeanette. 1993. *Written on the Body.* New York: Alfred A. Knopf.

Wittgenstein, Ludwig. 1998. *Philosophical Investigations.* Oxford: Blackwell.

Wolf, Eric R. 1966. *Peasants.* Englewood Cliffs, NJ: Prentice-Hall.

Wood, John C. 1999. *When Men Are Women.* Madison: University of Wisconsin Press.

Woodward, Mark R. 1985. Healing and Morality: A Javanese Example. *Social Science and Medicine* 21 (9): 1007–21.

Young, Alan. 1980. An Anthropological Perspective on Medical Knowledge. *Journal of Medicine and Philosophy* 5 (2): 102–16.

———. 1982. The Anthropologies of Illness and Sickness. *Annual Review of Anthropology* 11:257–85.

Zollinger, H. 1847. Het Eiland Lombok. *Tijdschrift van Nederlandsch-Indies* 2:177–205, 301–83.

Index